Perfect Health Diet

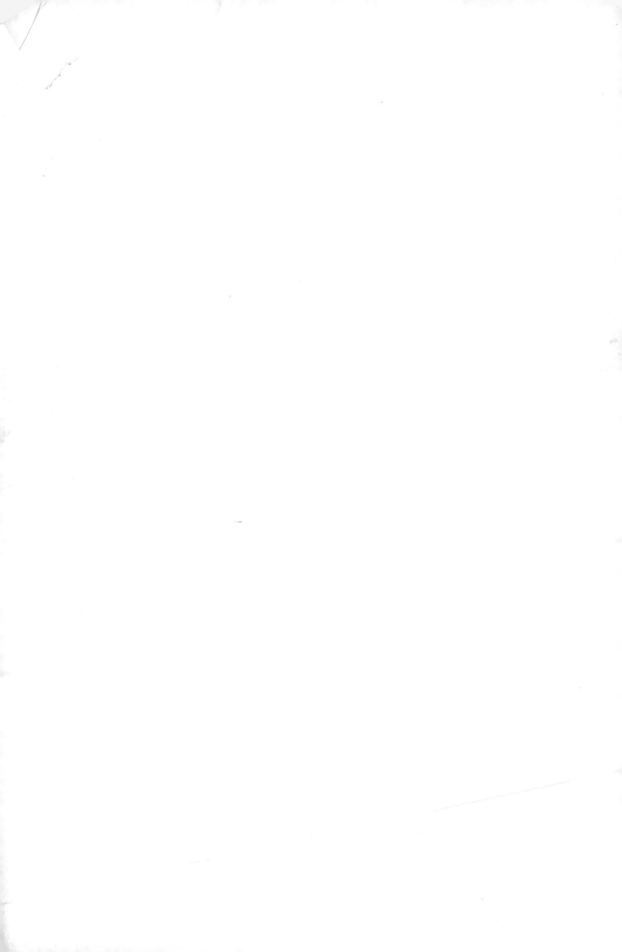

PerfectHealthDiet

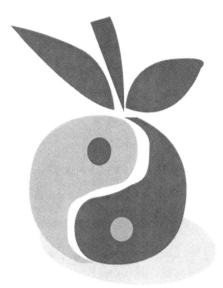

Four Steps to
Renewed Health, Youthful Vitality,
and
Long Life

PAUL JAMINET, PH.D.,
and
SHOU-CHING JAMINET, PH.D.

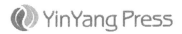 YinYang Press

Published by

YinYang Press, 393 Broadway #15,

Cambridge, Massachusetts, 02139.

www.yinyangpress.com

The authors acknowledge with gratitude the contributions of Monika Chas, who designed the cover and logo, and Seo Jung Sa and Seo Hong Sa, who drew illustrations.

For further information, please visit

www.perfecthealthdiet.com

ISBN: 978-0-9827209-0-5
Library of Congress Control Number: 2010938153

Table of Contents

Preface

We are two scientists who ate poorly and ignored a gradual decline in our health. But by age forty we had developed disturbing health problems:

- Paul had a chronic condition with rosacea, physical sluggishness, neuropathy, memory loss, and impaired mood.

- Shou-Ching had painful endometriosis, ovarian cysts, and uterine fibroids; allergies; constipation, acid reflux, and abdominal bloating.

Doctors were of little help. By 2005 we decided we had to learn how to be healthy. That year, we began experimenting with a low-carb Paleo diet.

Paul rapidly became leaner and stronger. Shou-Ching's allergies and digestive problems cleared. Clearly there was something to this diet.

But a series of unexpected problems appeared. Paul's cognitive and neuropathic issues worsened and at one point he developed scurvy. There were potential pitfalls in low-carb diets as well. We researched and experimented, adding nutritional supplements and fine-tuning the diet.

In 2009, Paul traced his remaining problems to a chronic bacterial infection; a course of antibiotics cleared it. Our health kept getting better; we began to feel like we were in our twenties again.

Now we would like to share what we have learned.

A Theory of Disease, Health, and Aging

We believe that disease and ill health are caused by the interplay of three factors: food toxins; malnourishment; and chronic infections by bacteria, viruses, fungi, and protozoa. All three of these factors can be (and must be!) addressed by diet.

Given the proper diet, the human body has amazing recuperative powers. We believe that the Perfect Health Diet, in combination with appropriate nutritional supplementation and antimicrobial therapies, will:

- **Prevent and mitigate or cure** the common diseases of aging – **cancer, heart disease and stroke, diabetes, and obesity**.

- **Cure or slow progression of autoimmune and chronic diseases.**

- **Maintain youthful vitality and good health** to a ripe old age.

We believe that diets like the Perfect Health Diet will work a revolution in medicine. Most of the chronic and degenerative diseases that afflict modern society are caused by bad diets and cannot be cured until the diet is fixed. Much of what people consider "aging" is, in fact, infectious disease aggravated by a bad diet. Scientists have overlooked the microbial origin of chronic diseases because antibiotics and other drugs are ineffective under western diets. Yet when the diet is healthy, many diseases spontaneously cure, and antibiotic drugs work wonders.

This medical revolution must be preceded by a rethinking of dietary science. Conventional dietary advice is largely mistaken. Emerging science – and the experience of millions who have adopted "Paleo" style diets – is now correcting those errors.

Who This Book Is Written For

The first draft of this book, written in 2008, was for friends and family, to help them with their health problems.

By 2010, after curing our own chronic health conditions, we were determined to share what we'd learned with the public. We have written for three groups:

- **Healthy people** who want to optimize their health and fitness, and remain young and energetic through the longest possible life;

- **Chronic disease sufferers**, both elderly and middle-aged, who suffer needlessly from diseases wrongly thought to be incurable.

- **Doctors and scientists** who want to find a more effective way to treat their patients.

It's not easy to write for all three audiences. We want to be persuasive to our fellow scientists and doctors, so we have presented extensive footnotes to the medical literature. Like scientists, chronic disease patients are often sophisticated skeptics, keen to "prove all things, and hold fast that which is good." But we also want the book to be easy to read and helpful for people who just want to know, "What should I do to live a long, healthy life?"

We've tried to make it easy for casual readers to find the main take-aways. The book is divided into "Steps," which explain the logic behind our advice, and intervening "Ideas" sections, which give practical guidance.

> *Within the "Steps" sections, more esoteric science is placed in text boxes like this one. Feel free to skip or skim these boxes.*

Casual readers can skip the science boxes and pay close attention to the "Summary" sections interspersed in the "Steps."

Readers can find further discussions at our blog, *www.perfecthealthdiet.com*. We'll strive to answer any questions we receive there.

Best wishes, dear reader. May our insights help you attain Perfect Health!

Introduction: Getting Started

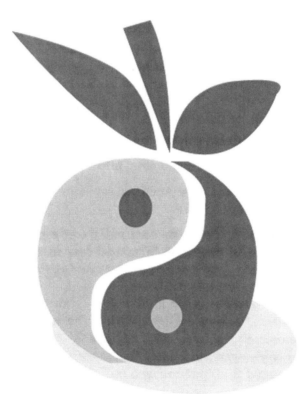

The Perfect Health Diet in One Page

The Perfect Health Diet is, by calories, a low-to-moderate-carb (20%) high-fat (65%) moderate-protein (15%) diet. However, by weight, the diet is about 65% plant foods, 35% meats and oils.

DO eat:

About 20% of total calories (~400 carb calories per day) from starchy tubers, rice, fruits and berries. Eat as many vegetables as you like; but don't count any calories from vegetables. Be sure to include seaweed (for iodine). In total, you might eat ~1.5 lb plant foods.

About 80% of total calories (~1600 calories per day) from <1 lb of fatty meats, seafood, and eggs, plus ~4 tbsp healthy oils and fats. Include salmon or other cold water fish for omega-3 fatty acids. Cook with butter, animal fats such as lard or tallow, coconut oil, and olive oil; snack on nuts, cheeses, and fruits. Use spices including salt.

Do NOT eat:

Grains and cereals (including wheat, oats, and corn but excluding rice) or any products made from them (including bread and pasta).

Sugar, corn syrup, or products containing them (soda, sweets).

Legumes (such as soybeans, kidney beans, pinto beans, or peanuts).

Omega-6-rich vegetable seed oils (such as soybean oil, corn oil, safflower oil, peanut oil, or canola oil).

These "do not eat" foods contain naturally toxic proteins; excessive fructose and omega-6 fats; and few nutrients.

AVOID:

Pasteurized milk, but DO eat fermented or fatty dairy foods: butter, cream, ice cream, sour cream, cheese, yogurt. Within the watery fraction of milk are dissolved biologically active cow hormones and potentially allergenic proteins; fatty and fermented dairy foods are safer. Raw milk proteins are more easily digested than pasteurized milk proteins.

Dry, lean meats which are protein-rich but fat-poor.

Finally, DO:

Supplement to optimize nutrition, with a daily multivitamin plus vitamins C, D3, and K2 and magnesium, selenium, iodine, copper, and chromium.

Practice intermittent fasting, for instance by restricting eating to an 8-hour window each day, or by taking longer "ketogenic fasts" with lots of coconut oil but no carbs or protein.

How to Construct a Perfect Diet

How does one's diet contribute to health? The perfect diet should:

- Provide a sufficiency of every nutrient.

- Deliver no toxins, and no excess nutrients for pathogens.

That way, all possible benefits from nutrition are obtained, and none of the detrimental effects from toxins or infection-promotion are experienced.

We believe that eating something close to the perfect diet is the key to long life and youthful vitality. A perfect diet prevents and, in some cases, cures the common diseases of aging (heart disease, cancer, dementia) and chronic diseases of middle age (autoimmune diseases, fatigue, acid reflux, graying hair, and many more).

We're here to show you how to eat the perfect diet.

"Good" Nutrients and "Bad" Nutrients

Nutrients are always beneficial at low doses. That is why they are called "nutrients."

But not all nutrients are beneficial at high doses. In fact, at very high doses most nutrients become toxic.

THE ECONOMICS OF NUTRITION

We can borrow some good ways of thinking about nutrition from economics. Economists think about how factors of production, like workers and capital goods, cooperate to produce a healthy economy. This is rather like how nutrients cooperate to produce a healthy body.

The most important concept we can borrow is that of *declining marginal benefits*:

- In economics, this means that the first worker a business hires does the most important work. The next laborer does the next most important work. And so on – each additional worker does less valuable work, until it doesn't make sense to hire anyone.

- In nutrition, this means that the greatest benefit comes from the first bit eaten of any nutrient. Each additional bit provides less benefit than the bit before. Eventually, the benefit from additional amounts approaches zero.

Declining marginal benefits applies to toxins as well as nutrients. It implies that the first bit eaten of any toxin has low toxicity. Each additional bit is slightly more toxic than the bit before. At high doses, the toxicity of each bit continues to increase, so that the toxin is increasingly poisonous.

Increasing marginal toxicity of toxins was first noticed by the medieval physician Paracelsus, who formulated the toxicologist's rule: "the dose makes the poison." At low doses, toxins are not dangerous; but at high doses they can be deadly.

Since most nutrients become toxins at high doses, we can draw for most nutrients a "marginal benefit curve" that looks like this:

Figure: Marginal Benefit Curve for Nutrients

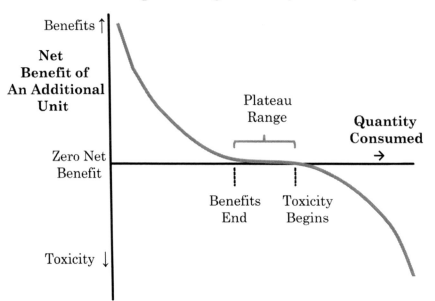

As the quantity consumed goes up, marginal benefits decrease, and go to zero at a point marked in the figure by the phrase "Benefits End."   As the quantity consumed increases further, marginal benefits turn negative at the point in the figure labeled "Toxicity Begins." A "good calorie" or "nutrient" at low doses becomes a "bad calorie" or "poison" at high doses.

There is an optimum quantity of most nutrients, located over the range in the curve where the marginal benefits are close to zero. This range, which we call the "**plateau range**," encompasses doses for which all the benefits of the nutrient are captured, but none of the toxicity.

The Perfect Health Diet is the one that gets every nutrient into its plateau range. It is defined by a single principle:

Eat so as to gain all possible benefits and no toxicity from food.

Three Steps to a Perfect Diet

We explain how to adopt these principle in three Steps.

Step One: Eat by *calories* 20% carbs – 65% fat – 15% protein, but by *weight* 65% plants – 35% animal foods.

Step One focuses on *macronutrients* – protein, carbs, fat, fiber – and how to get each into its plateau range.

Step One is a little more complicated than you might think, since there are four types of fats (short-chain fats, long-chain saturated and monounsaturated fats, omega-6 polyunsaturated fats, and omega-3 polyunsaturated fats) which have their own plateau ranges. Another complication is that carb calories come in a low-toxicity form (glucose) and a high-toxicity form (fructose). Also, calories can be derived from indigestible fiber, thanks to the help of gut bacteria.

Step One is followed by a brief section suggesting some tips that will help you get these macronutrients right. A few simple meal-construction principles make it easy to get all the macronutrients into their plateau range.

Step Two: Eat "Paleo," not toxic.

Unfortunately, not all foods are beneficial even at low doses. Some foods have toxins which outweigh their nutritional benefits even at the first bite. These foods should not be eaten.

Many of these toxic foods entered the human diet when farming was invented about 10,000 years ago. They are "Neolithic" but not "Paleolithic" foods. So getting rid of toxic foods is almost the same as eating a "Paleo" diet.

Step Two shows how to do this.

Step Three: Be well nourished.

Unfortunately, many modern foods are nutrient-poor. Foods alone may not be sufficient to get many vitamins and minerals into their plateau range. Therefore, it is important to supplement with selected vitamins and minerals.

It is not enough to rely on a multivitamin. Some nutrients, like magnesium or vitamin C, are too bulky to fit in a multivitamin; vitamin D must be tailored to individual needs; others, like vitamin K and iodine, are under-appreciated.

Step Three explains how to be well-nourished.

Step Four: From the Perfect Diet to Perfect Health

Executing the three steps will bring most people to the verge of Perfect Health. Steps One through Three will eliminate most autoimmune conditions, maximize the functioning of immune defenses, and heal wounded tissues.

To go the final step to perfect health requires a few additional practices:

- A healthy lifestyle, including adequate sleep, exercise, and occasional fasts and "ketogenic diet days" to build up immune defenses.

- Eliminating chronic infections by bacteria, viruses, fungi, and protozoa. Though little appreciated by doctors, chronic infections cause most diseases and eventually – because the immune system loses effectiveness with age – they debilitate almost everyone.

The good news is that the Perfect Health Diet improves immune function, enabling most diseases to be cured or delayed for decades. Step Four offers practical guidance for defeating diseases.

Following all four steps, we believe that nearly everyone will achieve great health and an exceptionally long life. And we have the centenarian stories to prove it!

Stumbling Blocks

For most people, the diet poses two stumbling blocks: giving up cereal grains, and eating more fat.

Giving up cereals like wheat, bread and pasta is the hardest step. Grains are convenient and easy (cereal for breakfast, a sandwich at lunch; beer and pasta at dinner). Worse, they are **addictive**. Grains like wheat contain natural opioids, which stimulate the same pleasure receptors as morphine and heroin.

But, as we'll see, giving up grains can deliver huge health benefits.

The other difficulty, eating more fat, shouldn't be hard: fat tastes great! But decades of anti-fat propaganda have made us fat-phobic: scared that eating fat will raise serum cholesterol and cause heart attacks or strokes.

Fat-phobia is a great mistake. Above about 600 calories per day, dietary carbs increase fat in the body – but only after poisoning the tissues they touch, and feeding any bacteria that intercept them. Excess carbs generate a bad lipid profile and contribute to heart disease, cancer, obesity, diabetes, and dementia. Switching to a fat-rich diet is a key step toward good health.

Fat-phobia does have some basis in fact. Omega-6 fats are toxic in excess. High-omega-6 diets, especially if also carb-rich and toxin-rich, quickly poison lab animals. (Resorting to omega-6-plus-grain-or-sugar diets is a favorite trick of diet researchers; it can wreck the health of mice in a few months – very convenient if you need to get a paper out quickly.) So it is important, if you don't want to go the way of those lab mice, to avoid omega-6-rich oils like soybean oil and corn oil.

We'll start with a Preview that looks at mammals and mother's milk for a few reasons to abandon fat-phobia and embrace a low (20% calories) carb high (65% calories) fat diet. The Preview is intended to persuade you that the diet makes sense, and is worth a try – and that it is worth reading the rest of the book. But remember:

The proof of the diet is in the eating.

If you try the diet, you will see your health improve. The trying may be hard ... but the rewards will be persuasive.

Preview: How Mice and Milk, Lions and Lambs Show the Way

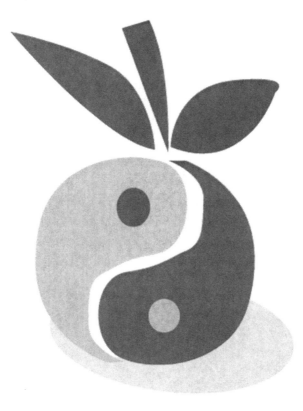

Four Reasons to Believe in a 20-65-15 Macronutrient Ratio

This macronutrient ratio is fundamental to good health. Yet most people are shocked by the idea of getting most calories from fat.

We'll go into the science in depth, but for now, we want to make you comfortable by offering four "plausibility arguments" for a high-fat diet:

1.   **These were the ratios eaten by our hunter-gatherer ancestors** from 2 million years ago until agriculture was invented 10,000 years ago. Evolution may have optimized human biology for this diet.

The Ancestral Human Diet

How do we know what our hunter-gatherer ancestors ate? We have evidence from modern hunter-gatherers and the skeletons of ancient humans and Neandertals.

Loren Cordain's analysis of the diets of 229 modern hunter-gatherers described in the *Ethnographic Atlas* of J.P. Gray, augmented by detailed data for 19 tribes, showed that modern hunter-gatherers obtain 65% of calories from animals and 35% from plants.[1] This translates to roughly a 35% carb – 50% fat – 15% protein ratio.

However, carb intake may have been elevated by the encroachment of civilization on hunting territories. Paleolithic hunter-gatherers seem to have relied more on animal foods. Isotope ratios and wear patterns on teeth show that *Australopithicus* 3-4 million years ago ate more meat than chimpanzees. By 2 million years ago, ancestral *Homo* were butchering meat with stone tools, and a meat-based diet enabled *Homo* to spread to northern latitudes 1.75 million years ago. By 30-50,000 years ago, Neandertals (hunting herbivores such as mammoths) and humans (hunting many species with an emphasis on fish) were top-level carnivores. Upper Paleolithic humans were higher-level carnivores than wolves and arctic foxes.[2]

In short, the Paleolithic diet, for which evolution optimized our bodies, probably consisted of 5% to 35% carb – 50% to 70% fat – 15% to 25% protein, with higher carbs near the equator and higher fat and protein at northern latitudes. The middle of the range is 20% carb – 60% fat – 20% protein.

[1] Cordain, Loren, "Implications of Plio-Pleistocene Hominin Diets for Modern Humans," pp 363-383 in Peter S. Ungar, ed., *Evolution of the human diet: the known, the unknown, and the unknowable*, New York: Oxford University Press, 2006.

[2] Ibid.; Richards MP, Trinkaus E. Out of Africa: modern human origins special feature: isotopic evidence for the diets of European Neanderthals and early modern humans. *Proc Natl Acad Sci* 2009 Sep 22; 106(38): 16034-9. *http://pmid.us/19706482.*

---

2.   **Mother's milk is a complete and perfect food for infants, and the perfect diet for adults must be similar**. Most milk calories are from fat, carbohydrate is the second source and protein is third.

Human Breast Milk and the Adult Diet

Human milk by calories is 39% carbs, 54% fat, and 7% protein; cow's milk is 29% carbs, 52% fat, and 19% protein.[1] We can trust that evolution has designed milk to provide infants and calves with optimal ratios.

How will the optimal adult diet differ from an infant's? The brain is the body's primary consumer of carbs, and the brain accounts for 50% of calorie consumption (10% of body weight) in infants but only 20% of calorie consumption (2% of body weight) in adults.[2] Since adults require less than half the carbs that infants do, the optimal adult carb intake is likely about 20% of total calories rather than the 39% of infants. Starting from the human milk ratios and changing half the carb calories to fat and protein, we get a ratio of **20% carb – 64% fat – 16% protein**.

[1] George DE, DeFrancesca BA. Human milk in comparison to cow milk. In: Lebenthals E, ed. *Textbook of gastroenterology and nutrition.* New York: Raven Press, 1989:239-61. Cf. *http://www.unu.edu/unupress/food/8F174e/8F174E04.htm.*

[2] Grande Covián F. Energy metabolism of the brain in children. *An Esp Pediatr.* 1979 Mar; 12(3):235-44. *http://pmid.us/443644.*

---

3. **You should eat what you are.** A lean human body, excluding water and minerals, is 56% fat and 44% protein by weight. This translates to 74% fat and 26% protein by calories. This suggests that fat and protein calories should be eaten in more or less a 74% to 26% ratio.

Composition of the Human Body

A relatively lean 154-lb "reference man" is composed of 42 kg water, 13.5 kg fats, 10.6 kg protein, and 3.7 kg minerals.[1]

Why does this indicate the optimal dietary composition? Two reasons:

First, in order to add new tissue, such as muscle, your diet needs to supply the ingredients – fat and protein in a 74-26 ratio. If 20% of the diet supplies carbs for the brain, while the rest is used to build tissue, then a 74-26 fat-to-protein ratio will make the whole diet **20% carb – 60% fat – 20% protein**.

Second, the human body is designed to cannibalize itself when there is a lack of food, consuming fats and protein from cells. Since summer drought and winter food scarcity must have been common, people would have evolved to remain healthy and capable of hunting through months with little or no food. This implies that a diet of 74% fat and 26% protein – the "cannibal diet" – must be generally healthy.

[1] Wang ZM et al. 1992, "The five-level model: a new approach for organizing body-composition research," *Am J Clin Nutr* 1992 Jul; 56(1): 19-28. *http://pmid.us/1609756.*

---

4. **Omnivorous animals prefer and thrive on low-carb high-fat diets.** Animals instinctively eat a mix of foods that is healthy. When scientists let mice choose their own food from an unlimited supply of carbs, fats, and protein, most strains chose to get a majority of calories from fat. When scientists allowed a mouse strain that develops obesity and diabetes on a 40% carb – 40% fat chow to choose its own diet, it chose a diet of 5.6% carb, 82.5% fat, and 12.0% protein and "proved highly resistant to the

development of obesity and diabetes." If mice are smart enough to avoid diabetes and weight gain by eating a high-fat low-carb diet, shouldn't humans be as wise?

In a study of 13 strains of mice, 9 chose to eat a majority of calories from fat, only 2 chose to eat more carb than fat calories.[1]

In the other study, wild-type FVB/N mice were compared with transgenic mice engineered to develop obesity and diabetes; the wild-type mice ate the proportions mentioned above, while the transgenic mice ate 2.2% carbs – 85.1% fat and "developed obesity [that was] ... less pronounced than on a high-fat and high-carbohydrate Western diet ... [and] did not become hyperglycemic; they showed decreased fed and fasted blood glucose levels."[2]

[1] Smith BK et al. "Macronutrient diet selection in thirteen mouse strains," *Am J Physiol Regul.* 2000; 278 R797–805. *http://pmid.us/10749765.*

[2] Ortmann S et al. "Self-selected macronutrient diet affects energy and glucose metabolism in brown fat-ablated mice," *Obesity Research* 2003 Dec; 11(12): 1536-44. *http://pmid.us/14694219.* Hat tip, Peter Dobromylskyj *http://high-fat-nutrition.blogspot.com/2007/10/physiological-insulin-resistance.html.*

All of these considerations point toward a macronutrient ratio of about 20% carbs, 65% fats, and 15% protein – the Perfect Health Diet ratios.

Why All Mammals Eat the Perfect Health Diet

When considering how much should be eaten of various nutrients, it's important to keep in mind how the body "pre-processes" foods in the digestive tract and liver before releasing them to the body.

The gut and liver alter food before nutrients are released to the body. The nutritional content of your *diet* is different from the nutritional content of your *food*!

Some great mistakes in the science of diet have resulted from forgetting this point. Scientists sometimes misinterpret their own studies for this reason!

How Digestion Transforms Nutrients

This table summarizes how nutrients are handled:

Food component	How handled
Fructose	Shunted to the liver for conversion (usually) to saturated fat and various intermediate toxins.
Glucose	Released to the bloodstream. Up to 500 calories per day are placed as liver or muscle glycogen. Excesses may be converted to saturated fat and stored in fat cells.
Protein	Released as amino acids to the bloodstream and taken up by cells throughout the body.
Short-chain fats	Shunted to the liver and metabolized there, often leading to release of ketone bodies.
Other fats	Released to the bloodstream and taken up by cells throughout the body.
Fiber/Vegetable matter	Eaten by gut bacteria, which release short-chain fats to the body as usable calories.

As a result of these transformations, the macronutrients that enter the bloodstream and reach body cells may be quite different from the macronutrients that entered the mouth:

- **Vegetables are a fat source.** Vegetables have all their official calories as carbs (glucose and fructose), but the amounts are low. Most vegetable carbohydrates are intercepted by gut bacteria, which digest vegetable fiber into short-chain fatty acids. Vegetarians may get up to 20% of calories from fats released by gut bacteria after fermentation of vegetable matter. (Gut bacteria can't eat the fats themselves because the gut lacks oxygen, which is required for fat metabolism.)

- **Most carbs are a fat source.** The average American gets 55% of calories from carbs, but most of these are converted to fat. On high-carb diets, fructose is converted directly to fat in the liver (if all goes well), and beyond about 15-20% of calories glucose is either converted to fat and stored in fat cells, or substitutes for fat as an energy source. Thus, that 55% of calories that enters the mouth as carbs may later end up in the body mostly as the 16-chain saturated fat palmitic acid.

Most people don't know that most of the carbs they eat become fat in the body. If they did, they might not be so shy about eating the fat directly.

Mammals Eat Different Foods … But the Same Diet

Mammals eat a wide range of different foods: cows and sheep eat grass; lions and wolves eat meat; gorillas eat fruit, and mice a mixed diet.

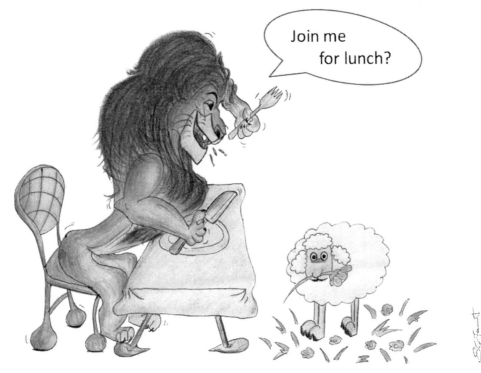

Lions and lambs don't eat the same diet … or do they?

But what if these differences are illusory? Have you noticed that:

- Cow's milk, indeed the milk of all mammals, has a similar macronutrient composition to human milk – with most calories as fat.

- All mammals have a body composition of equal amounts protein and fat by mass, and "cannibalize" themselves during starvation to obtain 74% of calories as fat and 26% of calories as protein.

This tells us that all mammals should flourish on a diet similar in composition to milk and muscle – mostly fat by calories. Yet cows and sheep and gorillas are vegetarians. Don't their diets have very little fat?

Yes – *before their food is transformed by the digestive tract*.

But after digestive transformation, as Barry Groves has pointed out[1], all mammals eat a close facsimile of the Perfect Health Diet – a diet dominated by saturated and monounsaturated fats, with only a few carbs.

CARNIVORE DIETS

Though wolves and dogs may obtain 5% of calories as fallen fruit, most wild carnivores obtain essentially all their energy from animal flesh.

You might think this makes for a protein-rich diet, but carnivores favor the fattier parts of their prey. Groves notes, "This is particularly noticeable with hyenas whose jaws and teeth are designed to break the long bones and skulls to get at the bone marrow and brain within, which are very high in fat."[2]

Assuming that carnivores feed on ruminants whose tissue fats are 20% polyunsaturated[3], carnivore macronutrient ratios are typically:

- <5% carbs
- 25% protein
- 56% saturated and monounsaturated fats
- 14% polyunsaturated fats

In carnivores the liver manufactures glucose from protein to meet the needs of neural and immune cells.

HERBIVORE DIETS

Ruminants have evolved special organs for bacterial digestion of plant foods. In these organs, bacteria scavenge every carb calorie, *leaving none for the animal*. As a by-product of carb digestion, the bacteria release volatile short-chain fats. These fats are transported to the liver, which uses them for energy and for fabrication of sugars, ketones, and fats for the rest of the body.

---

[1] Barry Groves, "Should all animals eat a high-fat, low-carb diet?" *http://www.second-opinions.co.uk/should-all-animals-eat-a-high-fat-low-carb-diet.html*.

[2] Barry Groves, "Should all animals eat a high-fat, low-carb diet?" *http://www.second-opinions.co.uk/should-all-animals-eat-a-high-fat-low-carb-diet.html*.

[3] Cordain L et al. Fatty acid analysis of wild ruminant tissues: evolutionary implications for reducing diet-related chronic disease. *Eur J Clin Nutr.* 2002 Mar;56(3):181-91. *http://pmid.us/11960292*.

Short-Chain Fats Are 70% of the Ruminant Diet, Carbs 0%

Dr. Richard A. Bowen summarizes how cattle, sheep, and goats get their energy:

> Volatile fatty acids (VFA) are produced in large amounts through ruminal fermentation and are of paramount importance in that they provide greater than 70% of the ruminant's energy supply....

> Within the liver, proprionate serves as a major substrate for gluconeogenesis, which is absolutely critical to the ruminant because almost no glucose reaches the small intestine for absorption.[1]

[1]   Bowen RA. "Digestive Physiology of Herbivores," *http://arbl.cvmbs.colostate.edu/hbooks/pathphys/digestion/herbivores/index.html.*

After processing by the digestive tract, ruminant macronutrient ratios are:

- 0% carbs

- 17% protein

- 80% saturated and monounsaturated fats – 70% short-chain, 10% long-chain

- 3% polyunsaturated fats

The liver converts short-chain fats to ketones and glucose to meet neuronal energy needs.

PRIMATE DIETS

Like other mammals, primates eat a wide range of diets: tarsiers are carnivorous, gorillas nearly herbivorous. But once again, by the time the diet leaves the digestive tract all primates eat remarkably similar diets.

Gorillas evolved in the forest and focused their diet on foliage – leaves, shoots, and stems – and fruit. To digest such a diet, they need bacteria. To house the bacteria, gorillas have a very long and large colon, much larger than that of humans.

A 1997 *Journal of Nutrition* article analyzed the diet of gorillas.[4] It turns out that 58% of gorilla calories come from short-chain fats released in the colon by bacteria after

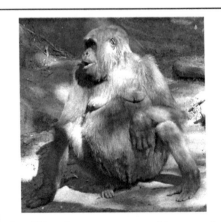

Gorillas ferment up to 50 pounds of vegetables per day in their big guts to obtain 58% of calories as short-chain fats.

---

[4] Popovich DG et al. The western lowland gorilla diet has implications for the health of humans and other hominoids. *J Nutr.* 1997 Oct;127(10):2000-5. *http://pmid.us/9311957.*

fermentation of plant fiber.   As a result, gorilla macronutrient ratios are approximately as follows:

- 16% carbs
- 20% protein
- 62% saturated and monounsaturated fats
- 2% polyunsaturated fats

Summary: Optimal Mammalian Macronutrient Ratios

Wild mammals, no matter what foods enter their mouths, provide their bodies with very similar macronutrients:

- 0% to 16% carbs.
- 15% to 25% protein.
- 56% to 77% saturated and monounsaturated fats
- 1% to 14% polyunsaturated fats

An equivalent diet for humans would have more carbs (to feed our larger brains). This predicts the optimal human diet to be about 20% carbs, 15% protein, 60% saturated and monounsaturated fat, and 5% polyunsaturated fat.

The Three Mammalian Dietary Strategies

Although mammals thrive on similar macronutrient ratios, we can tease out a few differences between omnivore, herbivore, and carnivore diets.

Each diet has a different strategy for meeting the body's glucose needs:

- **Omnivores** eat enough carbs to meet the body's glucose needs directly.
- **Herbivores** obtain little glucose from diet, but up to 70% of their energy needs from short-chain fats produced by bacterial fermentation. These short-chain fats are transformed in the liver to ketones which nourish neurons, substantially reducing the body's glucose needs.
- **Carnivores** obtain few or no carbohydrates from diet, and meet glucose needs by manufacturing glucose from protein.

The fact that these three strategies are all evolutionarily successful shows that they can all produce superb health in mammals. There are some implications for human diets:

- ***Most mammals satisfy glucose needs by manufacturing it in the liver***, not by eating it. This suggests there may be a health advantage to keeping glucose intake a little below the body's needs, and thereby keeping blood glucose levels low. *This is a clue to the benefits of low-carb (but not too low-carb!) diets.*

- ***Mammalian short-chain fat intakes cover a huge range – 0% to 70%.*** This tells us that short-chain fats are safe for humans, and that "ketogenic" diets in which a majority of calories are obtained from short-chain fats should be a feasible human dietary strategy. *This is good because ketogenic diets are therapeutic for some diseases.*

As we'll see when we look deeper into the literature on human diets, it turns out that the solution to the optimal human diet was there all along – in the zoo! Mammalian diets are a reliable guide to what we should be eating.

The Perfect Health Diet is a Mammalian Hybrid

The Perfect Health Diet is a hybrid of these three mammalian strategies:

- It *optimizes bodily nutrition* by giving humans the optimal mammalian macronutrient ratios.

- It *minimizes stress on the gut and liver* by providing food that needs relatively little transformation.

- It is *robust against dietary failure* by providing redundant sources of key nutrients, like glucose and ketones.

Key features of the Perfect Health Diet approach:

1. It follows the Omnivore Strategy in getting a significant number of calories directly from glucose, in the form of **safe starches like sweet potato, taro, and white rice**. Starch consumption of 200 to 400 calories per day meets half or more of the body's glucose needs and minimizes any risk the body may become glucose deprived.

2. It follows the Herbivore and Carnivore Strategies of **keeping blood glucose levels low** by limiting carbohydrate consumption to less than the human body's glucose needs of about 600 calories per day.

3. It follows the Herbivore Strategy of obtaining significant calories from **short-chain fats via coconut oil, dairy fat, and fermented plant fiber**. These short-chain fats are converted in the liver to ketones which nourish neurons and protect against glucose deficiency.

4. As with all natural mammalian diets, **60% of calories or so come from saturated and monounsaturated fats** – the safest calorie sources. Protein, glucose, and polyunsaturated fats, all of which are toxic in excess, are limited. Fructose, another toxin, is strictly limited.

The Ketogenic Diet: A Therapeutic Variant

Ketogenic diets are an implementation of a pure Herbivore Strategy. The human version of the Herbivore Strategy is to obtain nearly half of calories from short-chain fats, which may be obtained from coconut oil or created in the gut by fermentation of plant fiber.

Ketogenic diets are therapeutic for any disease in which elevated levels of glucose or glutamate are problematic, including:

- Epilepsy and some other brain conditions, probably including schizophrenia, bipolar disorder, depression, psychoses, and migraines.

- Solid tumor cancers.

- Diabetes, metabolic syndrome, and obesity.

- Bacterial infections and diseases caused by them, probably including atherosclerosis, Alzheimer's, Parkinson's, multiple sclerosis, Lyme disease, fibromyalgia, and many neuropathies.

We recommend a ketogenic version of the Perfect Health Diet for people with these diseases. To make the diet ketogenic, eat fewer carbs (about 200 calories per day, largely from fiber-rich safe starches like taro and sweet potato) and much more coconut oil.

Intermittent Ketogenic Fasting as Dietary Hygiene

We don't recommend the ketogenic diet as an everyday diet for healthy people: It lacks the redundancy and robustness of the Perfect Health Diet and is vulnerable to nutritional deficiencies. Nutritional needs on long-term ketogenic diets are still being worked out.

However, healthy people can get most of the benefits of ketogenic diets by engaging in occasional ketogenic fasts. This is basically a day of fasting in which you can eat as much coconut oil, heavy cream, fiber, and fermented vegetables – all sources of short-chain fats – as you like, but no carbs or protein of any kind.

Ketogenic fasts help kill bacteria, viruses, and cancer cells. Intermittent ketogenic fasting is therefore preventative for all the chronic diseases listed above.

Our Perfect Health Prescription

Here is the essence of the book in preview: We recommend following a hybrid mammalian strategy – the regular Perfect Health Diet – punctuated with a few Herbivore Strategy days – intermittent ketogenic fasts.

But what happens if you don't?

Why Bad Diets Wreck Human Health

Humans have evolved two major differences from other mammals:

- *We have a bigger brain, and therefore need more glucose and ketones.*

- *We have a smaller gut and liver, and therefore less ability to transform food.*

Here is a comparison of brain, liver, and gut sizes in humans and other primates:

Organ	% body weight, humans	% body weight, other primates
Brain	2.0	0.7
Liver	2.2	2.5
Gut	1.7	2.9

Source: Aiello LC, Wheeler P. The expensive tissue hypothesis: the brain and the digestive system in human and primate evolution. *Current Anthropology* 1995(Apr); 36(2):199-211.

The brain is the biggest determinant of glucose needs. While other primates need only about 7% of energy as glucose or ketones, humans need about 20%.

The Human Diet Has Little Margin for Error

Compared to other primates, humans have a 12% smaller liver and a 40% smaller gut. This means that:

- **Humans don't have the same ability to transform plant fiber into short-chain fats that other primates have.** Gorillas ferment so much plant fiber in their big colons that they get 58% of calories as short-chain fats; humans can generate only about 20% of calories from fiber.

- **Humans don't have the same ability to manufacture glucose in their livers from protein.** The smaller liver means less flexibility in the diet. While carnivores can meet their tiny glucose needs (5% to 10% of calories) in their big livers, humans with our small livers will struggle to meet our big glucose needs (20% of calories). This is why *humans should not attempt to follow a pure Carnivore Strategy.*

Wild animals can often maintain good health on a variety of diets. Ruminants can obtain fats either by eating fats (as calves do from their mother's milk) or by fermenting plants. Most mammals have big livers and small brains, so can easily manufacture needed glucose even if they never eat any. Most mammals have livers big enough to detoxify inappropriate diets.

Humans are different. Our small livers and digestive tracts won't let us vary our diet too far from what our body needs.

Human food intake has to closely match the body's needs of 65% fats, 20% carbs, 15% protein.

This means that compared to animals, human health is fragile. If we eat a bad diet, our liver and digestive tract won't make up for it. And our body will suffer.

Wild animals don't normally become obese, suffer heart attacks, get diabetes, develop cancer, or become senile. But humans do – if we eat the wrong diet.

The American Diet is SAD

Unfortunately very few people eat an optimal diet.

The macronutrient ratio of the typical American diet is 52% carbs, 33% fat, 15% protein.[5] Americans would have to shift about one-third of total calories from carb to fat to perfect their macronutrient ratios.

The American macronutrient ratio is almost identical to that of a McDonald's supersized cheeseburger, French fries, and soda value meal.[6] The "standard American diet" (or SAD) might as well consist of fast food.

Sadly, it is also almost identical to the 55% carb, 30% fat, 15% protein diet that for many years was recommended by the US government and groups like the American Heart Association.[7]

Our Diet Was SADDER

Why did our health go bad? We ate diets even worse than the standard American diet.

- Paul, first as a scientist and then as an Internet entrepreneur, got used to working busy 60 hour weeks and grabbing the most handy foods: French bread and cheese, and soda – lots of soda, for the caffeine and sugar rush.

- Shou-Ching was influenced by anti-fat and anti-meat nutritional advice from doctors and vegetarian friends, and worried that her father's premature death from stroke might indicate an inherited risk. So she avoided meat and eggs; soy, rice, and vegetable oils were staples of her diet.

---

[5] Cordain L et al. Origins and evolution of the Western diet: health implications for the 21st century. *Am J Clin Nutr* 2005 Feb; 81(2): 341-54. *http://pmid.us/15699220.*

[6] McDonald's value meal ratios calculated from *http://nutritiondata.com.*

[7] *http://www.health.gov/DietaryGuidelines/dga2005/document/html/chapter7.htm.*

We were both getting as much as 70% of calories from carbs, were deficient in nutrients, and were eating very high quantities of toxic foods: wheat and fructose in Paul's case, soy and vegetable oils in Shou-Ching's. We might have improved our health by eating exclusively at McDonald's.

So we were very far from practicing what we now preach. It was declining health that caused us to change our ways; and restored health that makes us advocates of the Perfect Health Diet.

Toward a Happier Future

A great mass of scientific evidence is converging on the Perfect Health Diet as the optimal way for humans to eat. We'll present much of that evidence in coming pages.

It's true that most nutritionists and doctors haven't yet accepted the inferences toward which this evidence points. But that's no surprise: long-held prejudices are hard to give up.

Max Planck said that scientific theories don't change because old scientists change their minds, they change because old scientists die.

So it may be with the science of nutrition. The evidence in favor of a diet like the Perfect Health Diet is becoming overwhelming; but it will take a few funerals yet before official recommendations are updated.

So much for our preview. From here, we'll leave mammals and examine the evidence in humans. Step One looks at the evidence underlying our macronutrient recommendations.

Step One to Perfect Health: Optimize Macronutrition

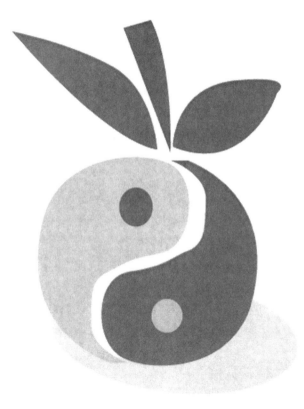

Protein

Except for some protein-deficient vegans and misguided bodybuilders, almost everyone eats a healthy amount of protein. People seem to naturally find protein tasty when they need it, bland when they don't, and gravitate to an optimal protein intake.

Protein Needs

If sufficient carbs are present in the diet, dietary protein needs are small. Even fast-growing infants don't need much protein: Human breast milk provides only 7% of calories as protein.

According to the US Dietary Reference Intake, adult women should obtain 46 gm (184 calories) per day of protein, and adult men 56 gm (224 calories) per day.[8] These values represent less than 10% of calories for most adults.

Reasons for Extra Protein

Either carb restriction or athletic goals may argue for higher protein intakes.

If carbs are restricted without short-chain fat provision (the "Carnivore Strategy"), up to 400 calories of protein may be consumed in the manufacture of glucose and ketones.

Even on a zero-carb diet, however, the body has no ability to use more than 600 calories per day of protein. During the one-year Bellevue All-Meat Trial in 1928, Vilhjalmur Stefansson ate an average of 2,650 calories a day, 2100 from fat and 550 from protein; Karsten Andersen averaged 2,620 calories a day, 2,110 from fat and 510 from protein.[9] On a zero-carb diet, 550 protein calories seems sufficient.

Only a few – very few! – protein calories can support rapid muscle growth. The protein content of muscle is 16.4%[10], so adding 26 pounds of muscle per year requires only 5 gm (20 calories) of protein per day.

In the normal range of protein intakes, controlled trials have not been able to detect any additional muscle gains from higher protein consumption.[11]

---

[8] http://en.wikipedia.org/wiki/Protein_(nutrient).

[9] McClellan WS, Du Bois EF. Clinical calorimetry XLV. Prolonged meat diets with a study of kidney function and ketosis. *Journal of Biological Chemistry*, 1931, 87:651–668. Hat tip Charles Washington, *http://blog.zeroinginonhealth.com/?p=397*.

[10] Janney NW. The protein content of muscle. *J. Biol. Chem.* 1916 25(2): 185-188. *http://www.jbc.org/content/25/2/185.full.pdf*.

Why do athletes think extra protein helps them add muscle? Two reasons:

- *Eating more calories* – whatever the source, whether fat, protein, or carb – builds muscles.[12] Many bodybuilders overfeed on protein. However, overfeeding with fats and starches would be just as effective.

- *Signaling effects.* If protein intake is low, extra intake of certain amino acids – notably leucine, a branched-chain amino acid – will prevent muscle breakdown and stimulate muscle growth. Leucine supplementation increases muscle growth in pigs on a low protein diet by 61%, and prevents muscle loss on low protein diets.[13]

Whey protein, which contains high levels of branched-chain amino acids including leucine and which also helps to heal the gut, disrupt biofilms, and promote probiotic gut flora, is therefore an attractive supplemental food.[14]

Two Reasons to Limit Protein

AMMONIA POISONING

Too much dietary protein can lead to poisoning by ammonia, which forms from leftover nitrogen when proteins are metabolized. The threshold for production of toxic levels of ammonia may be as low as 600 to 800 protein calories per day. The body's ability to convert ammonia to urea peaks with a protein intake of 230 g/day (920 calories per day), indicating that ammonia levels must be rising rapidly at that level of protein intake.[15]

---

[11] Lemon PW et al. Protein requirements and muscle mass/strength changes during intensive training in novice bodybuilders. *J Appl Physiol.* 1992 Aug;73(2):767-75. *http://pmid.us/1400008.* See also Hoffman JR et al. Effect of protein intake on strength, body composition and endocrine changes in strength/power athletes. *J Int Soc Sports Nutr.* 2006 Dec 13;3:12-8. *http://pmid.us/18500968.*

[12] Stearns RL et al. Effects of ingesting protein in combination with carbohydrate during exercise on endurance performance: a systematic review with meta-analysis. *J Strength Cond Res.* 2010 Aug;24(8):2192-202. *http://pmid.us/20683237.*

[13] Yin Y et al. Supplementing L-leucine to a low-protein diet increases tissue protein synthesis in weanling pigs. *Amino Acids.* 2010 May 15. [Epub ahead of print] *http://pmid.us/20473536.* Jitomir J, Willoughby DS. Leucine for retention of lean mass on a hypocaloric diet. *J Med Food.* 2008 Dec;11(4):606-9. *http://pmid.us/19053849.*

[14] Marshall K. Therapeutic applications of whey protein. *Altern Med Rev.* 2004 Jun;9(2):136-56. *http://pmid.us/15253675.* Krissansen GW. Emerging health properties of whey proteins and their clinical implications. *J Am Coll Nutr.* 2007 Dec;26(6):713S-23S. *http://pmid.us/18187438.*

[15] Rudman D et al. Maximal rates of excretion and synthesis of urea in normal and cirrhotic subjects. *J Clin Invest.* 1973 Sep;52(9):2241-9. *http://pmid.us/4727456.*

Explorer Vilhjalmur Stefansson, who spent the winter of 1906 living with Inuit on the Mackenzie River delta near the Arctic Ocean, tells of the danger of "rabbit starvation." This occurred in spring when stores of fat had run out and lean rabbits were the only food. When protein intake exceeds 45% of calories, nausea and diarrhea begin in days and death can follow in weeks.[16]

Rabbit starvation was reproduced in the Bellevue All-Meat Trial.[17]

Infants, especially pre-term infants, are much more sensitive to protein. Human breast milk is only 7% protein. Pre-term infants fed with 20% protein had more fever, lethargy, and poor feeding, and lower IQs at ages 3 and 6 years.[18] A slight increase in the protein content of formula, from 7% to 9%, is enough to make babies overweight at age 2.[19]

Pregnant mothers also need to limit protein to less than 20% of calories to avoid risks to their baby both perinatally and in later life.[20]

LONGEVITY AND OTHER HEALTH EFFECTS

In animal studies, protein restriction extends lifespan.[21] Experiments with individual amino acids have shown that methionine, which is ubiquitously present in food proteins, is particularly associated with shortened lifespan.[22]

---

[16] Speth JD, Spielmann KA. Energy source, protein metabolism, and hunter-gatherer subsistence strategies. *J of Anthropology and Archaeology*, 1983, 2:1–31.

[17] McClellan WS, Du Bois EF. Clinical calorimetry XLV. Prolonged meat diets with a study of kidney function and ketosis. *J. Biol. Chem.* 1931, 87:651–668.

[18] Goldman HI et al. Clinical effects of two different levels of protein intake on low-birth-weight infants. *J Pediatr.* 1969 Jun;74(6):881-9. *http://pmid.us/5781798*. Goldman HI et al. Effects of early dietary protein intake on low-birth-weight infants: evaluation at 3 years of age. *J Pediatr.* 1971 Jan;78(1):126-9. *http://pmid.us/5539071*. Goldman HI et al. Late effects of early dietary protein intake on low-birth-weight infants. *J Pediatr.* 1974 Dec;85(6):764-9. *http://pmid.us/4472449*.

[19] European Childhood Obesity Trial Study Group. Lower protein in infant formula is associated with lower weight up to age 2 y: a randomized clinical trial. *Am J Clin Nutr.* 2009 Jun;89(6):1836-45. *http://pmid.us/19386747*.

[20] See our post from July 12, 2010, *http://perfecthealthdiet.com/?p=196*, for details.

[21] Sun L et al. Life-span extension in mice by preweaning food restriction and by methionine restriction in middle age. *J Gerontol A Biol Sci Med Sci.* 2009 Jul;64(7):711-22. *http://pmid.us/19414512*. Miller RA et al. Methionine-deficient diet extends mouse lifespan, slows immune and lens aging, alters glucose, T4, IGF-I and insulin levels, and increases hepatocyte MIF levels and stress resistance. *Aging Cell.* 2005 Jun;4(3):119-25. *http://pmid.us/15924568*. Orentreich N et al. Low methionine ingestion by rats extends life span. *J Nutr.* 1993 Feb;123(2):269-74. *http://pmid.us/8429371*.

In addition to shortening lifespan, excess methionine can cause neural tube defects in developing babies[23] and atherosclerosis[24].

Protein Restriction, Autophagy, and Longevity

One mechanism by which protein restriction extends lifespan is by promoting a recycling process called autophagy.[1]

Proteins generally become useless after a time: they fold into the wrong shape, or they glycate with sugar, and no longer work.

These "junk proteins" gather in cells until a cleanup mechanism, autophagy, is triggered. When protein is scarce, cells turn on enzymes that digest junk proteins, recycling their amino acids. This cleanup improves cellular health. Autophagy is necessary for protein or calorie restriction to extend lifespan.[2]

[1] Jia K, Levine B. Autophagy is required for dietary restriction-mediated life span extension in C. elegans. *Autophagy.* 2007 Nov-Dec;3(6):597-9. *http://pmid.us/17912023.*

[2] Hansen M et al. A role for autophagy in the extension of lifespan by dietary restriction in C. elegans. *PLoS Genet.* 2008 Feb;4(2):e24. *http://pmid.us/18282106.*

Summary

Protein intake of 200 to 600 calories per day seems to be a healthy plateau range if sufficient carbs are eaten, but the plateau range becomes much narrower – a window around 500 to 600 calories – if carbs are restricted.

Within the plateau range, low protein intake may extend lifespan, and high protein intake may promote muscle gain.

---

[22] López-Torres M, Barja G. Lowered methionine ingestion as responsible for the decrease in rodent mitochondrial oxidative stress in protein and dietary restriction possible implications for humans. *Biochim Biophys Acta.* 2008 Nov;1780(11):1337-47. *http://pmid.us/18252204.*

[23] Dunlevy LP et al. Excess methionine suppresses the methylation cycle and inhibits neural tube closure in mouse embryos. *FEBS Lett.* 2006 May 15;580(11):2803-7. *http://pmid.us/16674949.*

[24] Troen AM et al. The atherogenic effect of excess methionine intake. *Proc Natl Acad Sci USA.* 2003 Dec 9;100(25):15089-94. *http://pmid.us/14657334.*

Carbs

Most plant foods are broken down in the digestive tract to indigestible fiber or to the simple sugars glucose and fructose.

Fructose is a poison at any dose: it reacts with proteins, creating toxins. To prevent such inappropriate "fructation" the body shunts fructose to the liver for disposal, mainly through conversion to fat. The conversion process, however, damages the liver, potentially causing metabolic syndrome.

So the potentially beneficial carbs are (1) those that digest to glucose or galactose, such as starch and milk sugars; and (2) indigestible fiber that feeds gut bacteria. In this chapter we consider sources of the "good sugars," glucose and galactose.

How Much Glucose Does the Body Need?

Glucose has three main uses in the body: It combines with proteins to form structural molecules called glycoproteins; it is an alternative fuel that cells can burn instead of fats; and it is a precursor for killing compounds ("reactive oxygen species" or ROS) made by immune cells.

A fasting person's daily glucose production has been measured at 8 µmol/kg/min, which for typical adults equals 120 to 160 grams, or 480-640 calories, per day.[25] We can get to a similar number for the body's glucose needs by adding up the body's specific uses of glucose.

GLUCOSE IN STRUCTURAL MOLECULES

Wet sugar is sticky and highly reactive. It likes to combine with proteins, and can do so in many ways. The human body has 20,000 genes, 200,000 proteins, but 2,000,000 glycoproteins, or compounds built up by combining proteins with sugars.

Interactions between cells are mediated by glycoproteins. Evolution of these sticky glycoproteins made multicellular life possible.

Some structural sugar compounds are highly abundant in the body:

- Mucin is one of the main components of mucus, and protects the gut and airways from pathogens and foreign matter. It is also a key part of tears and saliva.

- Hyaluronan lubricates joints and helps provide the scaffolding that shapes cells into tissues. Glucosamine and chondroitin sulfate are similar sugar-rich compounds important in connective tissue.

---

[25] Nair KS et al. Leucine, glucose, and energy metabolism after 3 days of fasting in healthy human subjects. *Am J Clin Nutr.* 1987 Oct;46(4):557-62. *http://pmid.us/3661473*.

Production of hyaluronan alone consumes 5 gm, or 20 calories, of glucose per day.[26] It is not known how much glucose is consumed in production of the other 2 million glycoproteins, but it probably exceeds 200 calories per day.

GLUCOSE AS FUEL FOR NEURONS

One often hears that glucose is the body's "primary fuel." This is quite mistaken.

It is true that all human cells can, if need be, metabolize glucose. But mitochondria, the energy producers in most human cells, prefer to burn fat. So in the body, fat is the preferred and primary fuel, except in specialist cells which lack mitochondria (red blood cells) or avoid fat metabolism (neurons).

Normal glucose-as-a-fuel consumption is dominated by neurons. The brain and nerves require about 20 calories per hour, waking or sleeping. These 480 daily calories can be provided by either glucose alone, or by a mix of glucose and ketone bodies (which are derived from fats or protein). So daily glucose consumption by the brain and nerves will be somewhere between 150 and 480 calories, depending on ketone availability.

GLUCOSE FOR MUSCLE GLYCOGEN

In addition to the cells like neurons and red blood cells that routinely consume glucose, muscles consume glucose in the form of glycogen during intense exertion. Glycogen is made of long chains of glucose compounded with a pyrophosphate group, and is energy rich because it can readily donate phosphate groups to restore adenosine triphosphate (ATP).

What Is Glycogen, and How Much Can The Body Hold?

Glycogen is a storage molecule composed of long chains of glucose-6-phosphate – the high-energy version of glucose, ready to contribute a phosphate to restore ATP, the molecule that powers protein functions. Liver glycogen is a reservoir from which glucose can be drawn as needed to maintain blood sugar levels; muscle glycogen provides energy for intense athletic exertion.

Glycogen makes up 1-2% of the mass of muscle, or about 300-500 gm. The liver has another 70-100 gm of glycogen, which it uses to manage blood glucose.[1]

[1] Wikipedia, "Glycogen," *http://en.wikipedia.org/wiki/Glycogen.*

Muscle glycogen usage is a relatively small drain on glucose. Highly trained runners utilize about 50 glycogen calories per mile. Highly trained cyclists cycling

---

[26] Stern R. Hyaluronan catabolism: a new metabolic pathway. *Eur J Cell Biol.* 2004 Aug;83(7):317-25. *http://pmid.us/15503855.*

at 70% of maximum oxygen utilization (an intense pace) utilize about 500 calories of glycogen per hour.[27]

Ordinary folk, exercising at low intensity for shorter periods of time, need very few extra glucose calories to maintain muscle glycogen levels. Someone who exercises 20 minutes per day at moderate intensity probably uses less than 50 glycogen calories.

Carb Loading for Endurance Athletes

When endurance athletes run out of muscle glycogen, it is known as "hitting the wall." Endurance athletes can maximize stored muscle glycogen by "carb loading." About 3 weeks before an event, the athlete adopts a zero-carb diet and continues to train intensively, depleting muscle glycogen. This causes muscle cells to enlarge their glycogen storage reservoirs. A few days before the event, the athlete begins to eat starch. About 3000 calories of starch is needed to fill muscle glycogen reservoirs. Caffeine aids the process.[1]

[1] Pedersen DJ et al. High rates of muscle glycogen resynthesis after exhaustive exercise when carbohydrate is coingested with caffeine. *J Appl Physiol.* 2008 Jul;105(1):7-13. *http://pmid.us/18467543.*

GLUCOSE AS A KILLING AGENT

One reason most cells prefer fats to glucose as an energy source is that fats burn cleanly, while glucose, when it is metabolized for energy, produces reactive oxygen species (ROS). These dangerous molecules can damage or destroy cells.

The destructiveness of ROS has been put to use by the immune system. Immune cells called macrophages can metabolize glucose to produce abundant ROS, which are used to kill pathogens like bacteria and fungi.

Under normal circumstances the immune system probably isn't doing a lot of killing, and doesn't consume much glucose. However, people with chronic infections, especially with fungi or protozoa, may need extra glucose.

ENDOGENOUS GLUCOSE PRODUCTION

Against these glucose needs must be set the glucose that is produced routinely by the body as a consequence of the metabolism of fats.

Fats are stored in the body as either phospholipids, which consist of two fatty acids joined by a glycerol backbone to a phosphate group and an organic molecule like choline or inositol, or triglycerides, which consist of three fatty acids and a glycerol backbone. Phospholipids make up cell membranes, while triglycerides are a storage form of fats.

---

[27] Burke LM et al. Effect of fat adaptation and carbohydrate restoration on metabolism and performance during prolonged cycling. *J Appl Physiol.* 2000 Dec;89(6):2413-21. *http://pmid.us/11090597.*

When fatty acids are consumed for energy, the glycerol backbones are released. Two glycerols make one molecule of glucose. Recycling of glycerol from fats helps to meet the body's glucose needs, since fats in food enter the body already attached to glycerol backbones.

A typical triglyceride provides about 12% of calories as glycerol, 88% as fatty acids. Eating 2400 calories per day on the Perfect Health Diet, in which 65% of calories are derived from triglycerides or phospholipids, will generate about 200 calories per day of glucose from the glycerol in food fats.

Summary: The Body's Glucose Needs

Although the precise magnitude of the various quantities is uncertain, it appears that the body's daily glucose consumption is about 150-480 calories for brain and nerves, 200-300 calories for glycoproteins such as mucin, 100 calories for muscle glycogen and immune, intestinal, and kidney cell use, offset by about 200 calories of glucose produced in the course of fat burning. In elite athletes, glucose needs are increased by 50 to 100 calories per hour of training.

For most people, something like 400-650 daily glucose calories must be obtained from the diet, manufactured from protein, or replaced with ketones.

Three Ways to Meet Glucose Needs

Figuring out the lower end of the "plateau range" for dietary glucose is complicated by the fact that there are three strategies to meet the body's glucose needs, each of which may be beneficial for different people:

1. **The Omnivore Strategy:** Eat enough calories per day of starch or glucose to meets the body's needs directly.

2. **The Herbivore Strategy:** Eat a ketogenic diet full of short-chain saturated fats which the liver metabolizes to ketone bodies. These can replace up to 330 calories per day of glucose consumption by the brain and nerves, reducing dietary glucose needs to a minimal level.

3. **The Carnivore Strategy:** If the supply of glucose and short-chain fats is insufficient to meet the body's needs, then the liver will manufacture glucose and ketones from protein. During starvation; the body gets the protein from muscle. The Carnivore Strategy is to eat enough protein (600 calories per day) to meet the body's glucose needs.

The Omnivore Strategy is the one most people follow: anyone who eats a high-carb diet will follow it willy-nilly.

The Herbivore Strategy, or ketogenic diet, mimics the diet of gorillas and ruminants, who obtain 58%-70% of calories from short-chain fats produced by bacteria in their digestive tracts. In humans, this strategy requires consuming a large amount of coconut oil – at least 12 tablespoons per day – plus fiber. As we mentioned earlier and will discuss further in Step Four, ketogenic diets are therapeutic for diseases such as epilepsy, diabetes, cancer, and bacterial infections.

The Carnivore Strategy often produces rapid short-term weight loss – it is the secret behind the "induction phase" of Dr. Atkins's diet for weight loss. In this strategy, protein is substituted for carbs, so that the liver can manufacture glucose and ketone bodies from protein:

- Glucose is made from the "glucogenic amino acids": glycine, serine, valine, histidine, arginine, cysteine, proline, alanine, glutamate, glutamine, apartate, asparagines, methionine.

- Ketones are made from the "ketogenic amino acids." Leucine and lysine are ketogenic but not glucogenic; threonine, isoleucine, phenylalanine, tryptophan, and tyrosine are both glucogenic and ketogenic.

Omnivore and Herbivore Strategies will do fine on 200 calories per day protein, but a Carnivore Strategy might require up to 600 calories per day.

Dangers of Glucose Deprivation

We are opposed to a pure Carnivore Strategy diet for these reasons:

1. **Stress on the liver.** We do not believe in forcing the liver to do unnecessary work. Forcing the liver to spend resources and oxygen to manufacture glucose may divert it from other health-improving tasks.

2. **Toxicity and reduced longevity.** Conversion of protein to glucose generates ammonia as a toxic by-product. We believe in minimizing toxin levels. The high protein intake needed to implement this strategy is associated with shortened lifespan.

3. **Risk of glucose deprivation**. While a healthy and well-nourished body can usually manufacture enough glucose to meet bodily needs, this is not a certainty. There are many reasons why the liver may be unable to manufacture adequate glucose, including:

    a. Vitamin deficiencies or liver disease may impair the liver's ability to manufacture glucose.

    b. Infections, especially fungal infections, or athletic training may increase glucose needs.

Potential symptoms of bodily glucose deprivation include:

- Impaired immune function, particularly against fungal infections. Such infections are most likely to appear in the skin, urinary tract and vagina, digestive tract, sinuses and mouth.

- Loss of mucus production, resulting in dry eyes, dry mouth, dry sinuses, and most importantly a dry and unprotected intestinal tract. In this state pathogens can more easily occupy the gut, while digestive enzymes may digest not only food but also the cells of the intestinal lining.

- Reduced glycoprotein production, compromising the integrity of cellular junctions and barriers such as the intestinal barrier and blood-brain barrier. This can allow pathogenic bacteria to invade the body and the brain, precipitating chronic disease.

- Impaired recycling of vitamin C, resulting in vitamin C and glutathione deficiencies. In the absence of vitamin C supplementation, this can cause impaired immune function, slow healing of wounds, unexplained weight loss, constipation, and oxidative damage such as prematurely graying hair.

In addition, an absence of plant foods can create deficiencies in nutrients like potassium and vitamin C. Potassium deficiency aggravates the ammonia poisoning which the Carnivore Strategy's reliance upon protein produces.[28]

Many people have run into trouble on very low-carb diets:

- While experimenting with vegetables as his only plant food, Paul developed dry eyes and dry mouth; chronic fungal infections; and scurvy.

- On the very low-carb Optimal Diet, there have been elevated rates of gastrointestinal cancers, probably due to mucus deficiencies.[29]

It seems that chronic infection may produce an immediate glucose deficiency, and that even in the absence of infections mucus deficiencies may lead to long-term gastrointestinal problems such as cancers.

Our Recommended Minimum Intake of Carbs

We recommend avoiding any risk of glucose deprivation. This can be achieved by:

- Eating at least 200 carb calories per day, to reduce the amount of glucose the liver must manufacture.

- Eating at least 600 calories per day of carbs and protein. This will ensure that insofar as protein is used to manufacture glucose, the body will not need to cannibalize muscle to obtain it.

- Including coconut oil and fiber in the diet, so that the liver can manufacture ketones from short-chain fats to make up any slack.

Most carb calories should come in the form of "safe starches" – from foods like rice, sweet potato, and taro. These provide glucose without fructose.

Perils of Too Much Glucose

Now we'll look at the damage that comes from eating too many carbohydrates.

---

[28] Hess DC et al. Ammonium toxicity and potassium limitation in yeast. *PLoS Biol.* 2006 Oct;4(11):e351. *http://pmid.us/17048990*.

[29] *http://high-fat-nutrition.blogspot.com/2010/08/back-comments-section-of-uric-acid-post.html*.

Two sources of damage are important:

- **Hyperglycemia** ("too much sugar"): Sugar poisoning inflicts the damage.
- **Hyperinsulinemia** ("too much insulin"): Insulin, a hormone that helps dispose of excess glucose, inflicts the damage.

What we'll find is that glucose in excess of bodily needs has toxic effects:

Sugar is a poison. In excess, it ruins health.

The Perils of Hyperglycemia

Ideally, blood glucose levels should remain in a stable range, between about 85 to 105 mg/dl. After eating carbohydrates, blood glucose should rise into the 120s to 140s, and fall back to the normal range in a few hours.

Eating near the body's glucose needs of 600 calories per day will tend to minimize average blood glucose levels.

As people increase carb consumption above the body's glucose needs, they become reliant on slow disposal mechanisms like fat formation, and average blood glucose levels go up.

If the liver and pancreas are poisoned by toxins like fructose, omega-6 fats, and wheat, insulin resistance may develop and blood glucose levels rise even further.

NERVE DAMAGE OCCURS WHEN BLOOD SUGARS RISE OVER 140 MG/DL

In a study of patients with peripheral neuropathy of unknown origin, neurologists found that many people who don't have diabetes nevertheless have "diabetic neuropathy" – nerve damage from excess glucose. Moreover, when given a glucose tolerance test, how high blood sugars rose over 140 mg/dl was correlated with severity of the neuropathy.[30]

This is interesting because most people's blood glucose levels rise above 140 mg/dl after a carb-rich meal. So most people are probably poisoning their nerves, little by little, every day.

The MONICA study showed that 13% of non-diabetics whose blood sugar rises over 140 mg/dl after a carb-rich meal have nerve damage.[31]

---

[30] Singleton JR et al. Increased prevalence of impaired glucose tolerance in patients with painful sensory neuropathy. *Diabetes Care*. 2001 Aug;24(8):1448-53. *http://pmid.us/11473085*. Hat tip Jenny Ruhl, *http://www.phlaunt.com/diabetes/14045678.php*.

[31] Ziegler D et al. Prevalence of polyneuropathy in pre-diabetes and diabetes is associated with abdominal obesity and macroangiopathy: the MONICA/KORA Augsburg Surveys S2 and S3. *Diabetes Care*. 2008 Mar;31(3):464-9. *http://pmid.us/18039804*.

HYPERGLYCEMIA DESTROYS THE ORGANS OF DIABETICS

In diabetics, organ damage arises from glucose toxicity, primarily due to uncontrolled glycation of proteins by excess blood sugar.[32] Elevated blood glucose causes neuropathy (nerve damage), nephropathy (kidney damage), retinopathy (eye damage), and cardiovascular disease.[33]

HYPERGLYCEMIA INCREASES MORTALITY

A useful measure of average blood glucose levels over the past month is "hemoglobin A1c," or HbA1c. This measures how much of the hemoglobin on red blood cells is glycated. It is possible to achieve HbA1c levels below 5%, but many people on high-carb diets develop HbA1c levels above 7%. HbA1c is an index of glucose poisoning: sugar glycates proteins indiscriminately, so the level of hemoglobin glycation indicates the severity of protein glycation generally.

The EPIC (European prospective investigation into cancer) study measured HbA1c values in 4462 men and 5570 women aged 45 to 79, and then followed patients, tracking death rates, for an average of six years.[34] They found that men with HbA1c levels above 7% were **5 times more likely to die** then men with HbA1c levels below 5%, and women with higher HbA1c levels were **12.5 times more likely to die**!

It was a simple and powerful relationship: the higher HbA1c, the more likely was death.

Most of the deaths were due to heart disease. The risk of heart attacks was increased 7.5-fold in the men and 9.5-fold in the women by high HbA1c. Blood sugar levels were an incredibly effective indicator of heart disease risk.

If you want to avoid a heart attack, keep blood sugar low.

The table below summarizes the results.

---

[32] Rossetti L. Glucose toxicity: the implications of hyperglycemia in the pathophysiology of diabetes mellitus. *Clin Invest Med*. 1995 Aug;18(4):255-60. *http://pmid.us/8549010*. Mooradian AD, Thurman JE. Glucotoxicity: potential mechanisms. *Clin Geriatr Med*. 1999 May;15(2):255. *http://pmid.us/10339632*.

[33] The Diabetes Control and Complications Trial Research Group. The effect of intensive treatment of diabetes on the development and progression of long-term complications in insulin-dependent diabetes mellitus. *N Engl J Med*. 1993 Sep 30;329(14):977-86. *http://pmid.us/8366922*. UK Prospective Diabetes Study (UKPDS) Group. Intensive blood-glucose control with sulphonylureas or insulin compared with conventional treatment and risk of complications in patients with type 2 diabetes (UKPDS 33). *Lancet*. 1998 Sep 12;352(9131):837-53. *http://pmid.us/9742976*

[34] Khaw KT et al. Association of hemoglobin A1c with cardiovascular disease and mortality in adults: the European prospective investigation into cancer in Norfolk. *Ann Intern Med*. 2004 Sep 21;141(6):413-20. *http://pmid.us/15381514*.

Table: HbA1c levels in 1995 in men and women aged 45 to 79 and subsequent CVD events and mortality 1995 to 2003.

	HbA1c <5%	HbA1c 5.0-5.4%	HbA1c 5.5-5.9%	HbA1c 6.0-6.4%	HbA1c 6.5-6.9%	HbA1c >7%
Coronary heart disease events, men	3.8%	6.4%	8.7%	10.2%	16.7%	28.4%
Coronary heart disease events, women	1.7%	2.1%	3.0%	7.3%	9.6%	16.2%
CVD events, men	6.7%	9.0%	12.1%	15.2%	25.0%	34.8%
CVD events, women	3.3%	3.8%	5.4%	9.8%	13.7%	36.8%
All-cause mortality, men	3.8%	5.5%	7.5%	9.9%	19.0%	18.5%
All-cause mortality, women	2.0%	2.7%	4.4%	6.4%	6.8%	25.0%

BLOOD GLUCOSE LEVELS DETERMINE STROKE RISK

The Whitehall study gave a glucose tolerance test to 19,019 men and then tracked their mortality for 38 years. It turned out that the risk of stroke rose in linear fashion with blood glucose level 2 hours after consuming 50 g (200 calories) glucose. Stroke mortality was lowest with a reading of 83 mg/dl. For every 18 mg/dl above that level, there was a 27% increase in stroke mortality.[35]

---

[35] Batty GD et al. Post-challenge blood glucose concentration and stroke mortality rates in non-diabetic men in London: 38-year follow-up of the original Whitehall prospective cohort study. *Diabetologia*. 2008 Jul;51(7):1123-6. *http://pmid.us/18438641*.

DIETARY CARBS AND HEART ATTACKS

The EPIC study showed that blood glucose levels, indicated by HbA1c, are responsible for most cardiovascular disease. We might expect, therefore, to see an association between high-carb diets and cardiovascular disease.

The question was investigated by a mammoth long-term U.S. study, the Nurse's Health Study. A 2006 report in the *New England Journal of Medicine* summarized the effects of carbohydrate composition on the nurses' health.[36] The researchers followed 98,462 women who completed a 1980 diet questionnaire, and split the women into ten equal-sized groups based on the fraction of calories obtained from carbohydrates. For simplicity we'll just compare the bottom and top deciles:

- The bottom decile obtained 58.8% of calories from carbohydrates and 26.9% from fat. Let's call this the "high-carb group."

- The top decile obtained 36.8% of calories from carbohydrates and 39.9% from fat. Let's call this the "moderate-carb group."

Compared to our recommendation of 20% carbs, the moderate-carb group has a carb excess of 17% of total calories, the high-carb group of 39%.

Now, in general, the moderate-carb group did not take good care of their health. They were more likely to smoke (26% smoked, compared to 17% of the high-carb group) and to avoid exercise (the moderate-carb group got 20% less exercise than the high-carb group). (They also drank a lot of coffee.)

But the rate of coronary heart disease cases was 0.131% in the high-carb group and 0.092% in the moderate-carb group. The high-carb group smoked less and exercised more, but their chance of a heart attack was 42% higher!

DIETARY CARBS CAUSE THE ATHEROGENIC BLOOD LIPID PROFILE

It's well known that a bad blood lipid profile – high triglycerides, low HDL, and high levels of "small, dense" LDL – is a risk factor for heart disease.

What's less commonly appreciated is that the bad blood lipid profile is almost entirely determined by excess carbohydrate consumption.

A series of studies by the group of Dr. Ronald Krauss grouped people by the carbohydrate fraction of their diet and measured their blood lipids, classifying them as "atherogenic" or "non-atherogenic." This was the result[37]:

---

[36] Halton TL et al. Low-carbohydrate-diet score and the risk of coronary heart disease in women. *N Engl J Med.* 2006 Nov 9;355(19):1991-2002. *http://pmid.us/17093250.*

[37] Krauss RM. Atherogenic lipoprotein phenotype and diet-gene interactions. *J Nutr.* 2001 Feb;131(2):340S-3S. *http://pmid.us/11160558.*

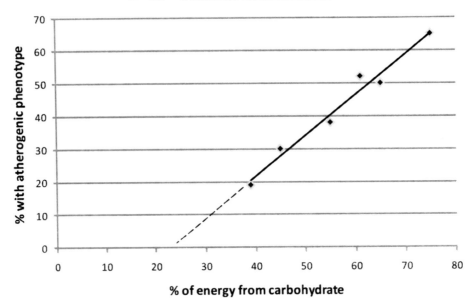

Figure: Percentage of people with atherogenic blood lipid profiles as a function of carbohydrate fraction of the diet.

A fit to the data suggests that atherogenic lipid profiles should disappear with carb consumption of 25% of energy or less. For a diet of 2400 calories per day, this corresponds to 600 carb calories per day.

The conclusion is obvious: if you want a good lipid profile, with low triglycerides, high HDL, and negligible "small, dense" LDL, keep dietary carbs below 600 calories per day.

It's not a coincidence, we think, that 600 calories is exactly the body's daily glucose need. Any carb intake above this level has to be disposed of, ideally through fat conversion. While this disposal is taking place, glucose levels are unnecessarily elevated and glucose toxicity is damaging health.

Hyperglycemia Worsens the Outcome of Every Health Condition

Just as in the EPIC patients, so too in critically ill patients in hospitals: the higher blood glucose levels, the more likely is death. ***This is true no matter what the health problem.***

More importantly, ***lowering blood glucose reduces the chance of death or poor outcome.*** Here are two summaries of the evidence:

> **High blood glucose levels** have been **associated with morbidity and poor outcome** in critically ill patients, **irrespective of underlying pathology**. In a large, randomised, controlled study the use of insulin therapy to maintain **normoglycaemia** for at least a few days **improved survival and**

reduced morbidity of patients who are in a surgical intensive care unit (ICU).[38]

Hyperglycemia is a common feature of the critically ill and **has been associated with increased mortality**.... Maintaining **normoglycemia** with intensive insulin therapy **improves survival rates and reduces morbidity** in prolonged critically ill patients in both surgical and medical intensive care units (ICUs), as shown by 2 large randomized controlled studies.[39]

These trials reduced blood glucose with drugs. A low-carb diet would have reduced blood glucose without drugs, and produced even better results.

HYPERGLYCEMIA PROMOTES BACTERIAL INFECTIONS AND MANY DISEASES

Chronic infections with parasitic bacteria aggravate or cause a host of diseases. The parasitic bacteria *Chlamydophila pneumoniae* has been associated with cardiovascular disease, Alzheimer's, multiple sclerosis, arthritis, and rosacea. The bacterial genus *Nocardia* has been associated with Parkinson's, and *Borrelia burgdorferi* with Lyme disease. Chronic fatigue appears to be caused by Human Gamma Retrovirus. Most chronic diseases, including autoimmune diseases, are probably caused by parasitic bacterial, viral, or protozoal infections.

Bacteria cannot use fats for fuel: they are dependent upon glucose and its metabolites like pyruvate and lactate. Hyperglycemia delivers more glucose into cells, enabling parasitic bacteria to feed and multiply.

HYPERGLYCEMIA PROMOTES CANCER PROGRESSION

Cancer cells, like bacteria, cannot burn fats: if mitochondria in cancer cells are allowed to burn fats, the cell dies.

So cancer cells are dependent on glucose for energy. This is known as the Warburg Effect, after Otto Warburg, its discoverer.

Higher blood glucose levels provide more fuel to tumor cells, stimulate their proliferation, and hasten the progression of cancer. If high blood glucose induces cells to start burning glucose, it may actually *cause* cancer by switching them from normal metabolism to tumor cell metabolism.

A Swedish study followed 64,597 people for 10 years and found that people who had fasting blood sugars over 110 mg/dl or who scored over 160 mg/dl two hours

---

[38] Vanhorebeek I, Langouche L. Molecular mechanisms behind clinical benefits of intensive insulin therapy during critical illness: glucose versus insulin. *Best Pract Res Clin Anaesthesiol.* 2009 Dec;23(4):449-59. *http://pmid.us/20108584.*

[39] Vanhorebeek I et al. Intensive insulin therapy in the intensive care unit: update on clinical impact and mechanisms of action. *Endocr Pract.* 2006 Jul-Aug;12 Suppl 3:14-22. *http://pmid.us/16905512.*

after a glucose tolerance test had much higher rates of cancer. The cancers most frequently induced by high blood sugars were cancers of the pancreas, endometrium, urinary tract, and malignant melanoma.[40]

In contrast, ketogenic diets which keep blood glucose levels low and provide ketone bodies to mitochondria have shown remarkable effectiveness at slowing cancer progression. In vitro, ketone bodies have been shown to sometimes restore mitochondria to health, triggering cancer cell death. Ketogenic diets have been shown in clinical trials to slow the progress of brain cancer, and clinical trials for other cancers are in progress.

In short, keeping blood glucose levels low, and mixing in some ketone bodies, may help prevent cancer or slow the progression of established cancers.

Benefits of Low Insulin

Insulin is released whenever carbs or protein are eaten. One calorie of protein releases about half as much insulin as one calorie of carbs. In the case of protein, the insulin is accompanied by another hormone, glucagon.

Insulin, however, is not benign. Insulin is firmly linked to shortened lifespan and elevated risk of heart disease, cancer, and mental degeneration.

Minimizing insulin prevents disease and lengthens lifespan.

INSULIN HASTENS AGING; LOW-INSULIN DIETS EXTEND LIFESPAN

Animals live 20-30% longer on low-insulin diets than on high-insulin diets. They are also healthier and more energetic throughout their lives.

Since insulin is released when carbs or protein are eaten, the most promising life-extension strategy is to reduce carb and protein consumption – either by eating a fat-rich diet or by overall calorie restriction.

Calorie restriction increases the life span of mice, rats, and monkeys, and cuts the risk that monkeys will die of cancer or heart problems. Here's a passage from a recent summary of a study linking insulin to aging:

> Tatar and his team found that insulin ... directly regulates tissue aging. The principle: Keep insulin levels low and cells are stronger, staving off infection and age-related diseases such as cancer, dementia and stroke.... [A] growing body of evidence [is] linking low insulin levels to increased longevity. In recent years, scientists have

---

[40] Stattin P et al. Prospective study of hyperglycemia and cancer risk. *Diabetes Care.* 2007 Mar;30(3):561-7. *http://pmid.us/17327321.*

found that mice and other animals live longer when they eat a low-calorie diet, which reduces insulin production.[41]

INSULIN WEAKENS DEFENSES AGAINST INFECTION

The body's first line of defense against pathogens is its "anti-microbial peptides" – small molecules that kill bacteria, viruses, and fungi. Insulin suppresses production of antimicrobial peptides, making the body vulnerable to infections.[42]

INSULIN HARDENS THE ARTERIES

In recent years doctors have found a precise way of assessing the risk of heart attack: the coronary artery calcium score. Calcium belongs in bones and teeth, not arteries. Calcification makes tissues hard; arteries should be supple, able to expand and contract with every heartbeat.

Calcified arteries predict cardiovascular disease. In diabetics, every doubling of the calcium score increases the risk of heart disease or stroke by about 32%.[43]

A study of 25,253 Californians and 10,377 Tennesseeans who had calcium scores and were then followed for an average of 6.8 years showed how calcium score affects death rates in the general population.[44] Survival rates were:

Calcium Score	Survival Rate
0-10	99.4%
11-100	97.8%
101-400	94.5%
401-1000	93.0%

[41] "Insulin plays central role in aging," *ScienceDaily*, June 4, 2004, *http://www.sciencedaily.com/releases/2004/06/040603064935.htm*.

[42] Becker T et al. FOXO-dependent regulation of innate immune homeostasis. *Nature*. 2010 Jan 21;463(7279):369-73. *http://pmid.us/20090753*. See also: "Hungry immune guardians are snappier," EurekaAlert, *http://www.eurekalert.org/pub_releases/2010-01/uob-hig011910.php*.

[43] Elkeles RS et al. Coronary calcium measurement improves prediction of cardiovascular events in asymptomatic patients with type 2 diabetes: the PREDICT study. *Eur Heart J*. 2008 Sep;29(18):2244-51. *http://pmid.us/18573867*.

[44] Budoff MJ et al. Long-term prognosis associated with coronary calcification: observations from a registry of 25,253 patients. *J Am Coll Cardiol* 2007;49:1860-1870. *http://pmid.us/17481445*. Hat tip: Dr. William Davis, *http://heartscanblog.blogspot.com/2008/09/add-boston-globe-to-list-of-heart-scan.html*.

1001+	76.9%

What causes arterial walls to become calcified? Insulin plays a role.

In test tubes either glucose or insulin can convert human vascular smooth muscle cells to osteogenic (bone secreting) cells. When this happens in the body, these cells secrete calcium phosphate into the vascular lining and try to turn arterial walls into bone. A recent paper concludes: "insulin can exert pro-atherosclerotic effects and promote vascular calcification."[45]

Hardening of the arteries proceeds faster if insulin is assisted by high blood sugar. This seems to be why diabetes patients, who are prone to both high insulin and high blood sugar, experience rapid calcification of arteries.[46]

INSULIN IMPAIRS THE MIND

Insulin is a signaling molecule in the brain. When insulin is released into the blood to deal with a high-carb diet, some gets into the brain and causes neurons to expose fewer insulin receptors, making them "insulin resistant."

Insulin resistance in the brain has negative effects. In rats, high insulin diets reduce synaptic connections and impair learning.[47] Insulin resistance in the brain promotes amyloid aggregation and Alzheimer's disease.[48]

BUT A LITTLE INSULIN IS A GOOD THING

Insulin levels should be low; but insulin is not a demon. There is no need to drive insulin levels to zero.

Evolution is very efficient: every molecule in the human body is put to as many uses as possible. Insulin is no exception. For millions of years human ancestors have eaten daily meals containing protein or carbs, triggering the release of insulin into the blood for a few hours per day. Insulin seems to have become a handy hormone, a molecule that could be used to stimulate housekeeping functions which are best performed only a few hours per day.

---

[45] Fadini GP et al. The good and the bad in the link between insulin resistance and vascular calcification. *Atherosclerosis*. 2007 Aug; 193(2): 241-4. *http://pmid.us/17606264*.

[46] Chen NX et al. High glucose increases the expression of Cbfa1 and BMP-2 and enhances the calcification of vascular smooth muscle cells. *Nephrol Dial Transplant*. 2006 Dec; 21(12): 3435-42. *http://pmid.us/17005530*.

[47] Stranahan AM et al. Diet-induced insulin resistance impairs hippocampal synaptic plasticity and cognition in middle-aged rats. *Hippocampus*. 2008;18(11):1085-8. *http://pmid.us/18651634*.

[48] Zhao WQ, Townsend M. Insulin resistance and amyloidogenesis as common molecular foundation for type 2 diabetes and Alzheimer's disease. *Biochim Biophys Acta*. 2009 May; 1792(5): 482-96. *http://pmid.us/19026743*.

One such function is the recycling of vitamin C, which is stimulated by insulin. Type I diabetics never release insulin; as a result vitamin C is not recycled and "tissue scurvy" is a serious threat. It's not uncommon for Type I diabetics to develop osteoporosis due to a lack of vitamin C.[49] Similarly, people on near-zero-carb diets may easily develop scurvy.[50]

The Upper Limit of the Plateau Range for Carbs

We saw earlier that blood lipid profiles become excellent when carb intake is limited to 600 calories per day – the level of the body's daily glucose needs.

This coincidence suggests that we should look closely at how excess glucose is disposed of, and why having to dispose of an excess may be dangerous.

SAFE GLUCOSE DISPOSAL BY FILLING GLUCOSE RESERVOIRS

Small amounts of glucose can be stored as liver and muscle glycogen. This is the healthiest, quickest, and safest way to dispose of excess blood glucose.

Glycogen storage capacity is limited to about 300-500 grams in skeletal muscle and 70-100 grams in the liver. Glycogen stores are never allowed to become fully depleted (unless one "hits the wall" in a marathon), and so glycogen reservoirs can rarely accommodate much glucose.[51]

High-intensity exercise depletes glycogen, and so elite athletes can usually safely dispose of their big bowl of rice.

But ordinary people who eat a high-carb diet will tend to keep their glycogen reservoirs full. In practice, this disposal mechanism is probably limited to a few hundred calories at most.

CONVERSION TO FAT

The body's adipose (fat) cells are fat storage reservoirs. They are able to convert glucose to fat, or store fats manufactured from glucose by the liver.

---

[49] Qutob S et al. Insulin stimulates vitamin C recycling and ascorbate accumulation in osteoblastic cells. *Endocrinology.* 1998 Jan;139(1):51-6. *http://pmid.us/9421397.* See also May JM et al. Human erythrocyte recycling of ascorbic acid: relative contributions from the ascorbate free radical and dehydroascorbic acid. *J Biol Chem.* 2004 Apr 9;279(15):14975-82. *http://pmid.us/14752116.*

[50] Willmott NS, Bryan RA. Case report: Scurvy in an epileptic child on a ketogenic diet with oral complications. *Eur Arch Paediatr Dent.* 2008 Sep;9(3):148-52. *http://pmid.us/18793598.*

[51] Acheson KJ et al. Glycogen storage capacity and de novo lipogenesis during massive carbohydrate overfeeding in man. *Am J Clin Nutr.* 1988 Aug;48(2):240-7. *http://pmid.us/3165600.*

The body can convert carbs to fat only at a slow rate: in a day, the body can convert about 475 grams of carbs into 150 grams of fat.[52] This is a glucose disposal rate of about 20 grams (80 calories) per hour.

This gives an idea of what a carb-rich meal does to blood glucose. The average American eats about 900 excess carb calories per day. If these have to be disposed of by conversion to fat at a rate of 80 calories per hour, then the average American must have elevated blood glucose (and insulin, to drive the conversion process) for about 12 hours per day.

So, if you're converting excess carbs to fat, you're not only expanding your waistline – you're also experiencing elevated blood glucose and the impaired health that comes with it.

DIRECT METABOLISM OF GLUCOSE IN CELLS THAT NORMALLY BURN FAT

If blood glucose levels become dangerously high, then the pancreas won't wait for adipose cells to remove it. Instead, it will secrete even more insulin in an attempt to force the body's cells to shift fuels from fat to glucose.

This is undesirable. Direct metabolism of glucose creates reactive oxygen species (ROS) which damage the cell. The presence of glucose in the cell feeds intracellular bacterial infections. Moreover, using glucose as a fuel switches the cell to metabolic pathways characteristic of cancer and diabetes, and probably promotes development of these diseases.

Ideally, most cells should never metabolize glucose directly – they should obtain all energy either from fats or from glucose-6-phosphate peeled off in a controlled way from glycogen.

SUMMARY: THERE ARE NO GOOD GLUCOSE DISPOSAL PATHWAYS

Above the body's daily glucose needs, which we earlier estimated at 450-600 calories, there are no healthy ways to dispose of excess glucose. The healthier disposal pathway, conversion to fat, is slow, so high-carb eating inevitably leads to elevated blood sugars and resulting glucose toxicity.

One is always better off stopping glucose consumption at the limit of bodily needs. Consuming saturated fat instead of carbs reaches the same endpoint, but without the intermediate toxicity from elevated blood glucose.

It's healthier to eat *fat* than to eat *carbohydrates that get converted to fat*.

---

[52] Acheson KJ et al. Glycogen storage capacity and de novo lipogenesis during massive carbohydrate overfeeding in man. *Am J Clin Nutr.* 1988 Aug;48(2):240-7. *http://pmid.us/3165600.*

So, it's desirable to eat no more carbohydrates than your body can use. Glucose-to-fat conversion begins somewhere around intakes of 500 to 600 carb calories per day. Beyond that level, carbs become an unhealthy source of calories.

Summary: The Healthy Plateau Range for Carbs

In short, the plateau range for carbs seems to be between about 200 calories per day, on the low side, and the body's glucose utilization – probably around 500 to 600 calories per day – on the high side.

Eating within this plateau range is the "hybrid mammalian" diet strategy – part Omnivore Strategy, in that most glucose needs are met by dietary carbs, but part Herbivore/Carnivore Strategy in that the liver is forced to manufacture some glucose and ketones to meet the body's needs.

Eating within this plateau range keeps blood glucose levels low, since there is generally room in liver glycogen to store a carb-rich meal. This strategy avoids both the impaired health and shortened lifespan of elevated blood glucose and insulin, and the impaired immune function and other risks of glycogen deprivation.

Some people may wish to bias their diets toward one end or the other of the plateau range:

- **Those who wish to become pregnant** may wish to eat at the high end of the plateau range – perhaps 600 calories per day – since a slight carb excess promotes fertility. **Athletes** may also benefit from eating at the high end of the plateau range in order to maintain muscle glycogen stores.

- Those at risk for diseases for which a Herbivore Strategy is therapeutic – such as **chronic bacterial infections, diabetes, cancer, or mental illness** – may benefit from a mildly "ketogenic" approach that keeps carb intake near 200 carb calories per day.

But for most people, we would suggest occupying the middle of the plateau range at about 400 carb calories per day. The great majority of carb calories should be obtained from starch sources like sweet potatoes, taro, and white rice; the rest from fruits and berries. Don't count vegetables as a carb source – they are a fiber (and therefore a fat) source.

An Introduction to Fats

Before we discuss their role in diet, it may be desirable to review the role of fats in the body. Fats are important: They are a structural part of every cell and the preferred fuel of mitochondria.

What Are Fats Anyway?

The simplest kind of fat is a fatty acid. This is composed of a stem with the chemical formula –COOH, called a carboxyl group, attached to a chain of carbon atoms. Each carbon atom comes with three hydrogen atoms if it is the last carbon atom in the chain (the "omega" carbon), or if it is in the middle of the chain either one or two hydrogen atoms. If the mid-chain carbons have two hydrogens they are considered to be "saturated"; if they have one (and therefore form a double bond with the next carbon in the chain) they are considered to be "unsaturated."

A chain that is wholly saturated is straight, and the resulting fatty acid is "saturated" (a SaFA). Any unsaturated point in the chain creates a floppy bend in the chain. If there is one such bend in the chain, the fatty acid is said to be "monounsaturated" (a MUFA). If there are two or more floppy bends in the chain, the fatty acid is said to be "polyunsaturated" (a PUFA). Humans use two types of PUFAs, omega-6 and omega-3.

Figure: Fatty acids. Left: The 4-carbon saturated fatty acid butyric acid. Right: The The 18-carbon omega-6 polyunsaturated fatty acid linoleic acid.

In PUFAs the double bonds are typically separated by 3 carbons, as in linoleic acid above. The "omega-6" designation means that the first double bond appears 6 carbons from the "omega" carbon, the last carbon in the chain. The body also uses "omega-3," "omega-7," and "omega-9" fatty acids.

Most fats in the body are found in triglycerides, a storage form of fat, or phospholipids, the structural form of fat found in cell membranes:

- A triglyceride has three fatty acids attached to a glycerol backbone, as shown in the figure below. Triglycerides are insoluble in water.

- A phospholipid is like a triglyceride, but the third fatty acid is replaced by a a phosphate group and an organic molecule like choline or inositol. The phosphate and organic molecule are water-soluble; this allows the phospholipid to mix with water.

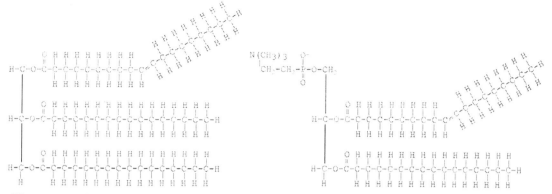

Figure: Left: A triglyceride. The glycerol backbone is joined by three fatty acids: in this case, two palmitic acids and one oleic acid. Right: A phospholipid. A water soluble organic molecule, in this case choline, attaches via a phosphate group to glycerol in place of the third fatty acid.

In cell membranes, phospholipids arrange themselves in a bilayer, with fatty acids in the middle and the water-soluble head groups on both sides.

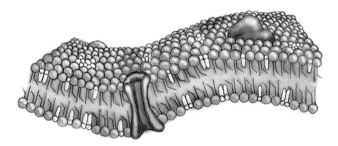

Figure: A portion of a cell membrane, showing a phospholipid bilayer threaded by a few proteins.

FATTY ACID TRANSPORT

Free fatty acids are insoluble in water and tend to bind to molecules (become "esterified"); this reactivity makes them potentially toxic. So most fatty acids are packed into triglycerides or phospholipids, and carried in the blood by transporter proteins.

Particles containing a transporter protein plus transported fats are called lipoproteins. Most people are familiar with LDL ("low-density lipoprotein") and HDL ("high-density lipoprotein"). These particles have the shape of a baseball: a core of fats and cholesterol, wrapped in a phospholipid monolayer for water solubility (like the skin of the baseball), with the transporter protein wrapped around the surface (like the seams of a baseball) to provide structure and the ability to interact with receptors on cell membranes. Here is what a healthy LDL particle looks like:

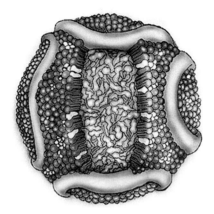

Figure: An LDL particle. Each particle contains about 1500 molecules of cholesterol bound to fatty acids in an oily core (red), surrounded by a coat containing about 800 phospholipid molecules (purple), 500 cholesterol molecules (yellow), and one molecule of apoprotein B100 (blue).

This is a healthy LDL particle because it has a lot of fat and cholesterol, making it large and buoyant. When LDL lacks fat and cholesterol, it becomes small and dense (because protein is denser than fat). Such "small, dense LDL," or sdLDL, is associated with heart disease because the transporter protein is exposed to glycation and oxidation. So sdLDL becomes oxidized or oxLDL, which contributes to formation of "foam cells" and atherosclerotic plaques.

When a cell wants to acquire fats or cholesterol, it expresses LDL receptors on its membrane. The apoprotein B100 molecule of LDL attaches to these LDL receptors, and the LDL particle is absorbed into the cell by a process called endocytosis.

Assessing The Body's Fat Needs

In the Preview, we presented a few principles for identifying the optimal macronutrient ratio. These principles included:

- **Eat a diet similar to mother's milk.** The ideal nutrition for adults is probably not far from the ideal nutrition for infants.

- **Eat what you are.** Eat to provide your body with the nutrients it would need to rebuild itself.

These principles ought to apply to fatty acid ratios as well as to the carb-fat-protein ratio. Let's see what fatty acid ratios they prescribe.

Fatty Acid Ratios of Human Breast Milk

The table below shows the fatty acid ratios from human breast milk at day 16 after delivery for two groups of mothers: in the left column, Japanese mothers of healthy babies[53], in the right column, American mothers of babies born 2 months premature[54].

Fatty acid	Name	Japanese healthy	American premature
4:0,6:0,8:0,10:0,12:0	Short-chain	10.4%	8.9%
14:0	Myristic	6.6%	8.8%
16:0	Palmitic	21.5%	19.2%
18:0	Stearic	6.0%	6.1%
16:1	Palmitoleic	4.2%	3.4%
18:1	Oleic	32.1%	37.4%
18:2 n6	LA	13.3%	11.9%
18:3 n6	GLA	0.1%	0.0%
20:3 n6	DGLA	0.4%	0.4%
20:4 n6	AA	0.4%	0.6%
18:3 n3	ALA	1.4%	1.2%
20:5 n3	EPA	0.2%	0.1%
22:5 n3	DPA	0.3%	0.1%
22:6 n3	DHA	1.0%	0.4%

[53] Jensen RG. Lipids in human milk. *Lipids*. 1999 Dec;34(12):1243-71. *http://pmid.us/10652985*. The short-chain fatty acids butyric and caprylic acid were not listed in Jensen's tables 8, 9, and 10 from which this data were drawn, and the fatty acids listed summed to 96.8% of total fats. Butyric and caprylic acid constitute 5.4% of cow's milk fats (*http://nutritiondata.com*). To account for missing fats, we added to Jensen's data 3.1% of total fats as butyric and caprylic acid.

[54] Clandinin MT et al. Fatty acid utilization in perinatal de novo synthesis of tissues. *Early Hum Dev*. 1981 Sep;5(4):355-66. *http://pmid.us/7285840*.

Milk from these two groups of mothers is similar, except for the long-chain PUFA. Milk from mothers of premature babies has 60% *less* of the long-chain omega-3 fats EPA and DHA, but 50% *more* of the long-chain omega-6 fat AA. The ratio of AA to EPA+DHA was 0.34 in Japanese mothers of healthy children, but 1.2 in American mothers of premature children: *3.4-fold higher*.

As we'll see, the ratio of AA to EPA+DHA predicts mortality in adults; perhaps it also indicates which mothers will give birth prematurely.

Another notable aspect of breast milk is its high content of short-chain fatty acids. This suggests that our diet should include short-chain fats.

We can sum up these fatty acids in terms of the four main fatty acid groups – SaFA, MUFA, and omega-6 and omega-3 PUFA. The result is:

Fatty acid	Japanese healthy	American premature
SaFA	44.6%	43.3%
MUFA	37.6%	41.0%
Omega-6 PUFA	14.6%	13.5%
Omega-3 PUFA	3.1%	2.2%

Since evolution will have striven to give infants the best possible nutrition, these percentages must be fairly close to the optimal dietary fatty acid mix.

EAT WHAT YOU ARE

Studies reporting human fatty acid abundances normally draw samples from blood or adipose tissue, not the whole body. However, Loren Cordain's group has provided us with fatty acid profiles of elk, deer, antelope and other species.[55] Here it is:

Fatty acid	Antelope	Mule Deer	Elk	Pasture-fed steer
SaFA	43.4%	45.2%	41.0%	43.5%
MUFA	29.7%	35.1%	33.0%	40.3%
Omega-6	22.4%	17.2%	22.4%	7.1%

[55] Cordain L et al. Fatty acid analysis of wild ruminant tissues: evolutionary implications for reducing diet-related chronic disease. *Eur J Clin Nutr.* 2002 Mar;56(3):181-91. *http://pmid.us/11960292.*

Omega-3	4.5%	5.0%	3.6%	3.2%

What's notable for our purposes is how closely these numbers resemble the fatty acid composition of human breast milk.

The seemingly high omega-6 to omega-3 ratio in wild animal muscle tissues is a bit misleading. As in human breast milk, most of the omega-6 PUFA is in the form of 18-carbon linoleic acid. Of the longer chain PUFAs, the AA to EPA+DHA ratio is 1.5 in deer muscle and 0.5 in deer brain – a little higher than the ratio in human breast milk, but not by much. Including all the longer-chain PUFAs, the ratio of omega-6 AA+DGLA to omega-3 EPA+DPA+DHA is 0.88 in deer muscle, 0.56 in deer brain. (Animal brains are omega-3 rich. Next time you're at a French restaurant, try calf's brains!)

Skeletal muscle is the single largest tissue contributor to body mass – accounting for about 30 kg of the typical man's weight and 20 kg of the typical woman's.[56] If we should eat what we are, then muscle fatty acid ratios are a good guide to optimal human dietary fatty acid ratios.

CONCLUSION: FIRST APPROXIMATION AT OPTIMAL FATTY ACID RATIOS

We can sort fatty acids into three functional groups:

- **Short-chain fatty acids:** These make up about 10% of human breast milk, but have no structural function in the body and so do not appear in animal muscle. Trusting in mother's milk as a guide, we'll tentatively pick 10% of fat calories (6.5% of total calories) as the optimal intake of short-chain fats.

- **Long-chain SaFA and MUFA:** These are the main structural fats of the human body and also the main energy-providing fats. They make up 75-80% of fats in cell membranes and breast milk. Tentatively, we'll pick 75-80% of fat calories (~50% of total calories) as an appropriate dietary intake of SaFA+MUFA.

- **Omega-6 and omega-3 PUFA.** These make up 10% to 25% of ruminant animal muscle fats and 15-18% of human breast milk fats. Most of these are in the form of omega-6 LA. Excluding LA, omega-6 and omega-3 PUFAs represent 3% to 5% of human breast milk. We'll tentatively pick 10-15% of fat calories (thus, 7-10% of total calories) as an appropriate level of PUFA.

Now let's refine these assessments by looking into the biomedical evidence.

---

[56] Wang Z et al. Whole-body skeletal muscle mass: development and validation of total-body potassium prediction models. *Am J Clin Nutr.* 2003 Jan;77(1):76-82. *http://pmid.us/12499326.*

The Dangerous Fats: PUFA

Omega-6 and omega-3 polyunsaturated fats (PUFA) are considered to be "essential" because, unlike SaFA and MUFA, they cannot be manufactured from glucose. They must be obtained from food.

What are "Essential" Fatty Acids?

Omega-6 and omega-3 polyunsaturated fats are termed "essential" fatty acids. But this word does NOT imply these fats are "desirable"!

"Essential" is a scientific term of art: it means that the human body cannot manufacture these fats from other foods, and so any omega-6 or omega-3 fats in the body must be obtained from diet. It says nothing about how many are needed. In fact, it implies THEY PROBABLY AREN'T NEEDED: if they were important, the body would have evolved a way to make them. Truly necessary fats, like saturated and monounsaturated fats, can be manufactured from carbohydrates and protein.

Chapter Preview

Omega-6 polyunsaturated fats are healthful in modest amounts – at the levels contained in meat, fish, and eggs – but become toxic in excess.

Many Americans get over 10% of dietary calories from omega-6 fats, 20 times the biological need. The ratio of omega-6 to omega-3 fats in the tissues of Americans is nine times the optimum. This omega-6 excess has been linked to a host of diseases, including heart disease, cancer, and mental illness, and increased mortality. [57]

A few simple rules will bring PUFA levels near the optimum:

Vegetable seed oils (and foods prepared with them) should be eliminated. Cooking and salad oils should be low in omega-6 fats: butter, coconut oil, and beef tallow are best, olive oil next best.

Meats low in omega-6 like beef, lamb, and salmon should be preferred.

Sufficient oily fish – about a pound of salmon per week – should be eaten to balance omega-3 and omega-6 tissue levels.

For those who dislike salmon, an alternative is to eat meat and eggs from pastured naturally-fed animals rather than from penned grain-fed animals. Pastured naturally fed animals have healthy omega-6 to omega-3 ratios, alleviating the need for additional omega-3. However, if you like salmon, sardines, or other

---

[57] Lands WE. Dietary fat and health: the evidence and the politics of prevention: careful use of dietary fats can improve life and prevent disease. *Ann N Y Acad Sci.* 2005 Dec;1055:179-92. *http://pmid.us/16387724.*

omega-3-rich fish, it's not necessary to buy meat from pastured naturally fed animals. We eat conventional supermarket meats.

What's the Dispute About?

For decades now, scientists and doctors have been debating the optimal levels of dietary PUFA, and to what degree PUFA-rich foods and oils should be included in the diet.

The PUFA debate is entangled with several other controversies: the debate over the "lipid hypothesis," which blames cholesterol and saturated fat for heart disease, and the debate over high-carb versus low-carb diets.

Despite the sound and fury, however, there is actually considerable scientific consensus about PUFA.

CONSIDERABLE AGREEMENT ON OPTIMAL AMOUNTS

Consider these official recommendations, ordered from high to low in their PUFA recommendation. In all cases the 18-carbon fatty acid LA is expected to provide over 90% of omega-6 fats:

- The U.S. Dietary Guidelines advise an omega-6 intake of 5% to 10% of energy, plus 0.6 to 1.2% of energy from omega-3 ALA, plus 8 ounces per week of oily fish such as salmon for EPA+DHA.[58]

- The European Union recommends an omega-6 fatty acid intake of 4-8% of calories and an omega-3 intake of 2 g/day (1% of calories) of omega-3 ALA and 200 mg/day (0.1% of calories) of EPA and DHA.[59]

- The Japan Society for Lipid Nutrition recommends omega-6 intake of 3-4% of energy and omega-3 intake of 2.6 g/day (1.2% of energy), including at least 1 g/day (0.5% of energy) EPA+DHA.[60]

- A panel of scientists convened by the International Society for the Study of Fatty Acids and Lipids and the US Office of Dietary Supplements

---

[58] Department of Health and Human Services and Department of Agriculture. *Dietary Guidelines for Americans: The Report of the Dietary Guidelines Advisory Committee on Dietary Guidelines for Americans, 2005.* *http://www.health.gov/DietaryGuidelines/dga2005/report/default.htm.*

[59] European Commission Directorate General for Health and Consumer Protection. *Eurodiet: Nutrition and Diet for Healthy Lifestyles in Europe.* 2001. *http://ec.europa.eu/health/ph_determinants/life_style/nutrition/ report01_en.pdf/.*

[60] Hamazaki T, Okuyama H. The Japan Society for Lipid Nutrition recommends to reduce the intake of linoleic acid. A review and critique of the scientific evidence. *World Rev Nutr Diet.* 2003;92:109-132. *http://pmid.us/14579687.*

recommended that adults obtain 4.4-6.7 g/day (2-3% of calories) of omega-6 fatty acids, 2.2 g/day (1% of calories) of omega-3 ALA, and 0.65 g/day (0.3% of calories) of omega-3 EPA+DHA.[61]

It's worth noting the common ground:

(1) No one thinks that PUFA should constitute more than 10% of calories. These are not intended to be a leading source of energy.

(2) The omega-3 recommendations cluster around 1% of calories from ALA and 0.5% of calories from EPA+DHA.

(3) The recommended omega-6 consumption varies by only a factor of 3 (2-3% of calories at the low end, 5-10% at the high end). An intake of 4% of calories from omega-6, plus 1-2% from omega-3, would be within the recommended range for the EU and Japan and only slightly below the US and above the ISSFAL ranges.

Our own recommendation is in line with those from Japan and the ISSFAL/USODS workshop group: 2-4% of energy from omega-6 fats, and 1.5 g/day (0.7% energy) of EPA+DHA from fish (equivalent to 1 pound of salmon per week). We have no specific recommendation for the omega-3 ALA.

CARB VS. FAT DEBATE AND FOOD RECOMMENDATIONS

Should one seek out high-PUFA foods, or avoid them?

This may depend on how many carbs are consumed:

- On very low-fat diets like the Ornish diet, which recommends getting only 10% of calories from fat, getting 5% of calories from PUFA would require eating fats that average 50% PUFA. This means fats should come from vegetable oils – soybean oil, corn oil, safflower oil, flaxseed oil – and that meats, especially red meats which are low in PUFA, should be avoided. This diet has little concern for getting adequate SaFA or MUFA, because it is a high-carb diet and the vast majority of carb calories are converted in the body to SaFA and MUFA.

- On low-carb diets like the Perfect Health Diet, fats provide 65% of total calories, so to limit PUFA to 5% of total calories (omega-6 ~3%, omega-3 ~1.5%) requires elimination of vegetable oils. SaFA and MUFA rich oils and foods, such as beef, lamb, salmon, butter, and coconut oil, become the focus of the diet.

So the debate over whether to eat PUFA-rich foods is in large part a debate over what should be the primary calorie source – fats or carbs.

---

[61] Simopoulos AP et al. Workshop statement on the essentiality of and recommended dietary intakes for Omega-6 and Omega-3 fatty acids. *Prostaglandins Leukot Essent Fatty Acids*. 2000 Sep;63(3):119-21. *http://pmid.us/10991764*.

GETTING TO THE PUFA PLATEAU RANGES

For Perfect Health, what we care about is getting the *amount* of each nutrient into its "plateau range." Three key issues determine the plateau ranges of omega-6 and omega-3 PUFA:

1. How much of each PUFA must be eaten to avoid a deficiency?

2. At what level of consumption does each PUFA become toxic?

3. What omega-6 to omega-3 ratio optimizes health?

PUFA Deficiency: Not a Concern

PUFA deficiency conditions are extremely rare. It is so difficult to induce PUFA deficiencies that it took decades to prove a human need for PUFA.[62]

The need for PUFA was originally discovered in the 1920s by feeding rats lifelong fat-free diets. On zero-PUFA diets, rats grew more slowly.

In humans, the main symptom of an omega-6 deficiency is a dry scaly skin rash. In the 1940s and 1950s, it was common to feed infants a fat-free milk formula – skim milk with sugar. After some months, these infants developed eczema which could be cured by providing lard, which is about 10% PUFA. Other possible effects of an omega-6 deficiency are impaired growth of infants, susceptibility to infection, and slow wound healing.[63]

Evidence showing that PUFA deficiencies were possible in adults came from the period when intravenous nutrition did not provide fats:[64]

- Two cases of omega-6 deficiency arose in 1969 and 1970 in people who had much of their intestines surgically removed and who were placed on fat-free intravenous feeding for months.

- A case of omega-3, but not omega-6, deficiency arose in a girl who in 1982 underwent a series of surgeries after a gunshot wound in the abdomen. After 5 months of intravenous feeding with safflower oil as the only fat – which has abundant omega-6 but negligible omega-3 – she developed an omega-3 deficiency, characterized by episodes of numbness, tingling, weakness, inability to walk, leg pain, psychological disturbances and blurred vision.

---

[62] Holman RT. The slow discovery of the importance of omega 3 essential fatty acids in human health. *J Nutr.* 1998 Feb;128(2 Suppl):427S-433S. *http://pmid.us/9478042.*

[63] Jeppesen PB et al. Essential fatty acid deficiency in patients receiving home parenteral nutrition. Am J Clin Nutr. 1998;68(1):126-133. *http://pmid.us/9665106.*

[64] Holman RT. The slow discovery of the importance of omega 3 essential fatty acids in human health. *J Nutr.* 1998 Feb;128(2 Suppl):427S-433S. *http://pmid.us/9478042.*

A small amount of dietary PUFA relieves a deficiency:

- Omega-6 deficiencies are eliminated by 1-2% of calories as LA if the diet has no omega-3,[65] and by just 0.3% of calories as LA if the diet has over 1% omega-3.[66] Thus, a little omega-3 in the diet reduces the requirement for omega-6.

- Omega-3 deficiency can be relieved, bringing DHA in the liver to normal levels, by eating as little as 0.2% of calories as omega-3 fats.[67]

Omega-6 fats constitute 2% or more of most modern foods, so on practical diets it is impossible to become clinically deficient in omega-6 fats, unless some medical condition such as cystic fibrosis prevents fat digestion. Absolute omega-3 deficiencies are also rare.

PUFA Toxicity

Although it is not widely known, a huge body of evidence from animal studies has established that both omega-6 and omega-3 PUFA are toxic in high doses – and even more toxic when combined with sugar, grains, or alcohol.

THE DEVIL'S DIET

Most of the animal studies of the last 30 years that reported negative health effects from a "high-fat diet" have similar diets. Typical ratios are:

- 40% of calories from carbs (often sugar and wheat flour),
- 40% of calories from omega-6-rich fats (often soybean or corn oil),
- 20% of calories as protein.

Now this is not a very "high fat" diet – it is low in fat compared to the Perfect Health Diet, for instance; it is similar in macronutrient ratios to the South Beach Diet, the Zone Diet, and other popular diets.

However while human diets are relatively low in toxins – the South Beach Diet urges removal of sugars and refined grains; the Zone Diet of omega-6 fats – the "high fat diet" of animal studies is a **maximum toxicity diet**, consisting almost entirely of toxic foods – sugar, grains, and omega-6 fats.

---

[65] Kris-Etherton P et al. The debate about n-6 polyunsaturated fatty acid recommendations for cardiovascular health. *J Am Diet Assoc.* 2010 Feb; 110(2): 201-4. *http://pmid.us/20102846.*

[66] Cunnane SC. Problems with essential fatty acids: time for a new paradigm? *Prog Lipid Res.* 2003 Nov;42(6):544-68. *http://pmid.us/14559071.*

[67] See Figure 1 of Holman RT. The slow discovery of the importance of omega 3 essential fatty acids in human health. *J Nutr.* 1998 Feb;128(2 Suppl):427S-433S. *http://pmid.us/9478042.*

As we'll see, omega-6 fats and sugar are a dangerous combination, as omega-6 fats are prone to oxidation when sugar is present. Since blood sugar levels are elevated much of the day on a 40% carb diet, this macronutrient mix is able to create large quantities of oxidized omega-6 PUFA.

SATURATED FATS ELIMINATE THE NEGATIVE EFFECT OF A "HIGH-FAT DIET"

In the animal studies, substituting saturated fat for the soybean oil or corn oil eliminates the negative health effects. The healthiest oils are coconut oil and butter, which have very low omega-6 levels and are high in saturated fats. Saturated fats are immune to the oxidizing effect of sugars.

Here is a sampling of studies in which PUFA destroy and SaFA rescue the health of lab animals:

- Our favorite study compared a high-carb corn oil diet (62% of calories as carbs, 21% as corn oil, 17% as protein) with a low-carb diet with fats given either as coconut oil or butter (17% of calories as carbs, 71% as coconut oil or butter, 12% as protein). We like this study because the low-carb diets were so similar to the Perfect Health Diet. Mice eating the coconut oil and butter diets maintained healthy livers despite nutrient deficiencies that normally induce liver disease, while mice on the high-carb corn oil diet developed severe disease.[68]

- Researchers induced fatty liver disease in mice by feeding diets deficient in key nutrients. One diet provided 34% of calories as corn oil, the other as coconut oil.   (Corn oil is 57% omega-6 PUFA, while coconut oil is 2% omega-6 PUFA and 92% SaFA.) The mice fed corn oil had severe liver damage, but "histological scores demonstrated significantly less steatosis, inflammation and necrosis in SAFA-fed mice of all mouse strains."[69]

- Researchers induced liver disease by feeding mice a combination of alcohol and omega-3-rich fish oil. They then stopped the alcohol and split the mice into two groups, one fed fish oil plus glucose, the other SaFA-rich palm oil plus glucose. Livers of the fish oil group failed to recover, but the palm oil

---

[68] Romestaing C et al. Long term highly saturated fat diet does not induce NASH in Wistar rats. *Nutr Metab (Lond).* 2007 Feb 21;4:4. *http://pmid.us/17313679.* Hat tip Chris Masterjohn, *http://blog.cholesterol-and-health.com/2009/10/maternal-intake-of-saturated-fat-causes.html.*

[69] Rivera CA et al. Toll-like receptor-2 deficiency enhances non-alcoholic steatohepatitis. *BMC Gastroenterol.* 2010 May 28;10(1):52. [Epub ahead of print] *http://pmid.us/20509914.*

group "showed near normalization." The researchers hailed SaFA as "*a novel treatment for liver disease.*"[70]

- Mice fed 27.5% of calories as alcohol developed severe liver disease and metabolic syndrome when given a corn oil diet, but no disease at all when given a SaFA-rich cocoa butter diet. (The first line of this paper reads, "*The protective effect of dietary saturated fatty acids against the development of alcoholic liver disease has long been known*" – yet somehow this knowledge has eluded many doctors.)[71]

- Scientists induced liver disease in mice by feeding alcohol plus corn oil. They then substituted a saturated-fat rich mix based on beef tallow and coconut oil for 20%, 45%, and 67% of the corn oil. The more saturated fat, the healthier the liver.[72]

The pattern is obvious: give sugar, wheat, or alcohol in combination with either omega-6 or omega-3 PUFA, and mice develop fatty liver and metabolic syndrome. Give a diet without PUFA, and the liver does fine.

Omega-6 Fats and Obesity

Fatty liver and metabolic syndrome are not the only health problems caused by excess PUFA. Obesity is another.

In both rodents and humans, weight increases as omega-6 consumption increases.

In one study, rats were divided into three groups receiving diets identical in fat, protein, and carbohydrate calories, but differing in the source of the fats: one group received beef tallow (low in omega-6), another olive oil (moderate in omega-6), and the third safflower oil (very high in omega-6). Relative to the tallow group, rats in the olive oil group saw a 7.5% increase in total body weight, and the safflower group saw a 12.3% increase.[73]

In another study, 782 men were kept on calorie-controlled diets for five years. They were split into two groups, one consuming animal fats and the other omega-

---

[70] Nanji AA et al. Dietary saturated fatty acids: a novel treatment for alcoholic liver disease. *Gastroenterology.* 1995 Aug;109(2):547-54. *http://pmid.us/7615205.*

[71] You M et al. Role of adiponectin in the protective action of dietary saturated fat against alcoholic fatty liver in mice. *Hepatology.* 2005 Sep;42(3):568-77. *http://pmid.us/16108051.*

[72] Ronis MJ et al. Dietary saturated fat reduces alcoholic hepatotoxicity in rats by altering fatty acid metabolism and membrane composition. *J Nutr.* 2004 Apr;134(4):904-12. *http://pmid.us/15051845.*

[73] Pan DA, Storlien LH. Dietary Lipid Profile Is a Determinant of Tissue Phospholipid Fatty Acid Composition and Rate of Weight Gain in Rats. *J Nutr.* 1993 Mar;123(3):512-9. *http://pmid.us/8463854.* Hat tip Stephan Guyenet, *http://wholehealthsource.blogspot.com/2008/12/vegetable-oil-and-weight-gain.html.*

6-rich vegetable oils. The vegetable oil consuming group had steady gains in body fat and weight compared to the animal fat group; in later years of the study, the vegetable oil group averaged about 5% or 8 pounds more weight.[74]

Immune Function, Allergies, and Asthma

Omega-6 fats are generally considered to be inflammatory, and they are. Inflammation stimulates the immune response. However, in excess, omega-6 fats actually suppress the immune system. They also distort the immune response.[75] This distortion of the immune response is doubly bad:

- The response to extracellular pathogens becomes exaggerated, leading to **allergies**.[76] Young children seem to be especially vulnerable: higher levels of omega-6 fats in mother's milk are associated with **runny nose, asthma, and skin rashes**.[77]

- The response to intracellular viruses and bacteria is weakened. This presumably increases the likelihood of diseases associated with intracellular infections, such as **atherosclerosis, Alzheimer's, multiple sclerosis, Lyme disease, Parkinson's**, and other **diseases of aging**.

Omega-6 Fats and Mental Illness

Vegetable oil consumption is associated with depression, mental illness, and high rates of violence. We'll cite papers demonstrating such links later, in our discussion of omega-6 to omega-3 balance, but for now, since a picture is worth a thousand words, let's look at an intriguing correlation.

---

[74] Dayton S et al. Composition of lipids in human serum and adipose tissue during prolonged feeding of a diet high in unsaturated fat. *J Lipid Res.* 1966 Jan;7(1):103-11. *http://pmid.us/5900208.* Hat tip Stephan Guyenet, *http://wholehealthsource.blogspot.com/2008/12/vegetable-oil-and-weight-gain.html.*

[75] Mizota T et al. Effect of dietary fatty acid composition on Th1/Th2 polarization in lymphocytes. *JPEN J Parenter Enteral Nutr.* 2009 Jul-Aug;33(4):390-6. *http://pmid.us/19221048.* Harbige LS. Fatty acids, the immune response, and autoimmunity: a question of n-6 essentiality and the balance between n-6 and n-3. *Lipids.* 2003 Apr; 38(4): 323-41. *http://pmid.us/12848277.*

[76] Chilton FH et al. Mechanisms by which botanical lipids affect inflammatory disorders. *Am J Clin Nutr.* 2008 Feb;87(2):498S-503S. *http://pmid.us/18258646.*

[77] Lowe AJ et al. Associations between fatty acids in colostrum and breast milk and risk of allergic disease. *Clin Exp Allergy.* 2008 Nov;38(11):1745-51. *http://pmid.us/18702657.* Wijga AH et al. Breast milk fatty acids and allergic disease in preschool children: the Prevention and Incidence of Asthma and Mite Allergy birth cohort study. *J Allergy Clin Immunol.* 2006 Feb;117(2):440-7. *http://pmid.us/16461146.*

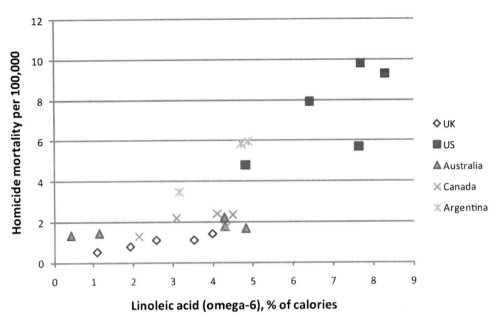

Figure: Homicide mortality versus consumption of omega-6 linoleic acid, plotted for 1961, 1970, 1980, 1990, and 2000 in five countries. Within each country, homicide rates go up as linoleic acid consumption goes up.[78]

Throughout the industrialized world, omega-6 consumption has increased sharply since 1960 due to increasing use of vegetable oils. Joseph Hibbeln, Levi Nieminin, and William Lands had the idea of comparing omega-6 consumption to rates of violence. They found, across a panel of five countries for which good data was available, two patterns:

- The more omega-6 a country consumed, the higher its homicide rate. The US, with the highest omega-6 consumption thanks to agricultural subsidies for soybeans and corn, had the highest homicide rate.

- As omega-6 consumption increased between 1960 and 2000, each country saw an increase in its homicide rate.

Omega-6 Fats and Digestive Health

The incidence of digestive ailments scales with consumption of omega-6 fatty acids. The EPIC study found that those in the highest quartile of consumption of

[78] Hibbeln JR et al. Increasing homicide rates and linoleic acid consumption among five Western countries, 1961-2000. *Lipids.* 2004 Dec;39(12):1207-13. *http://pmid.us/15736917.* Hat tip Stephan Guyenet, *http://wholehealthsource.blogspot.com/2008/09/omega-ratio.html.*

linoleic acid, the omega-6 fat in vegetable oils, have 2.5 times the risk of ulcerative colitis as those with the lowest consumption.[79]

Omega-6 Fats and Cancer

Omega-6-rich oils promote cancer progression and metastasis. For instance, corn oil but not saturated fat stimulates the progression of prostate cancer.[80]

When mice with implanted tumors were fed a diet high in linoleic acid, the omega-6 fat in vegetable oils, they experienced a rate of metastasis four times higher than mice fed oleic acid, a monounsaturated fat.[81]

Evidence For PUFA Toxicity From Clinical Trials

We know of 8 randomized intervention trials that substituted PUFA, largely from omega-6-rich vegetable oils, for SaFA-rich dairy or animal fats. Here they are, ordered from high to low propensity for the PUFA dieters to die:

Rose Corn Oil Trial. This study is interesting because it was the only trial to supply PUFA in a form – corn oil – that does not contain omega-3 fats. (Most other trials used soybean oil, which is 7% omega-3.) Compared to the control diet, butter, milk, eggs, fatty meats, sausage, and ice cream were restricted and replaced by 80 g/day of corn oil. Study participants had previously suffered a heart attack. Two years later, 5 of 28 corn oil dieters (18%) had died and 48% had had a serious cardiac event; but only 1 of 26 control dieters (4%) had died and 25% had had a second heart attack. Rose et al. concluded that corn oil "cannot be recommended as a treatment of ischemic heart disease" because it is "most unlikely to be beneficial, and it is possibly harmful." The death rate was 364% higher in the PUFA group.[82]

The Anti-Coronary Club Program. The high-PUFA group of 814 men 40 to 59 years old was recruited from the public at large through radio and newspapers (subjects with history of coronary heart disease were excluded). A control group of 463 men was recruited from patients visiting a Cancer Detection Clinic. The experimental diet replaced butter with a high-PUFA margarine, and whole milk

---

[79] IBD in EPIC Study Investigators et al. Linoleic acid, a dietary n-6 polyunsaturated fatty acid, and the aetiology of ulcerative colitis: a nested case-control study within a European prospective cohort study. *Gut.* 2009 Dec;58(12):1606-11. *http://pmid.us/19628674.*

[80] Lloyd JC et al. Effect of Isocaloric Low Fat Diet on Prostate Cancer Xenograft Progression in a Hormone Deprivation Model. *J Urol.* 2010 Apr;183(4):1619-24. *http://pmid.us/20172549.*

[81] Le TT et al. Coherent anti-Stokes Raman scattering imaging of lipids in cancer metastasis. *BMC Cancer.* 2009 Jan 30;9:42. *http://pmid.us/19183472.*

[82] Rose GA et al. Corn oil in the treatment of ischaemic heart disease. *Br Med J.* 1965 Jun 12;1(5449):1531-3. *http://pmid.us/14288105.*

by skim milk; PUFA was increased from 4% to 10% of energy and SaFA reduced from 16% to 9% of energy. Clinical outcomes were assessed four years after each man began the study. In total, there were 27 deaths in the high-PUFA group (9 from coronary heart disease), 6 deaths in the control group (none from coronary heart disease. The death rate was 3.3% in the high-PUFA group and 1.4% in the control group.[83] The Anti-Coronary Club had become the Pro-Mortality Club: those in the PUFA arm were 156% more likely to die.

Sydney Diet-Heart Study. This study included 458 men aged 30-59 with coronary heart disease. After five years, 39 (18%) of the 221 high-PUFA dieters, but only 28 (12%) of the 237 controls, had died. The death rate was 49% higher in the high-PUFA group.[84]

Minnesota Coronary Survey. This was a 4.5 year study of 9057 patients in six Minnesota mental hospitals and a nursing home. The study compared a control diet with 18% SaFA and 5% PUFA to one with 9% SaFA and 15% PUFA. There were 269 deaths on the PUFA diet and 248 deaths on the control diet; over the full 4.5 year study period, those on the PUFA diet were about 9% more likely to die than those on the control diet. The difference was not considered significant.[85]

Los Angeles Veterans Administration Study. This study included 846 veterans with average age 65 at the start of the study, 422 in the control diet and 424 receiving a high-PUFA diet. Omega-6 LA constituted 4% of calories in the control and 14.9% of calories in the high-PUFA diet. At the end of the 8-year trial, death rates were slightly higher in the high-PUFA group. There were 7 cancer deaths among the high-PUFA group, 2 among the control group.[86] A later retrospective search found 31 cancer deaths among the high-PUFA group and 17 among the controls.[87] The number of smokers was much larger in the control diet

---

[83] Christakis G et al. Effect of the Anti-Coronary Club program on coronary heart disease. Risk-factor status. *JAMA*. 1966 Nov 7;198(6):597-604. *http://pmid.us/5953429/*

[84] Woodhill JM et al. Low fat, low cholesterol diet in secondary prevention of coronary heart disease. *Adv Exp Med Biol*. 1978;109:317-30. *http://pmid.us/727035*.

[85] Frantz ID Jr et al. Test of effect of lipid lowering by diet on cardiovascular risk. The Minnesota Coronary Survey. *Arteriosclerosis*. 1989 Jan-Feb;9(1):129-35. *http://pmid.us/2643423*.

[86] Dayton S et al. Controlled trial of a diet high in unsaturated fat for prevention of atherosclerotic complications. *Lancet*. 1968 Nov 16;2(7577):1060-2. *http://pmid.us/4176868*.

[87] Pearce ML, Dayton S. Incidence of cancer in men on a diet high in polyunsaturated fat. *Lancet*. 1971 Mar 6;1(7697):464-7. *http://pmid.us/4100347*.

group than in the high-PUFA group[88]; perhaps the excess of deaths in the high-PUFA group would have been larger had the number of smokers been equal.

Oslo Diet-Heart Study. Of 412 men who had previously suffered a heart attack, 206 were placed on a control diet and 206 on a diet low in animal fat and high in vegetable oils and seafood and supplied by the doctors with "considerable quantities of Norwegian sardines canned in cod liver oil."[89] After 11 years, 101 of the vegetable/fish oil group and 108 of the control group had died; the difference was not considered significant. Fatal heart attacks were lower in the vegetable/fish oil group, but cancer and infectious disease deaths were higher.[90] The confounding effect of the omega-3 fish oil, which improved the omega-3 to omega-6 tissue ratio, makes this study a poor test of PUFA toxicity.

Medical Research Council Trial. This studied 393 Englishmen who had previously suffered heart attacks. 194 men were kept on their normal diets, while 199 were placed on a diet in which animal fat, biscuits and cakes were reduced and 3 oz (85 g) soybean oil taken daily. Participation periods varied from 2 years up to 6¾ years. During the trial, there were 31 deaths on the normal diet, 25 from heart disease, and 28 deaths on the soybean diet, 27 from heart disease. These differences were not considered significant.[91]

The Finnish Mental Hospital Study. This study was neither randomized nor blinded, but it is widely cited because it is the only trial to (appear to) show a significant benefit for the high-PUFA diet group. It is also unique in having a cross-over design. The study took place in two Finnish mental hospitals, hospital N and hospital K. It lasted from 1959 to 1971. For the first 6 years, hospital N had the high-PUFA diet, hospital K the control diet. For the last 6 years, hospital N served the control diet, hospital K the high-PUFA diet. The control diet was the normal hospital diet; the high-PUFA diet replaced milk by a mixture of soybean oil with skim milk ("filled milk") and butter with a high-PUFA margarine.[92]

---

[88] Dayton S et al. A controlled clinical trial of a diet high in unsaturated fat. Circulation 1969; 40(suppl):1–63.

[89] Leren P. The effect of plasma cholesterol lowering diet in male survivors of myocardial infarction: a controlled clinical trial. *Acta Med Scand Suppl.* 1966;466:1-92. *http://pmid.us/5228820.*

[90] Leren P. The Oslo diet-heart study: eleven-year report. *Circulation* 42 (1970) 935–942. *http://pmid.us/5477261.*

[91] Medical Research Council, Controlled trial of soya-bean oil in myocardial infarction. *Lancet.* 1968 Sep 28;2(7570):693-9. *http://pmid.us/4175085.*

[92] Miettinen M et al. Effect of cholesterol-lowering diet on mortality from coronary heart-disease and other causes. A twelve-year clinical trial in men and women. *Lancet.* 1972 Oct 21;2(7782):835-8. *http://pmid.us/4116551.* Turpeinen O et al. Dietary prevention of coronary heart disease: the Finnish Mental Hospital Study. *Int J Epidemiol.* 1979

The published reports associated deaths with the patient's diet at the time of his death. So if a patient at hospital N ate the high-PUFA diet for six years, returned to the normal hospital diet and died the next day, his death was associated with the normal diet, not the PUFA diet. Using this method, the death rate on the PUFA diet was 40.8 per thousand person-years, compared to 47.2 on the normal diet – a 14% decrease on the PUFA diet.

However, if one believes that major causes of death like heart disease and cancer have long incubation periods, and depend on the diet eaten for many years previously, then an alternative method of analysis makes more sense. The Finnish doctors fortunately measured adipose tissue levels of omega-6 LA over the last six years of the study, and this lets us estimate tissue levels throughout the study at each hospital. The result is as follows:

Table: *Estimated adipose tissue levels of omega-6 LA in patients*

	Hospital N (diet then control)	Hospital K (control then diet)
Year 0	10.2%*	10.2%*
Year 2	19.7%*	10.2%*
Year 4	32.4%*	10.2%
Year 6	32.0%*	10.2%*
Year 6/0	26.9%†	10.2%†
Year 8/2	17.6%†	19.7%†
Year 10/4	13.3%†	32.4%†
Year 12/6	9.8%†	32.0%†
12-Yr Average	**20.4%†**	**17.3%†**

†Table 1, Meittinen et al 1972. *Estimated.

Jun;8(2):99-118. *http://pmid.us/393644*. Miettinen M et al. Dietary prevention of coronary heart disease in women: the Finnish mental hospital study. *Int J Epidemiol.* 1983 Mar;12(1):17-25. *http://pmid.us/6840954*. Hat tip Stephan Guyenet, *http://wholehealthsource.blogspot.com/2009/07/finnish-mental-hospital-trial.html*.

Here we see that the patients in Hospital N had a higher average PUFA level over the 12-year study than the patients in Hospital K. Over the 12 years, their average tissue levels of LA were about 20% higher.

This is interesting, because Hospital N experienced a higher death rate than Hospital K. The death rate at Hospital N was 46.8 per thousand person-years, that at Hospital K was 36.4 per thousand person years. By this method of analysis, the high-PUFA Hospital N had a death rate 28% higher than the low-PUFA Hospital K.

So, was a high-PUFA diet associated with more deaths or fewer deaths? It depends on how long-lasting are the ill-effects of PUFA.

SUMMARY OF THE CLINICAL TRIALS

Among the eight intervention trials, the high-PUFA diet appears clearly harmful in three, possibly harmful in two others, clearly superior in none:

- In three – the Rose Corn Oil Study, Anti-Coronary Club Program, and Sydney Diet-Heart Study – the PUFA diet seemed clearly harmful, raising death rates 364%, 156%, and 49%, respectively.

- In two – the Minnesota Coronary Survey and the LA Veterans Administration Studies – the PUFA diet raised the death rate by less than 10%. The increases were not considered significant.

- The Oslo Diet-Heart Study saw 6.5% fewer deaths in the PUFA+fish oil arm, a difference that was not considered significant. Given the powerful ability of fish oil to suppress cardiac mortality, it seems plausible that the PUFA arm would have seen higher death rates than the control if it had not included a large amount of fish oil.

- The Medical Research Council Study saw 3, or 10%, fewer deaths on its PUFA arm, but 2 (8%) more cardiac deaths. These differences were judged to be insignificant, and that judgment is supported by the unexpectedness of this pattern: in other studies the PUFA arm saw higher overall mortality but reduced cardiac mortality.

- The Finnish Mental Hospital Study was beset by an inappropriate crossover design which clouds the results. If PUFA only affects mortality at the moment it is consumed, then the PUFA diet lowered mortality; if PUFA has long-term detrimental effects, then the PUFA diet increased mortality.

Overall, these results seem consistent with the existence of mortality-increasing PUFA toxicity in diets with omega-6 LA at 10% to 15% of calories. High-LA dieters seem especially prone to dying from cancer.

Balancing Omega-6 and Omega-3 PUFA: Introduction

Dr. William E. Lands and collaborators did much to elucidate the optimal ratio of omega-6 to omega-3 fats. His work was helpful because it separated the EFA puzzle into two more tractable issues: how tissue abundances affect health, and how dietary intake affects tissue abundances.

In humans and other animals, the most biologically active PUFAs are the long PUFAs: principally, the 20-carbon omega-6s **arachidonic acid (AA)** and **dihomo-gamma-linolenic acid (DGLA)**, the 20-carbon omega-3 **eicosapentaenoic acid (EPA)**, and the 22-carbon omega-3 **docosahexaenoic acid (DHA)**. In the body, AA, DGLA, and EPA are precursors to eicosanoids; EPA and DHA are precursors to compounds called resolvins; and DHA is a structural fat in the brain, nerves, and retina.

How Tissue Fatty Acids Are Measured

Throughout this chapter, tissue abundances are measured from plasma phospholipids or red blood cell membranes. Blood samples are used because they are easily obtained from patients. Autopsies have shown that blood fatty acid abundances closely mimic human organ abundances.[1]

[1] Holman RT. The slow discovery of the importance of omega 3 essential fatty acids in human health. *J Nutr.* 1998 Feb;128(2 Suppl):427S-433S. *http://pmid.us/9478042.*

Biochemistry of Omega-6 and Omega-3 Balance

Polyunsaturated fatty acids are fragile: they react easily with oxygen. Nature has turned the fragility of polyunsaturated fats to its advantage by using oxidized PUFA as signaling molecules, called **eicosanoids**. When a cell is damaged, enzymes release PUFA from the cell membrane and turn them into eicosanoids. The eicosanoids trigger inflammation that brings in the immune system to help fight pathogens or remove toxins.

Some of the most popular drugs in the world – aspirin and ibuprofen – work by preventing omega-6 fats from being turned into eicosanoids.

An excess of omega-6 fatty acids can be toxic in two ways:

- **Too many inflammatory eicosanoids:** High tissue omega-6 levels, especially combined with a deficiency of omega-3, generate too many omega-6-derived eicosanoids and trigger chronic inflammation. Excessive omega-6 eicosanoid production is associated with heart attacks, stroke, arrhythmia, arthritis, asthma, headaches, menstrual cramps, inflammation, tumor metastases and osteoporosis.[93]

- **Abnormal reactions:** With excess omega-6 fats around, the body loses control of their modification. Free radicals can oxidize the fragile omega-6

---

[93] Lands WE. Dietary fat and health: the evidence and the politics of prevention: careful use of dietary fats can improve life and prevent disease. *Ann N Y Acad Sci.* 2005 Dec;1055:179-92. *http://pmid.us/16387724.*

fats, a process called "lipid peroxidation." If the resulting lipid hydroperoxides are not quickly scavenged by the antioxidant glutathione and catalyst glutathione peroxidase, they can turn into highly toxic compounds called aldehydes. Aldehydes are highly reactive with DNA, proteins, and phospholipids.[94] For instance, aldehydes react with apolipoprotein B (the protein of LDL) to create oxidized-LDL, a major contributor to atherosclerosis.[95]

Omega-3 fats also are intentionally oxidized by the body into eicosanoids. But the omega-3 eicosanoids moderate the effect of omega-6 eicosanoids. They are therefore an antidote to some forms of omega-6 toxicity.

How Omega-3 Fats Moderate Omega-6 Toxicity

Eicosanoids made from the omega-6 AA are generally inflammatory. However, derivatives of the omega-3 fats tend to be anti-inflammatory:

- Eicosanoids derived from the omega-3 EPA moderate the inflammatory signaling of the omega-6-derived eicosanoids.
- Docosanoids derived from the omega-3 DHA help to terminate inflammation.

The optimal omega-6 to omega-3 ratio in tissue

Cardiovascular disease risk seems to be especially influenced by the omega-6 to omega-3 ratio in tissue. Dr. William E. Lands has studied this relationship, illustrated in the figure below.[96]

---

[94] Catalá A. Lipid peroxidation of membrane phospholipids generates hydroxy-alkenals and oxidized phospholipids active in physiological and/or pathological conditions. *Chem Phys Lipids.* 2009 Jan;157(1):1-11. *http://pmid.us/18977338.*

[95] Holvoet P et al. Association of high coronary heart disease risk status with circulating oxidized LDL in the well-functioning elderly: findings from the Health, Aging, and Body Composition study. *Arterioscler Thromb Vasc Biol.* 2003 Aug 1;23(8):1444-8. *http://pmid.us/12791672.* Holvoet P. Oxidized LDL and coronary heart disease. *Acta Cardiol.* 2004 Oct;59(5):479-84. *http://pmid.us/15529550.*

[96] Lands WE. Dietary fat and health: the evidence and the politics of prevention: careful use of dietary fats can improve life and prevent disease. *Ann N Y Acad Sci.* 2005 Dec;1055:179-92. *http://pmid.us/16387724.* Lands WE, *http://efaeducation.nih.gov/sig/personal.html.* Hat tip Stephan Guyenet, *http://wholehealthsource.blogspot.com/2008/09/omega-fats-and-cardiovascular-disease.html.*

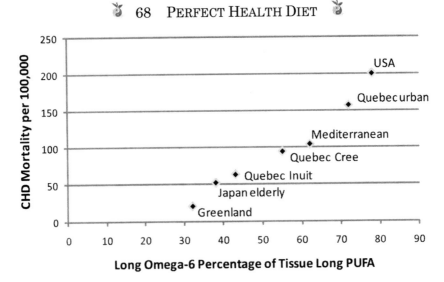

Figure: The horizontal axis is the percentage of long (20-carbon or longer) PUFA in tissue that are omega-6, not omega-3. The greater the omega-6 fraction, the higher the cardiovascular mortality rate.

Coronary heart disease mortality depends on the balance between long omega-6 and long omega-3 PUFA in tissues. Heart disease mortality rises as the omega-6 fraction rises and the omega-3 fraction decreases, and approaches zero when long tissue PUFAs are 72% omega-3, 28% omega-6. Total mortality is also minimized at about the same tissue ratio of 72% long omega-3, 28% long omega-6.[97]

Tissue abundances of most Americans (see "USA" in the upper right) are less than 25% long omega-3, more than 75% long omega-6. This tissue omega-6 to omega-3 ratio is about 9-fold higher than the optimum: It should be 3:1 in favor of omega-3, but instead is 3:1 in favor of omega-6. This mistake alone more than triples America's cardiovascular mortality relative to Japan's.

More Benefits of a Low Omega-6 to Omega-3 Ratio

Although we have focused on the cardiovascular benefits of a low omega-6 to omega-3 ratio, scientists have identified benefits to other parts of the body:

- Reducing the omega-6 to omega-3 ratio improves bone mineral density.[98]

[97] Hibbeln JR et al. Healthy intakes of n-3 and n-6 fatty acids: estimations considering worldwide diversity. *Am J Clin Nutr.* 2006 Jun;83(6 Suppl):1483S-1493S. *http://pmid.us/16841858.*

[98] Watkins BA et al. Dietary ratio of n-6/n-3 PUFAs and docosahexaenoic acid: actions on bone mineral and serum biomarkers in ovariectomized rats. *J Nutr Biochem.* 2006 Apr;17(4):282-9. *http://pmid.us/16102959.* Watkins BA et al. Dietary ratio of (n-6)/(n-3) polyunsaturated fatty acids alters the fatty acid composition of bone compartments and

- Reducing the omega-6 to omega-3 ratio relieves depression.[99]

- Reducing the omega-6 to omega-3 ratio decreases anger and anxiety, reduces aggression, and reduces suicidal behaviors and self-harm.[100]

- A low omega-6 to omega-3 ratio improves recovery from sepsis and operations and shortens stay in intensive care units.[101]

Clinical Trials Support a Low Omega-6 to Omega-3 Ratio

Perhaps the most successful clinical trial ever at reducing mortality was the Lyon Diet Heart Study. This study compared the American Heart Association Step One diet (a high-carb, high-vegetable-oil diet) with a Mediterranean diet that was low (less than 7 g/day) in omega-6 and high in omega-3 due to a supplement providing 2 g/day of ALA. The result: a striking reduction in all-cause mortality, heart attacks, and cancer.

After a mean follow-up of 27 months, the number of cardiac deaths was 16 on the AHA diet, 3 on the Lyon diet; the number of all-cause deaths was 20 on the AHA

biomarkers of bone formation in rats. *J Nutr.* 2000 Sep;130(9):2274-84. *http://pmid.us/10958824.*

[99] Nemets B et al. Addition of omega-3 fatty acid to maintenance medication treatment for recurrent unipolar depressive disorder. *Am J Psychiatry.* 2002 Mar;159(3):477-9. *http://pmid.us/11870016.* Su KP et al. Omega-3 fatty acids for major depressive disorder during pregnancy: results from a randomized, double-blind, placebo-controlled trial. *J Clin Psychiatry.* 2008 Apr;69(4):644-51. *http://pmid.us/18370571.* Su KP et al. Omega-3 fatty acids in major depressive disorder. A preliminary double-blind, placebo-controlled trial. *Eur Neuropsychopharmacol.* 2003 Aug;13(4):267-71. *http://pmid.us/12888186.* Stoll AL et al. Omega 3 fatty acids in bipolar disorder: a preliminary double-blind, placebo-controlled trial. *Arch Gen Psychiatry.* 1999 May;56(5):407-12. *http://pmid.us/10232294.* Hat tip Stephan Guyenet, *http://wholehealthsource.blogspot.com/2008/09/omega-ratio.html.*

[100] Buydens-Branchey L et al. Associations between increases in plasma n-3 polyunsaturated fatty acids following supplementation and decreases in anger and anxiety in substance abusers. *Prog Neuropsychopharmacol Biol Psychiatry.* 2008 Feb 15;32(2):568-75. *http://pmid.us/18060675.* Hamazaki T et al. The effect of docosahexaenoic acid on aggression in young adults. A placebo-controlled double-blind study. *J Clin Invest.* 1996 Feb 15;97(4):1129-33. *http://pmid.us/8613538.* Zanarini MC, Frankenburg FR. omega-3 Fatty acid treatment of women with borderline personality disorder: a double-blind, placebo-controlled pilot study. *Am J Psychiatry.* 2003 Jan;160(1):167-9. *http://pmid.us/12505817.* Hallahan B et al. Omega-3 fatty acid supplementation in patients with recurrent self-harm. Single-centre double-blind randomised controlled trial. *Br J Psychiatry.* 2007 Feb;190:118-22. *http://pmid.us/17267927.*

[101] Heller AR et al. Omega-3 fatty acids improve the diagnosis-related clinical outcome. *Crit Care Med.* 2006 Apr;34(4):972-9. *http://pmid.us/16484909.*

diet, 8 on the Lyon diet.[102] At 4 years follow-up, there had been 19 cardiac deaths on the AHA diet, 6 on the Lyon diet; 24 total deaths on the AHA diet, 14 on the Lyon diet; 17 cancer cases and 4 cancer deaths on the AHA diet, 7 cancer cases and 3 cancer deaths on the Lyon diet.[103]

Another clinical trial which tested increased dietary omega-3 was the Diet and Reinfarction Trial (DART), which enrolled 2,033 British men who had previously suffered a heart attack. In this trial a fish group tripled their omega-3 intake from 0.6 g EPA per week to 2.4 g. This group saw a significant reduction in heart attacks and in all-cause deaths: 9.3% of the fish group died, 12.8% of the control group.[104]

Keep Omega-6 Below 4% of Energy For Good Tissue Ratios

Some scientists have questioned whether omega-6 PUFA in the form of LA significantly affects the tissue omega-6 to omega-3 ratio. Their reasoning is that tissue levels of AA, the 20-carbon omega-6 which is precursor to the most inflammatory eicosanoids, plateau once LA consumption reaches 1-2% of calories and rise slowly with further LA consumption. The body seems to avoid converting LA into AA once the AA level is adequate.

However, this is not the end of the story. Intake of 1-4% of calories as LA has little effect upon other fatty acids, but above 4% of calories, LA suppresses tissue levels of omega-6 DGLA and omega-3 EPA. DGLA is a long omega-6 fat, but one that moderates the inflammatory effects of AA. Due to this effect, LA consumption above 4% of energy increases AA:DGLA and AA:EPA ratios with inflammatory effects.[105]

---

[102] de Lorgeril M et al. Mediterranean diet, traditional risk factors, and the rate of cardiovascular complications after myocardial infarction: final report of the Lyon Diet Heart Study. *Circulation.* 1999 Feb 16;99(6):779-85. *http://pmid.us/9989963.*

[103] de Lorgeril M et al. Mediterranean dietary pattern in a randomized trial: prolonged survival and possible reduced cancer rate. *Arch Intern Med.* 1998 Jun 8;158(11):1181-7. *http://pmid.us/9625397.*

[104] Burr ML et al. Effects of changes in fat, fish, and fibre intakes on death and myocardial reinfarction: diet and reinfarction trial (DART). *Lancet.* 1989 Sep 30;2(8666):757-61. *http://pmid.us/2571009.* Hat tip Stephan Guyenet, *http://wholehealthsource.blogspot.com/2008/10/dart-many-lessons-learned.html.*

[105] Angela Liou Y, Innis SM. Dietary linoleic acid has no effect on arachidonic acid, but increases n-6 eicosadienoic acid, and lowers dihomo-gamma-linolenic and eicosapentaenoic acid in plasma of adult men. *Prostaglandins Leukot Essent Fatty Acids.* 2009 Apr;80(4):201-6. *http://pmid.us/19356914.*

Above 4% of calories, LA has been shown to reduce EPA and DHA levels in pregnant mothers.[106]   In piglets, 1.2% LA consumption with adequate omega-3 leads to healthy brain development, but increasing LA to 10.7% of calories deprives brains of DHA and compromises neurodevelopment.[107]

4% of calories as omega-6 LA is a threshold of toxicity: above this level omega-3 tissue levels are suppressed.

But there is another reason to balance omega-6 and omega-3 at low dietary intakes: omega-3 fats are themselves toxic at high doses.

More Evidence for Low PUFA: Omega-3 Toxicity

Both omega-3 and omega-6 PUFA are susceptible to oxidation and both produce liver damage when combined with sugar or alcohol. However, in addition to this shared toxicity from lipid peroxidation, omega-3 PUFA have their own forms of toxicity.

BLEEDING AND STROKE

High omega-3 intake, especially of EPA and DHA, prolongs bleeding times and may increase the risk of stroke. In Greenland Eskimos with very high intakes of EPA+DHA (6.5 g/day, equivalent to about 5 pounds of salmon per week), an increased incidence of hemorrhagic stroke has been observed.[108]

However, intakes of less than 3 g/day, the level Generally Recognized as Safe by the US government, are unlikely to result in bleeding or stroke.[109]

EARLY AGING AND SHORTENED LIFESPAN

There is also evidence of long-term dangers from high omega-3 intake. One study showed that when pregnant rats are given excessive doses of omega-3 fats, their offspring have shortened life span and greater neural degeneration in old age. The

---

[106] Friesen RW, Innis SM. Linoleic acid is associated with lower long-chain n-6 and n-3 fatty acids in red blood cell lipids of Canadian pregnant women. *Am J Clin Nutr.* 2010 Jan;91(1):23-31. *http://pmid.us/19923368.*

[107] Novak EM et al. High dietary omega-6 fatty acids contribute to reduced docosahexaenoic acid in the developing brain and inhibit secondary neurite growth. *Brain Res.* 2008 Oct 27;1237:136-45. *http://pmid.us/18710653.*

[108] Institute of Medicine. *Dietary Reference Intakes for Energy, Carbohydrate, Fiber, Fat, Fatty Acids, Cholesterol, Protein, and Amino Acids.* Washington, D. C.: National Academies Press; 2002. See page 493: *http://www.nap.edu/openbook.php?record_id=10490&page=493.*

[109] Kris-Etherton PM et al. Fish consumption, fish oil, omega-3 fatty acids, and cardiovascular disease. *Circulation.* 2002 Nov 19;106(21):2747-57. *http://pmid.us/12438303.*

authors concluded, "both over- and under-supplementation with omega-3 FA can harm offspring development."[110]

FISH OIL CAPSULES (BUT NOT FISH) ARE TOXIC

Fish are eaten within days of being killed, and refrigerated until cooking; so their omega-3 oils remain fresh. However, fish oil capsules tend to be stored at room temperature for long periods of time. Fish oil in capsules must often become rancid, since omega-3 fats are so easily oxidized.

It is interesting that fish consumption has an excellent record in clinical trials, but fish oil capsule supplements do not. In the Diet and Angina Randomized Trial (DART-2), 3114 men with stable angina were followed for 3-9 years. There was a control group, a group advised to eat oily fish, and a group taking 3 fish oil capsules daily. There was a significant increase in sudden cardiac death among the subgroup taking fish oil capsules.[111]

What Was the Paleolithic Omega-6 to Omega-3 Ratio?

How would Paleolithic omega-6 to omega-3 tissue ratios compare to those of modern societies – Greenland Inuit at 30% long omega-6, Japanese at 50%, Mediterranean Europeans at 60%, and Americans at 80%?[112]

Dr. Artemis Simopoulos has estimated the dietary omega-6 to omega-3 ratio of Paleolithic man at 1:1.[113] Wild animal tissues typically have omega-6 to omega-3 ratios between 1:1 and 2:1 if LA is included and around 0.5:1 if only long-chain fats are considered. Long omega-3 fats are abundant in tissues prized by Paleolithic man, such as brain and bone marrow. For instance, in bone marrow, 92% of fats are saturated or monounsaturated, 5.7% are omega-6 and 2.3% omega-3.[114]

---

[110] Church MW et al. Excess omega-3 fatty acid consumption by mothers during pregnancy and lactation caused shorter life span and abnormal ABRs in old adult offspring. *Neurotoxicol Teratol.* 2010 March - April;32(2):171-181. *http://pmid.us/19818397.*

[111] Burr ML et al. Lack of benefit of dietary advice to men with angina: results of a controlled trial. *Eur J Clin Nutr.* 2003 Feb;57(2):193-200. *http://pmid.us/12571649.*

[112] Lands WE. Commentary on the workshop statement. Essentiality of and recommended dietary intakes for Omega-6 and Omega-3 fatty acids. Prostaglandins Leukot Essent Fatty Acids. 2000 Sep;63(3):125-6. *http://pmid.us/10991766.*

[113] Simopoulos AP. Evolutionary aspects of omega-3 fatty acids in the food supply. Prostaglandins Leukot Essent Fatty Acids. 1999 May-Jun;60(5-6):421-9. *http://pmid.us/10471132.*

[114] Cordain et al. Fatty acid analysis of wild ruminant tissues: evolutionary implications for reducing diet-related chronic disease. *Eur J Clin Nutr.* 2002 Mar;56(3):181-91. *http://pmid.us/11960292.*

If fats were 50% of calories in the Paleolithic and derived entirely from bone marrow, then omega-6 fats would be 3% of energy and omega-3 fats 1.2% of energy, right in line with our recommendations.

Chimps Eat Bone Marrow and Brain Too

Paleolithic humans were not alone in favoring the brain and bone marrow. As anthropologist Craig Stanford notes, "chimpanzees value fat above all else in the carcasses of their prey. We infer this from their preference for the brain and the bone marrow, two of the most fat-rich body parts."[1]

[1] Stanford, Craig B. (1999) *The Hunting Apes: Meat Eating and the Origins of Human Behavior*, Princeton: Princeton University Press. Full text online: *http://press.princeton.edu/books/stanford/*. Quote is from page 152.

In the Early Upper Paleolithic when *Homo sapiens* was populating Eurasia, the human diet was dominated by fish and marine foods, the richest sources of omega-3 fats. The Paleolithic diet was free of omega-6-rich plant foods, such as grains and legumes. Fruits, vegetables, and tubers, which were part of the diet, have low omega-6 levels.

So it seems likely that many Paleolithic humans attained an omega-6 to omega-3 tissue ratio as good as that of modern Japanese.

Dietary Intakes For The Optimal Tissue Ratio

What should you eat to obtain the optimal tissue omega-6 to omega-3 ratio?

Different cultures around the world have widely different omega-6 and omega-3 intakes. This has allowed scientists to develop a formula relating tissue abundances of long PUFAs to dietary intake of the various PUFAs.[115] An Excel calculator is available online.[116]

The short-chain plant-derived PUFAs LA and ALA have little direct use in the body; but they do serve as a reservoir from which longer-chain PUFAs can be manufactured. Typically, only a fraction of these short PUFAs are converted to the long PUFAs which control mortality risk.

In practice, for most people, three fatty acids determine tissue abundances of the long-chain PUFAs:

- The 18-carbon omega-6 **linoleic acid (LA)** is the dominant omega-6 fat in most diets; internationally, LA is generally over 90% of dietary omega-6

---

[115] Lands WE et al. Maintenance of lower proportions of (n - 6) eicosanoid precursors in phospholipids of human plasma in response to added dietary (n - 3) fatty acids. *Biochim Biophys Acta*. 1992 Dec 10;1180(2):147-62. *http://pmid.us/1463766*.

[116] Lands, WE, *http://efaeducation.nih.gov/sig/dietbalance.html*.

fats, ranging from about 90% in Filipino diets to about 98% of the omega-6 in American diets. Much of the long-chain omega-6 fats (such as AA and DGLA) in tissue are derived from LA, not obtained directly from diet. The main dietary sources of LA are vegetable oils and baked or fried foods cooked with vegetable oils.

- Although the 18-carbon omega-3 alpha-linolenic acid (ALA) is a larger component of diet, tissue long-chain omega-3 levels depend mainly on dietary intake of the long-chain omega-3s **EPA, DPA and DHA**. This is partly because LA inhibits the conversion of ALA into long-chain omega-3s, so that at the high vegetable oil intakes of most Americans, the conversion rate of ALA into EPA is small.

Thus, two foods largely control the tissue omega-6 to omega-3 ratio: vegetable oils (supplying omega-6 LA) and cold-water fish (supplying long omega-3s). We can calculate the key tissue abundance ratio from just two inputs – LA intake as a fraction of total energy, and long omega-3 intake as a fraction of total energy. A graph of the results of this calculation is available online at the US National Institute of Health "EFA Education" site.[117]

The table below gives the salmon intake required at different LA intakes to achieve the optimal 28% long omega-6, 72% long omega-3 tissue ratio.

LA g/d (% of energy)	EPA+DPA+DHA g/d (% of energy)	Salmon lb/week
4.8 (2%)	1.8 (0.74%)	1.2
7.2 (3%)	2.6 (1.1%)	1.7
9.6 (4%)	3.5 (1.4%)	2.3
12.0 (5%)	4.4 (1.8%)	2.9

The conversion between grams and percent of calories is based on a diet of 2200 calories/day. The salmon estimate assumes 10.7 g EPA+DPA+DHA per pound of salmon, which is typical of farm-raised Atlantic salmon.

It is not feasible to obtain less than 2% of energy from LA eating agriculturally produced foods. Nor is it feasible to eat 3 pounds of salmon per week. The Japanese eat about 1.5 g of long omega-3s per day, equivalent to about 1 pound of salmon per week. Few people except the Inuit eat 3 pounds of cold-water fish in a week. So, this table covers the range of food intakes that are capable of optimizing tissue PUFA levels.

---

[117] Lands, WE, *http://efaeducation.nih.gov/sig/food2.html.*

To have an optimal omega-6 to omega-3 tissue ratio, most Americans would need big changes in diet:

- Americans now eat about 0.1 g/d of long omega-3. Eating 1 lb of salmon per week would increase the average American's EPA+DHA intake about 15-fold.

- Americans now eat about 36 g/d of LA, 8.9% of their 3770 calories.[118] This is up from about 12 g/d in 1909.[119] To get LA intake down to 7 g/d would require about a 5-fold reduction in omega-6 consumption.

To perfect their tissue omega-6 to omega-3 ratio, Americans should reduce omega-6 intake by a factor of 5 and increase EPA and DHA intake by a factor of 15.

Such big changes can be achieved, but only with the elimination of vegetable oils and foods prepared with them (including most commercial breads, doughnuts, cookies, crackers, chips, and French fries) and the inclusion of cold-water fish as a regular feature of the diet.

Conclusion

Many diseases – cardiovascular disease, mental and mood disorders, and immune disorders like allergies and asthma – are improved if enough fatty fish is eaten to create a 2.5 to 1 tissue ratio of long omega-3 to long omega-6 fats.

However, there is ample evidence that both omega-6 and omega-3 fatty acids become toxic above about 4% of calories.

We recommend aiming for dietary intake of about 3% omega-6, chiefly in the form of LA, plus sufficient omega-3 to balance tissue ratios. This can be achieved by:

- Eliminating omega-6-rich oils in favor of butter and coconut oil.

- Favoring low-omega-6 meats like beef, lamb, salmon, and other fish.

- Eating about 1 pound per week of salmon or other fatty fish to optimize the omega-3 to omega-6 ratio.

---

[118] U.S. Department of Agriculture, "Interactive Nutrient Content of the U.S. Food Supply," *http://65.216.150.146/NFSDatabase/QueNut.asp*, accessible from *http://www.cnpp.usda.gov/USFoodSupply.htm*. Hat tip Stephan Guyenet, *http://wholehealthsource.blogspot.com/2008/12/vegetable-oil-and-weight-gain.html*.

[119] U.S. Department of Agriculture, Interactive Nutrient Content of the U.S. Food Supply, accessible from *http://www.cnpp.usda.gov/USFoodSupply.htm*.

The Safe Fats: SaFA and MUFA

The macronutrients we've considered so far all become toxic above a threshold: protein above 600 calories per day, glucose above 600 calories per day, fructose at any dose, PUFA above 100 calories per day.

We've considered every macronutrient except SaFA and MUFA – and we have only about 1300 calories per day before toxicity effects begin.

What about athletes who consume very large calorie intakes – 5000, 8000, or 12,000 calories per day? Can they eat such large numbers of calories without experiencing macronutrient toxicity?

Yes: SaFA and MUFA are non-toxic, beneficial for that matter, even when eaten in very large amounts.

The body can use longer (14-carbon or more) SaFA and MUFA in nearly unlimited quantities:

- They are the core structural fats of the human body, making up 75-80% of the fatty acids in most cells.

- They are the primary energy source for most of the body, and a healthier form of energy than glucose.

They also have no known toxicity, even at very high doses, as long as metabolic damage or high insulin does not prevent fats from being utilized. This makes saturated and monounsaturated fats a benign source of calories.

As long as enough is obtained of other nutrients, it never hurts to eat more (saturated and monounsaturated) fat!

No Toxicity from Chemical Reactions

Since they are chemically stable, SaFA and MUFA are essentially non-toxic. The primary places in the body they are chemically modified are:

- In the liver primarily, SaFA and MUFA can be elongated and desaturated to transform particular fatty acids that are present in relative excess – typically, 16-carbon SaFAs created from carbs – into SaFA or MUFA that are relatively deficient.

- In mitochondria throughout the body, SaFA and MUFA are burned for calories, a process that steadily shortens them 2 carbons at a time until nothing is left but carbon dioxide and water.

Each of these transformations is benign, and creates no toxic products.

In contrast, the chemically fragile PUFA, whose extra carbon double bonds are easily altered by oxidation, glycation, or fructation, are frequently modified into toxic compounds in the body. Thus, PUFA, but not SaFA or MUFA, create oxidized LDL, a cause of atherosclerosis and heart disease.

Here is a variation of a table we showed earlier. In studies in 1996 and 1997, volunteers ate for 5 weeks each diets supplemented with four different kinds of fat: a SaFA-rich diet, a MUFA-rich diet, an omega-6-rich diet, and an omega-3-rich diet.[120] Levels of LDL oxidation after each period were:

Table: Levels of ox-LDL on various diets.

Diet	TBARS, 1996 study	TBARS, 1997 study
SaFA	1.15	0.89
MUFA	1.15	1.06
Omega-6	1.51	1.56
Omega-3	1.69	1.70

Notes: TBARS: thiobarbituric acid reactive substances in LDL, in nmol of MDA per mg of LDL protein.

In the PUFA-supplemented diets ox-LDL was increased by at least 30% compared to SaFA- or MUFA-supplemented diets. Overall, the amount of ox-LDL in the body was roughly proportional to the amount of PUFA. If the diets had continued beyond 5 weeks, the superiority of the SaFA- and MUFA-rich diets probably would have been even more impressive.

"Lipotoxicity" of Free Fatty Acids

There is another way that fatty acids can engage in chemical reactions: isolated fatty acids can bond to other molecules. The storage and structural forms of fats in the body, phospholipids and triglycerides, are stable, but free fatty acids (or NEFA, "non-esterified fatty acids") can and do bond to other molecules, potentially altering their function.

In healthy people this does not lead to problems: free fatty acids are burned in mitochondria soon after their release (or "lipolysis") from phospholipids or triglycerides, and free fatty acid levels are low. However, in people with damaged metabolisms, free fatty acid levels can become elevated even as mitochondria are blocked from burning fats by, for instance, high insulin levels. This excess of free fatty acids in cells can lead to "lipotoxicity."

---

[120] Mata P et al. Effect of Dietary Fat Saturation on LDL Oxidation and Monocyte Adhesion to Human Endothelial Cells In Vitro. *Arterioscler Thromb Vasc Biol.* 1996 Nov;16(11):1347-55. *http://pmid.us/8911273*. Mata P et al. Monounsaturated and polyunsaturated n-6 fatty acid-enriched diets modify LDL oxidation and decrease human coronary smooth muscle cell DNA synthesis. *Arterioscler Thromb Vasc Biol.* 1997 Oct;17(10):2088-95. *http://pmid.us/9351376*. Hat tip Stephan Guyenet, *http://wholehealthsource.blogspot.com/2009/08/diet-heart-hypothesis-oxidized-ldl-part.html*.

> ### "Lipotoxicity" of Free Fatty Acids (cont.)
>
> Elevated blood NEFA and clinical evidence for lipotoxicity, therefore, are the result of metabolic syndrome. For instance, in a study of NEFA and sudden cardiac death, only patients with metabolic syndrome died:
>
> > Increases in blood pressure and in levels of plasma glucose, insulin, and triglycerides are features of the metabolic syndrome (syndrome X). Besides an increase in NEFA, all of these variables were increased at inclusion in subjects who died suddenly during follow-up.[1]
>
> Since lipotoxicity arises from the metabolic derangements caused by high-carb diets and food toxicities from grains, vegetable oils, and fructose, we do not consider it evidence for the toxicity of *dietary* SaFA and MUFA. High SaFA and MUFA diets, by removing food toxins, are a crucial step in the restoration of healthy metabolic control and the elimination of lipotoxicity.
>
> [1] Jouven X et al. Circulating nonesterified fatty acid level as a predictive risk factor for sudden death in the population. *Circulation.* 2001 Aug 14;104(7):756-61. http://pmid.us/11502698.

Huge Storage Capacity

The body has large reservoirs for the storage of excess SaFA and MUFA. As structural elements of cells, these fatty acids constitute almost half the lean mass of the body. Tens of pounds of SaFA and MUFA, containing tens of thousands of calories, are stored in skeletal muscle alone. Adipose cells store further amounts.

These reservoirs are evolutionary valuable, because, as the preferred fuel of mitochondria, SaFA and MUFA are desirable things to have in storage. Note that a lean person has reservoirs of 15 kg (135,000 calories) of SaFA and MUFA, but glycogen stores are only about 70-100 g in the liver and 300-500 g in skeletal muscle – about 2000 calories total, or less than a day's energy. As a reserve for high-intensity exertion and management of blood glucose levels, this glycogen is not intended to be used for ordinary energy needs. During food scarcity, *it cannot be*, or a person would starve in a few days.

Clearly, SaFA and MUFA, not carbs, are what nature wants us to use as our primary energy source in times of food scarcity – and, for that matter, in times of food abundance. If glucose were a superior energy source, we would have evolved ways to store it in quantity, the way plants store starch.

If the body has the ability to store SaFA and MUFA equaling 100 days or more of total energy needs, then the body can safely handle even a large dietary excess of these fats.

Benefits of High SaFA and MUFA Consumption

In addition to its lack of toxicity, high dietary intake of SaFA and MUFA delivers several benefits:

(1) Improvements in lipid profiles, diminishing the risk of heart disease.

(2) An increase in muscle mass. Muscle is composed of equal weights of fat and protein. One way to store fat, without making individual cells excessively fatty, is to increase the number of cells. Muscle is the primary body component which grows in order to store excess fat.

(3) An increase in body temperature. High fat diets increase the levels of mitochondrial uncoupling proteins which cause fat to be burned for heat. High-fat diets, therefore, usually increase body temperature, which is likely to improve health.

Clinical trials further support the idea that SaFA and MUFA are the safest and most beneficial source of marginal calories.

Benefits of SaFA and MUFA: Improved Lipid Profiles

Saturated fat consumption improves lipid profiles:

- It increases levels of protective HDL cholesterol.

- It makes LDL particles larger and more buoyant, protecting them from glycation and oxidation. This is Dr. Ronald Krauss's "pattern A," the healthful pattern of LDL cholesterol-carrying particles.

As a result of its improvements to LDL particle size, saturated fat reduces the level of atherogenic oxidized-LDL.

Monounsaturated fat is also superior to carbohydrates and PUFA in its effect on lipid profiles. MUFA do not increase levels of small, dense LDL and ox-LDL, as carbohydrates and PUFA do.[121]

SaFA and MUFA also improve another blood lipid marker, triglyceride levels. Triglycerides are largely determined by carbohydrate consumption (as the liver converts excess glucose to triglycerides and pushes them into the blood) and insulin levels (as high insulin levels inhibit the removal of triglycerides from the blood). On the Perfect Health Diet, both glucose and insulin are kept low, and so fasting triglycerides are typically between 40 and 60 mg/dl – the healthiest levels.

Benefits of SaFA and MUFA: Increased Muscle Mass

Many people believe that excess calories are meant to be stored in adipose tissue, and that obesity is the result of "summer" storage of calories in preparation for a harsh "winter." We disagree.

---

[121] Berglund L et al. Comparison of monounsaturated fat with carbohydrates as a replacement for saturated fat in subjects with a high metabolic risk profile: studies in the fasting and postprandial states. *Am J Clin Nutr.* 2007 Dec;86(6):1611-20. *http://pmid.us/18065577.*

Summer is not meant to make people fat; it is meant to make people strong. Muscle is built up when food is abundant, and is scavenged when food is scarce. Muscle, by calories, is about 74% fat and 26% protein – just right to meet the body's glucose, protein, and fat needs after conversion of some protein to glucose. A typical adult male contains 30 kg (66 lb) of skeletal muscle – about 200,000 calories – enough to maintain life for 100 days without food.

By contrast, adipose tissue, which stores little protein, is an unbalanced nutrient reserve. Stored adipose fats would not extend the life of a starving man as long as an equal weight of muscle. Nor would abdominal flab be as useful as muscle in helping a hungry Paleolithic hunter obtain food. No, the natural storage reservoir of excess calories is muscle.

This is why it is so easy to add muscle on high-fat diets. A few minutes of intense exercise a week, and the muscles grow.

Bodybuilders and weightlifters have long known of the benefits of high-fat diets for muscle gain[122]:

- George Hackenschmidt, the "Russian Lion," drank 11 pints of milk per day. Milk is about 50% fat by calories, 90% SaFA and MUFA.

- Vince Gironda, the "Iron Guru," stated that nutrition was 85-90% of bodybuilding, and advocated eating 36 eggs per day. Eggs are 68% fat by calories, 83% SaFA and MUFA. Gironda sometimes ate 1/3 cup protein powder with a dozen eggs and 12 ounces of raw cream: this mix has about 740 protein and 1440 fat calories, for 66% fat.

- Casey Viator, who became Mr. America as a teenager, ate 2 dozen eggs and 2 gallons of raw milk per day.

Arnold Schwarzenegger recommended eating between 60 and 100 grams of carbohydrate per day – 240 to 400 calories, which necessarily requires obtaining the bulk of calories from fat.[123]

---

[122] Randy Roach, "Splendid Specimens: The History of Nutrition in Bodybuilding," Weston A. Price Foundation, Dec 13, 2004, *http://www.westonaprice.org/men/splendidspecimens.html*.

[123] *http://www.askmen.com/sports/bodybuilding_60/69b_fitness_tip.html*.

How High-Fat Diets Produce Muscle Gain

A few scientific studies indicate how high SaFA and MUFA intake cause muscle gain. For instance:

- Testosterone promotes muscle growth[1], and in men testosterone levels are proportional to dietary fat intake.[2]

- Higher-fat diets inhibit muscle breakdown, preserving muscle.[3]

- Growth hormone is the main muscle-promoting hormone and is released during fasting.[4] Fasting closely resembles the adoption of a Carnivore Strategy diet of 74% fat, 26% protein, 0% carbs. Eating a low-carb, high-fat diet, which reproduces the fasting pattern of gene expression, increases growth hormone release during the overnight fast. This dietary pattern also reduces hunger, causing people to spend more time in negative caloric balance, promoting growth hormone release.

Growth hormone is increased not only by a high-SaFA-and-MUFA diet, but also by consumption of shorter-chain (10- and 12-carbon) saturated fats.[5]

[1] Bhasin S et al. The effects of supraphysiologic doses of testosterone on muscle size and strength in normal men. *N Engl J Med.* 1996 Jul 4;335(1):1-7. *http://pmid.us/8637535.*

[2] Wang C et al. Low-fat high-fiber diet decreased serum and urine androgens in men. *J Clin Endocrinol Metab.* 2005 Jun;90(6):3550-9. *http://pmid.us/15741266.*

[3] Katorski B et al. Growth hormone effect on the role of fat in nitrogen metabolism. *Am J Physiol.* 1965 Nov;209(5):910-2. *http://pmid.us/5849491.*

[4] Moller N et al. Growth hormone and protein metabolism. *Clin Nutr.* 2009 Dec;28(6):597-603. *http://pmid.us/19773097.*

[5] Smith RG. From GH to Billy Ghrelin. *Cell Metab.* 2009 Aug;10(2):82-3. *http://pmid.us/19656485.*

Benefits of SaFA and MUFA: Higher Body Temperature

Low body temperature is unfortunately very common, chiefly due to endemic hypothyroidism compounded by poor mitochondrial function.

The problem is especially severe among the elderly, who tend to have a reduced body temperature[124] and during infections are less able to generate a curative fever.[125]

A high SaFA and MUFA diet won't cure hypothyroidism, but it will improve mitochondrial function and raise body temperature. Higher fat consumption leads

---

[124] Güneş UY, Zaybak A. Does the body temperature change in older people? *J Clin Nurs.* 2008 Sep;17(17):2284-7. *http://pmid.us/18705705.*

[125] Norman DC. Fever in the elderly. *Clin Infect Dis.* 2000 Jul;31(1):148-51. *http://pmid.us/10913413.*

to greater heat generation in mitochondria, quickened metabolism and a warmer body.

Higher body temperature improves comfort and cold tolerance. It is strongly associated with good health.

In one respect – its effect on pathogens – we can be confident that higher body temperature actually *causes* good health.   Many bacteria and viruses do not tolerate high body temperatures as well as our human cells. This is why fever is a part of the immune response to infection.

We believe that chronic parasitic infections are a primary cause of human aging and disease. Low body temperature helps these infections take root, while high body temperature helps defeat them.

Evidence from Clinical Trials and Prospective Studies

Ever since Ancel Keys accused saturated fat of causing heart disease, doctors have been suspicious of it. It's taken decades, and numerous clinical trials, for medical researchers to realize that the concern over SaFA was misplaced.

We've already reviewed randomized intervention trials comparing SaFA with PUFA. In our analysis, SaFA came out clearly healthier than PUFA in three trials, and as healthy as PUFA in the other five.

A recent meta-analysis of epidemiological and prospective cohort studies concluded:

> [T]here is no significant evidence for concluding that dietary saturated fat is associated with an increased risk of CHD or CVD.[126]

Another review concluded that dietary saturated fats are clearly superior to carbohydrates.[127] Here is a summary of its conclusion:

> Emphasis on reducing dietary saturated fat may miss the target of preventing cardiovascular disease (CVD) in the epidemic of obesity and associated metabolic disturbances, authors of a critical review of the issues concluded.
>
> Limiting intake of carbohydrates, particularly refined carbohydrates, offers the best hope for reducing the CVD burden associated with atherogenic dyslipidemia, Patty W. Siri-Tarino, PhD, of the Children's Hospital Oakland Research Institute in

---

[126] Siri-Tarino PW et al. Meta-analysis of prospective cohort studies evaluating the association of saturated fat with cardiovascular disease. *Am J Clin Nutr.* 2010 Mar;91(3):535-46. *http://pmid.us/20071648.*

[127] Siri-Tarino PW et al. Saturated fat, carbohydrate, and cardiovascular disease. *Am J Clin Nutr.* 2010 Mar;91(3):502-9. *http://pmid.us/20089734.*

California, and colleagues concluded in an article published in the *American Journal of Clinical Nutrition.*[128]

It's easy to see why reducing carbs works better than reducing saturated fat: the carbs get converted to saturated fat in the body, but only after poisoning the body with excess glucose and insulin.

If our belief is right, that SaFA and MUFA are benign and other macronutrients are toxic at common intake levels, then eating more SaFA and MUFA should *improve* health by displacing toxins from the diet.

New studies are starting to verify this. A Japanese study followed 58,453 Japanese adults, aged 40 to 79 at the start of the study, for 14.1 years.[129] Higher saturated fat intake was associated with:

- A 31% reduction in mortality from stroke.

- An 18% reduction in mortality from cardiovascular disease.

Conclusion

Saturated and monounsaturated fats, in their dietary and tissue storage forms as triglycerides or phospholipids, are chemically stable compounds with no toxicity.

They are therefore the healthiest macronutrients to eat in large quantities. Every other macronutrient becomes toxic in excess: glucose above about 600 calories per day, protein above about 600 calories per day, polyunsaturated fats above about 100 calories per day. But saturated and monounsaturated fats are safe in any amount.

As the dominant fats in animal and dairy foods, they are easy to obtain, and should constitute half or more of calories in healthy diets.

---

[128] Charles Bankhead, "Review Calls for Reevaluation of the Fat-CVD Link," MedPage Today, Feb 18, 2010, *http://www.medpagetoday.com/Cardiology/Atherosclerosis/18538.*

[129] Yamagishi K et al. Dietary intake of saturated fatty acids and mortality from cardiovascular disease in Japanese: the Japan Collaborative Cohort Study for Evaluation of Cancer Risk Study. *Am J Clin Nutr.* 2010 Oct;92(4):759-65. *http://pmid.us/20685950.*

Short-Chain Fats

Short-chain (12-carbon or fewer) fats make up about 58% of coconut oil, 54% of palm kernel oil (not palm oil), and 14% of butter.

Most people eat few short-chain fats. The best dietary sources were never part of the western diet, and butter has been displaced by vegetable oils.

If our estimated optimal level of 10% of fat calories (6.5% of total calories) as short-chain fats is correct, then most Americans are starved for these fats. But the deficiency could be easily made up: Two tablespoons (30 ml) of coconut oil provide about 140 calories of short-chain fats – about 6% of total calories for most people – just the right daily amount.

Let's look into the biomedical science and see if health really is improved by eating a little coconut oil.

Functions of the Short-Chain Fats

Short-chain fats are rarely incorporated into cell membranes. They are specially treated by the digestive system: Rather than being released into the blood as are most fats, short-chain fats are shunted to the liver via the portal vein. In the liver, short-chain fats are disposed of by oxidation.

Short-chain fats are the most "ketogenic" of all fats, meaning they are the most likely to be turned into ketone bodies and released into the blood.[130] This is why short-chain fats provide most of the calories in therapeutic ketogenic diets. Ketosis can be maintained with a higher level of carbohydrate consumption if short-chain fats are consumed.[131]

Short-chain fats appear to have three beneficial effects:

- As ketone bodies, they provide an alternative fuel for neurons that is neuroprotective. Ketone bodies also protect against cancer.

- Short-chain fats are antimicrobial: they kill or inhibit parasites, bacteria, viruses, and fungi.

- Short-chain fats stimulate some of the same pathways as niacin, leading to increased HDL and improved blood lipids.

Now for a closer look at each of these benefits.

---

[130] Young SJ, Renner R. Ketogenicity of soybean oil, coconut oil and their respective fatty acids for the chick. *J Nutr.* 1977 Dec;107(12):2206-12. *http://pmid.us/562929.*

[131] Liu YM. Medium-chain triglyceride (MCT) ketogenic therapy. *Epilepsia.* 2008 Nov;49 Suppl 8:33-6. *http://pmid.us/19049583.*

Neuroprotection

Ketones are an alternative energy source for neurons and protect them against glucose deprivation. Ketones also improve mitochondrial function, and relieve an excess of glutamate. Since many neurological disorders result from glucose starvation, defects in glucose metabolism, mitochondrial dysfunction, or glutamate excitotoxicity, it's no surprise that eating short-chain fats improves a variety of neurological disorders:

- Ketogenic diets protect neurons from glucose deprivation and excitotoxicity[132], from other types of injury[133], improve recovery from spinal injury[134], and prevent brain damage after heart attacks.[135]

- Ketogenic diets are therapeutic for epilepsy[136], Parkinson's disease[137], Alzheimer's[138], ALS[139], and infantile spasms (West syndrome).[140]

- Ketogenic diets improve behavior of children with autism[141], are anti-depressant[142], and may stabilize mood in bipolar disorder.[143] A ketogenic diet cured one case of schizophrenia.[144]

---

[132] Samoilova M et al. Chronic in vitro ketosis is neuroprotective but not anticonvulsant. *J Neurochem*. 2010 May;113(4):826-35. *http://pmid.us/20163521*.

[133] Maalouf M et al. The neuroprotective properties of calorie restriction, the ketogenic diet, and ketone bodies. *Brain Res Rev*. 2009 Mar;59(2):293-315. *http://pmid.us/18845187*.

[134] "Low-carb diet speeds recovery from spinal cord injury," *ScienceDaily*, Oct 22, 2009, *http://www.sciencedaily.com/releases/2009/10/091020162237.htm*.

[135] Tai KK et al. Ketogenic diet prevents cardiac arrest-induced cerebral ischemic neurodegeneration. *J Neural Transm*. 2008 Jul;115(7):1011-7. *http://pmid.us/18478178*.

[136] Kossoff EH. More fat and fewer seizures: dietary therapies for epilepsy. *Lancet Neurol*. 2004 Jul;3(7):415-20. *http://pmid.us/15207798*.

[137] Cheng B et al. Ketogenic diet protects dopaminergic neurons against 6-OHDA neurotoxicity via up-regulating glutathione in a rat model of Parkinson's disease. *Brain Res*. 2009 Aug 25;1286:25-31. *http://pmid.us/19559687*.

[138] Henderson ST et al. Study of the ketogenic agent AC-1202 in mild to moderate Alzheimer's disease: a randomized, double-blind, placebo-controlled, multicenter trial. *Nutr Metab (Lond)*. 2009 Aug 10;6:31. *http://pmid.us/19664276*. Costantini LC et al. Hypometabolism as a therapeutic target in Alzheimer's disease. *BMC Neurosci*. 2008 Dec 3;9 Suppl 2:S16. *http://pmid.us/19090989*.

[139] Zhao Z et al. A ketogenic diet as a potential novel therapeutic intervention in amyotrophic lateral sclerosis. *BMC Neurosci*. 2006 Apr 3;7:29. *http://pmid.us/16584562*. Barañano KW, Hartman AL. The ketogenic diet: uses in epilepsy and other neurologic illnesses. *Curr Treat Options Neurol*. 2008 Nov;10(6):410-9. *http://pmid.us/18990309*.

[140] You SJ et al. Factors influencing the evolution of west syndrome to lennox-gastaut syndrome. *Pediatr Neurol*. 2009 Aug;41(2):111-3. *http://pmid.us/19589458*.

We believe that short-chain fats should be a central part of the diet of anyone with a mental or neurological disorder.

Anti-Cancer

Ketones also help prevent cancer and slow its progression. Cancer cells are irretrievably dependent on glucose for energy; if they attempt to use ketones or fats for energy, they die. Ketogenic diets, which restrict glucose to cancer cells while feeding neurons with ketones, slow cancer progression.[145] Consumption of short-chain fats for ketone generation is, along with carb restriction, the key to these diets. A typical ketogenic diet used in therapy has 60% medium-chain fats, 10% longer fats, 10% carb, and 20% protein.[146]

Ketogenic diets are an effective therapy for brain cancer.[147]   Here is a representative case report:

> PET scans indicated a 21.8% average decrease in glucose uptake at the tumor site ... [The] patient exhibited significant clinical improvements in mood and new skill development during the study. She continued the ketogenic diet for an additional twelve months, remaining free of disease progression.[148]

---

[141] Evangeliou A et al. Application of a ketogenic diet in children with autistic behavior: pilot study. *J Child Neurol.* 2003 Feb;18(2):113-8. *http://pmid.us/12693778.*

[142] Murphy P et al. The antidepressant properties of the ketogenic diet. *Biol Psychiatry.* 2004 Dec 15;56(12):981-3. *http://pmid.us/15601609.*

[143] El-Mallakh RS, Paskitti ME. The ketogenic diet may have mood-stabilizing properties. *Med Hypotheses.* 2001 Dec;57(6):724-6. *http://pmid.us/11918434.*

[144] Kraft BD, Westman EC. Schizophrenia, gluten, and low-carbohydrate, ketogenic diets: a case report and review of the literature. *Nutr Metab (Lond).* 2009 Feb 26;6:10. *http://pmid.us/19245705.*

[145] Seyfried TN, Shelton LM. Cancer as a metabolic disease. *Nutrition & Metabolism* 2010, 7:7. *http://www.nutritionandmetabolism.com/content/pdf/1743-7075-7-7.pdf.*

[146] Nebeling LC, Lerner E. Implementing a ketogenic diet based on medium-chain triglyceride oil in pediatric patients with cancer. *J Am Diet Assoc.* 1995 Jun;95(6):693-7. *http://pmid.us/7759747.*

[147] Seyfried BT et al. Targeting energy metabolism in brain cancer through calorie restriction and the ketogenic diet. *J Cancer Res Ther.* 2009 Sep;5 Suppl 1:S7-15. *http://pmid.us/20009300.*

[148] Nebeling LC et al. Effects of a ketogenic diet on tumor metabolism and nutritional status in pediatric oncology patients: two case reports. *J Am Coll Nutr.* 1995 Apr;14(2):202-8. *http://pmid.us/7790697.*

Brain cancers are normally untreatable, so oncologists have been more open to therapeutic diets for this cancer. We believe that ketogenic diets will become a standard part of treatment for all solid tumor cancers.

Protection of the Gut and Liver Against Pathogens

Short-chain fatty acids and their monoglycerides (such as monolaurin, the monoglyceride of 12-carbon lauric acid, and monocaprin, the monoglyceride of 10-carbon capric acid) have antimicrobial actions against:

- Yeast and fungi.[149]

- Parasites such as giardia.[150]

- Bacteria including Salmonella[151], Propionibacterium (a cause of acne)[152], E. coli and Bacillus subtilis[153], Chlamydia[154], and H. pylori[155].

- Enveloped viruses including HIV, herpes, and cytomegalovirus.[156]

---

[149] Bergsson G et al. In vitro killing of Candida albicans by fatty acids and monoglycerides. *Antimicrob Agents Chemother.* 2001 Nov;45(11):3209-12. *http://pmid.us/11600381.* Liu S et al. Biological control of phytopathogenic fungi by fatty acids. *Mycopathologia.* 2008 Aug;166(2):93-102. *http://pmid.us/18443921.*

[150] Rayan P et al. The effects of saturated fatty acids on Giardia duodenalis trophozoites in vitro. *Parasitol Res.* 2005 Oct;97(3):191-200. *http://pmid.us/15991042.*

[151] Van Immerseel F et al. Medium-chain fatty acids decrease colonization and invasion through hilA suppression shortly after infection of chickens with Salmonella enterica serovar Enteritidis. *Appl Environ Microbiol.* 2004 Jun;70(6):3582-7. *http://pmid.us/15184160.* Gantois I et al. Butyrate specifically down-regulates salmonella pathogenicity island 1 gene expression. *Appl Environ Microbiol.* 2006 Jan;72(1):946-9. *http://pmid.us/16391141.*

[152] Nakatsuji T et al. Antimicrobial property of lauric acid against Propionibacterium acnes: its therapeutic potential for inflammatory acne vulgaris. *J Invest Dermatol.* 2009 Oct;129(10):2480-8. *http://pmid.us/19387482.*

[153] Zhang H et al. Antibacterial interactions of monolaurin with commonly used antimicrobials and food components. *J Food Sci.* 2009 Sep;74(7):M418-21. *http://pmid.us/19895490.*

[154] Bergsson G et al. In vitro inactivation of Chlamydia trachomatis by fatty acids and monoglycerides. *Antimicrob Agents Chemother.* 1998 Sep;42(9):2290-4. *http://pmid.us/9736551.*

[155] Sun CQ et al. Antibacterial actions of fatty acids and monoglycerides against Helicobacter pylori. *FEMS Immunol Med Microbiol.* 2003 May 15;36(1-2):9-17. *http://pmid.us/12727360.*

[156] Thormar H et al. Inactivation of enveloped viruses and killing of cells by fatty acids and monoglycerides. *Antimicrob Agents Chemother.* 1987 Jan;31(1):27-31.

Short-chain fatty acids seem to be benign toward probiotic bacteria, but suppressive of pathogens.

Dietary short-chain fatty acids are generally absorbed in the intestine and shunted to the liver, although some lauric acid enters the body.[157] As such they are likely to give most protection to the gut and liver. Still, protection of the gut and liver is important because:

- The gut is where most pathogenic bacteria enter the body, and biofilms in the gut may provide a reservoir that shelters pathogenic bacteria from the immune system and maintains chronic infections.

- Liver infections (or gut infections that spread bacterial toxins to the liver) may be a primary cause of metabolic disorders.

Indeed, so far as we know the entire benefit of dietary fiber comes through its conversion to short-chain fats by probiotic gut bacteria. It is the short-chain fats, not the fiber per se, that are beneficial.

Better Lipid Profiles and Reduced Heart Disease

Some doctors reject the idea that short-chain fats are cardioprotective. For example, Dr. Walter Willett in the September 2006 *Harvard Heart Letter* said that "coconut and coconut oil can't be considered heart-healthy foods" because "coconut oil substantially elevates LDL (bad) cholesterol" even though "coconut oil has a powerful HDL-boosting effect."[158]

With finer measurement of blood lipids using new techniques, however, it has been established that it is not LDL cholesterol that is dangerous, but "small, dense LDL" – LDL particles with insufficient fats and cholesterol around their lipoprotein. Small, dense LDL is vulnerable to protein glycation and conversion to oxidized LDL, which causes atherosclerotic plaque formation.[159] Having large, buoyant LDL particles with lots of fat and cholesterol protecting each lipoprotein is actually healthful.[160]

http://pmid.us/3032090. Isaacs CE. The antimicrobial function of milk lipids. *Adv Nutr Res.* 2001;10:271-85. *http://pmid.us/11795045.*

[157] Shorland FB et al. Studies on fatty acid composition of adipose tissue and blood lipids of Polynesians. *Am J Clin Nutr.* 1969 May;22(5):594-605. *http://pmid.us/5784563.*

[158] Willett WC. Ask the doctor. I have heard that coconut is bad for the heart and that it is good for the heart. Which is right? *Harv Heart Lett.* 2006 Sep;17(1):8. *http://pmid.us/17133658.*

[159] Austin MA et al. Low-density lipoprotein subclass patterns and risk of myocardial infarction. *JAMA.* 1988 Oct 7;260(13):1917-21. *http://pmid.us/3418853.*

[160] El Harchaoui K et al. Value of low-density lipoprotein particle number and size as predictors of coronary artery disease in apparently healthy men and women: the EPIC-

Tests for whether LDL is in the small, dense or large, buoyant form are expensive. However, a good proxy is the triglyceride to HDL ratio. When this is high, LDL particles are mostly in the small, dense form; when it is low, LDL particles are in the healthy, large, buoyant form.[161]

What do short-chain fats do? They reduce triglycerides[162], and they raise HDL – often doubling HDL levels to 100 mg/dl or higher[163]. Their effect on lipids – higher HDL, lower triglycerides, and very likely lower small dense LDL and lower Lp(a) – is unambiguously positive.

The heart's "hydraulic efficiency" is 28% higher on ketones than glucose, suggesting that short-chain fats may be therapeutic for heart disease.[164]

Epidemiological data supports the benefits of coconut oil:

- Among countries with reliable data, Sri Lanka has the highest intake of coconut oil and the lowest rate of ischemic heart disease.[165]

- Stroke and heart disease appear to be entirely absent among the islanders of Kitava, who obtain almost 20% calories from coconut oil.[166]

- Tokelau Islanders, who obtain 50% of calories from coconut oil, are similarly free of stroke and heart disease.[167]

Norfolk Prospective Population Study. *J Am Coll Cardiol.* 2007 Feb 6;49(5):547-53. *http://pmid.us/17276177.*

[161] Boizel R et al. Ratio of triglycerides to HDL cholesterol is an indicator of LDL particle size in patients with type 2 diabetes and normal HDL cholesterol levels. *Diabetes Care.* 2000 Nov;23(11):1679-85. *http://pmid.us/11092292.*

[162] Xue C et al. Consumption of medium- and long-chain triacylglycerols decreases body fat and blood triglyceride in Chinese hypertriglyceridemic subjects. *Eur J Clin Nutr.* 2009 Jul;63(7):879-86. *http://pmid.us/19156155.*

[163] See anecdotal reports at *http://drbganimalpharm.blogspot.com/2009/10/low-carb-paleo-nothings-impossible.html.*

[164] Veech RL. The therapeutic implications of ketone bodies: the effects of ketone bodies in pathological conditions: ketosis, ketogenic diet, redox states, insulin resistance, and mitochondrial metabolism. *Prostaglandins Leukot Essent Fatty Acids.* 2004 Mar;70(3):309-19. *http://pmid.us/14769489.*

[165] Kaunitz H. Medium chain triglycerides (MCT) in aging and arteriosclerosis. *J Environ Pathol Toxicol Oncol.* 1986 Mar-Apr;6(3-4):115-21. *http://pmid.us/3519928.*

[166] Lindeberg S et al. Haemostatic variables in Pacific Islanders apparently free from stroke and ischaemic heart disease--the Kitava Study. *Thromb Haemost.* 1997 Jan;77(1):94-8. *http://pmid.us/9031456.*

[167] Prior IA et al. The Tokelau Island migrant study. *Int J Epidemiol.* 1974 Sep;3(3):225-32. *http://pmid.us/4416612.* Stanhope JM et al. The Tokelau Island Migrant Study: serum lipid concentration in two environments. *J Chronic Dis.* 1981;34(2-3):45-55.

Coconut Oil Is Better Than Niacin for Cardioprotection

Recently scientists have been investigating the mechanisms by which dietary short-chain fats raise HDL and lower triglycerides. It turns out that short-chain fats stimulate some of the same pathways as niacin, another compound that raises HDL and lowers triglycerides. For instance, niacin and ketone bodies both stimulate the receptor GPR109A and through this receptor increase levels of adiponectin, a beneficial hormone.[1]

Niacin is much recommended by doctors, even though its conversion to niacinamide in the body can lead to flushing and liver toxicity. Coconut oil achieves the benefits of niacin with no flushing and no liver toxicity.

[1] Plaisance EP et al. Niacin stimulates adiponectin secretion through the GPR109A receptor. *Am J Physiol Endocrinol Metab.* 2009 Mar;296(3):E549-58. *http://pmid.us/19141678.* Ahmed K et al. GPR109A, GPR109B and GPR81, a family of hydroxy-carboxylic acid receptors. *Trends Pharmacol Sci.* 2009 Nov;30(11):557-62. *http://pmid.us/19837462.*

Weight Loss

Shorter-chain fats seem to strongly promote weight loss. In one study, 8 weeks taking the equivalent of 1 tbsp per day of coconut oil caused a significant decrease in body weight, waist size, and blood triglycerides.[168] In another, obese women who received 2 tbsp (30 ml) coconut oil per day slimmed their waist and increased HDL without an increase in LDL, while a comparison group receiving soybean oil did not slim their waist and had lower HDL with higher LDL and total cholesterol.[169]

And, of course, Polynesian islanders like the Kitavans and Tokelauans who eat a lot of coconut have always been noted for "their extreme leanness."[170]

Coconut oil leads to a naturally slim waist.

Short-Chain Fats are Safe

At the doses achievable in human diets, short-chain fats seem to be entirely safe.

---

http://pmid.us/7462380. Hat tip Stephan Guyenet, *http://wholehealthsource.blogspot.com/2009/01/tokelau-island-migrant-study.html.*

[168] Xue C et al. Consumption of medium- and long-chain triacylglycerols decreases body fat and blood triglyceride in Chinese hypertriglyceridemic subjects. *Eur J Clin Nutr.* 2009 Jul;63(7):879-86. *http://pmid.us/19156155.*

[169] Assunção ML et al. Effects of dietary coconut oil on the biochemical and anthropometric profiles of women presenting abdominal obesity. *Lipids.* 2009 Jul;44(7):593-601. *http://pmid.us/19437058.*

[170] Lindeberg S et al. Haemostatic variables in Pacific Islanders apparently free from stroke and ischaemic heart disease--the Kitava Study. *Thromb Haemost.* 1997 Jan;77(1):94-8. *http://pmid.us/9031456.*

There are no reports of toxicity from short-chain fats in human diets, even when they constitute the bulk of the diet:

- Ketogenic diets providing 60% of calories as short-chain fats have been safely followed for years by epilepsy and brain cancer patients.[171] Problems on ketogenic diets arise not from the fats, but from nutrient deficiencies – notably selenium[172] and vitamin C[173] deficiencies.

- Coconut oil delivered intravenously to people who cannot eat – "parenteral nutrition" –is comparable in safety to olive oil and fish oil and safer than soybean or safflower oil.[174]

Herbivore Strategy mammals typically obtain 60 to 70% of calories from short-chain fats – another argument that short-chain fats are safe.

Conclusion

Short-chain fats may significantly improve gut health, protect against infections and cancer, improve neurological function and reduce cardiovascular disease risk. They have no known negative effects.

It seems prudent to follow nature's recommendation and mimic the share of short-chain fats found in mother's milk – about 10% of fat calories or, if fats are 65% of total calories, about 6.5% of total calories.

---

[171] Kang HC et al. Safe and effective use of the ketogenic diet in children with epilepsy and mitochondrial respiratory chain complex defects. *Epilepsia.* 2007 Jan;48(1):82-8. *http://pmid.us/17241212.*

[172] Bank IM et al. Sudden cardiac death in association with the ketogenic diet. *Pediatr Neurol.* 2008 Dec;39(6):429-31. *http://pmid.us/19027591.*

[173] Willmott NS, Bryan RA. Case report: scurvy in an epileptic child on a ketogenic diet with oral complications. *Eur Arch Paediatr Dent.* 2008 Sep;9(3):148-52. *http://pmid.us/18793598.*

[174] Hardy G, Puzovic M. Formulation, stability, and administration of parenteral nutrition with new lipid emulsions. *Nutr Clin Pract.* 2009 Oct-Nov;24(5):616-25. *http://pmid.us/19841249.*

Fiber

Within the human body, bacteria outnumber human cells ten to one.[175] (Bacteria are small and add only a few pounds to our weight – lucky, or they would be hard to carry around!)

These bacteria can be friendly, or harmful:

- **Cooperative, "probiotic" bacteria** aid digestion, release nutrients, and guard the gut against more dangerous pathogens.

- **Uncooperative, "pathogenic" bacteria** steal food and nutrients, release toxins, and invade the body to cause infectious diseases.

A healthy person has about a thousand bacterial species in the gut; people with bowel disease typically have fewer, about 750 species, because pathogenic bacteria drive out some probiotic species.[176] The quality of one's gut bacteria plays a powerful role in one's health.

Two Ways to Change Your Gut Bacteria

Most probiotic supplements provide species of bacteria that flourish in infants who suckle breast milk; these are healthful species, but a small part of the adult gut microbiome. Such supplements are great for overcoming food poisoning, but for optimal health a wider range of species is necessary.

Fecal transplants – moving the stool from a healthy person into the colon of a sick person – are a superior probiotic. They provide all of the thousand or so bacterial species in the donor's colon. Fecal transplants have been startlingly effective at curing some bowel diseases, and may be a therapy of the future for conditions like obesity.[1]

[1] See our post, "Bowel Disease, Part IV: Restoring Healthful Gut Flora," July 27, 2010, *http://perfecthealthdiet.com/?p=269.*

Dietary fiber – plant matter that is indigestible to humans, but digestible by gut bacteria – helps determine the nature of one's gut bacteria. The *amount* of fiber determines *how many* bacteria live in the gut, and the *type* of fiber determines *which species* flourish.

Harmful Fiber

Some fiber, such as that in cereal grains, seems to be harmful. Grain fiber has two major problems. It contains toxic proteins such as gluten, which we will discuss in Step Two; and it contains roughage that can injure the intestinal wall.

---

[175] The Human Microbiome Project, NIH, *http://nihroadmap.nih.gov/hmp/.*

[176] Qin J et al. A human gut microbial gene catalogue established by metagenomic sequencing. *Nature.* 2010 Mar 4;464(7285):59-65. *http://pmid.us/20203603.*

Conventional medical opinion recommends whole grain fiber despite these issues. Dr. Paul L. McNeil explains:

> When you eat high-fiber foods, they bang up against the cells lining the gastrointestinal tract, rupturing their outer covering. What we are saying is this banging and tearing increases the level of lubricating mucus. It's a good thing.
>
> It's a bit of a paradox, but what we are saying is an injury at the cell level can promote health of the GI tract as a whole.[177]

This may be one of those clever ideas that, according to George Orwell, "only an intellectual could believe."

The claim has been tested in a single clinical trial – the Diet and Reinfarction Trial (DART), published in 1989. This study included 2,033 British men who had previously suffered a heart attack, and compared a high-fiber group with a control group. The high-fiber group ate whole grains and doubled their grain fiber intake from 9 to 17 grams per day.

The result? Deaths in the high fiber group were 22% higher over the two-year study – 9.9% of the control group died versus 12.1% of the high-fiber group.[178]

The Benefits of Butyrate

The gut is an anaerobic environment, meaning it lacks oxygen. That prevents bacteria from metabolizing fats, forcing them to rely on carbohydrates, which carry their own oxygen. As a byproduct of carbohydrate fermentation, bacteria generate short-chain fats such as propionate, butyrate and acetate. Since they cannot exploit these fats themselves, they are released to the body. Short-chain fats from gut bacteria are the primary energy source for certain intestinal cells called colonocytes[179], and may meet 5-10% of the whole body's caloric needs.[180]

The most important of these short-chain fats is butyrate, a 4-carbon saturated fat. Butyrate improves health in a remarkable number of ways:

---

[177] Quoted in *http://www.sciencedaily.com/releases/2006/08/060823093156.htm*. Hat tip Dr. Michael Eades, *http://www.proteinpower.com/drmike/uncategorized/a-cautionary-tale-of-mucus-fore-and-aft/*.

[178] Burr ML et al. Effects of changes in fat, fish, and fibre intakes on death and myocardial reinfarction: diet and reinfarction trial (DART). *Lancet.* 1989 Sep 30;2(8666):757-61. *http://pmid.us/2571009*. Hat tip: Stephan Guyenet, *http://wholehealthsource.blogspot.com/2008/10/dart-many-lessons-learned.html*.

[179] Andoh A et al. Role of dietary fiber and short-chain fatty acids in the colon. *Curr Pharm Des.* 2003;9(4):347-58. *http://pmid.us/12570825*.

[180] McNeil NI. The contribution of the large intestine to energy supplies in man. *Am J Clin Nutr.* 1984 Feb;39(2):338-42. *http://pmid.us/6320630*.

- **Prevents obesity.** Butyrate improves insulin sensitivity and prevents rats from becoming obese.[181] Perhaps what obese people need most is an infusion of butyrate-producing gut bacteria.

- **Heals the intestine.** Butyrate supplements or enemas have been used to treat Crohn's disease and ulcerative colitis.[182]

- **Improves gut barrier integrity.** Butyrate decreases intestinal permeability, preventing entry of toxins and pathogens to the body.[183]

- **Relieves constipation.** A rye fiber that increased butyrate production by 63% compared to wheat bran increased weekly defecations 1.4-fold, softened feces, and eased defecation.[184]

- **Helps prevent colon cancer.** Butyrate induces differentiation of cancer cells into normal types[185] and prevents cancer-causing mutations.[186] Its protection against colon cancer is enhanced by fish oil (DHA).[187]

- **Delays neurodegeneration.** Much like its cousins, the ketone bodies, butyrate improves nerve function and survival in mouse models of several neurological disorders, including Huntington's disease.[188]

---

[181] Gao Z et al. Butyrate improves insulin sensitivity and increases energy expenditure in mice. *Diabetes.* 2009 Jul;58(7):1509-17. *http://pmid.us/19366864.* Hat tip, Stephan Guyenet, *http://wholehealthsource.blogspot.com/2009/12/butyric-acid-ancient-controller-of.html,* for links to this and other papers cited below.

[182] Di Sabatino A et al. Oral butyrate for mildly to moderately active Crohn's disease. *Aliment Pharmacol Ther.* 2005 Nov 1;22(9):789-94. *http://pmid.us/16225487.* Scheppach W et al. Effect of butyrate enemas on the colonic mucosa in distal ulcerative colitis. *Gastroenterology.* 1992 Jul;103(1):51-6. *http://pmid.us/1612357.* Hat tip Stephan Guyenet, *http://wholehealthsource.blogspot.com/2009/12/butyric-acid-ancient-controller-of.html.*

[183] Suzuki T et al. Physiological concentrations of short-chain fatty acids immediately suppress colonic epithelial permeability. *Br J Nutr.* 2008 Aug;100(2):297-305. *http://pmid.us/18346306.*

[184] Holma R et al. Constipation Is Relieved More by Rye Bread Than Wheat Bread or Laxatives without Increased Adverse Gastrointestinal Effects. *J Nutr.* 2010 Mar;140(3):534-41. *http://pmid.us/20089780.*

[185] Whitehead RH et al. Effects of short chain fatty acids on a new human colon carcinoma cell line (LIM1215). *Gut.* 1986 Dec;27(12):1457-63. *http://pmid.us/3804021.*

[186] Scharlau D et al. Mechanisms of primary cancer prevention by butyrate and other products formed during gut flora-mediated fermentation of dietary fibre. *Mutat Res.* 2009 Jul-Aug;682(1):39-53. *http://pmid.us/19383551*

[187] Kolar SS et al. Docosahexaenoic acid and butyrate synergistically induce colonocyte apoptosis by enhancing mitochondrial Ca2+ accumulation. *Cancer Res.* 2007 Jun 1;67(11):5561-8. *http://pmid.us/17545640.*

- **Improves cardiovascular markers.** Butyrate supplementation in rats lowers blood cholesterol, triglycerides, and fasting insulin.

- **Reduces ill effects of diabetes.** Butyrate stabilizes blood glucose levels in diabetic rats.[189]

- **Reduces inflammation.** Butyrate downregulates inflammatory cytokines and calms the immune system.[190]

- **Fosters tissue healing.** Injection of butyrate along with hyaluronan and vitamin A into the hearts of rats that had suffered a heart attack "afforded substantial cardiovascular repair and recovery."[191]

Given all these benefits, one wonders why butyrate is not commonly available as a dietary supplement. It should be noted that butyrate makes up 3-5% of butter: yet more proof that nature has included in mother's milk the most nutritious ingredients.

(Probably) Healthful Fiber

Some berries combine fiber with antimicrobial agents that act against pathogenic bacteria, but not probiotic bacteria. Blueberries reduce the population of pathogenic bacteria while feeding probiotic bacteria. Blueberry husks taken with probiotics generate a rise in circulating butyrate in the blood, and blueberry fiber is more beneficial than rye or oat bran.[192]

"Resistant starch" is starch that is indigestible to human digestive enzymes. When starchy foods, like potato or taro or rice, are cooked, the starch is gelatinized to a form that is readily digested by human amylase; but if it is allowed to cool, some of this gelatinized starch re-forms into resistant starch.

---

[188] Ferrante RJ et al. Histone deacetylase inhibition by sodium butyrate chemotherapy ameliorates the neurodegenerative phenotype in Huntington's disease mice. *J Neurosci.* 2003 Oct 15;23(28):9418-27. *http://pmid.us/14561870.*

[189] Kumar C et al. Modulatory effect of butyric acid-a product of dietary fiber fermentation in experimentally induced diabetic rats. *J Nutr Biochem.* 2002 Sep;13(9):522. *http://pmid.us/12231422.*

[190] Säemann MD et al. Anti-inflammatory effects of sodium butyrate on human monocytes: potent inhibition of IL-12 and up-regulation of IL-10 production. *FASEB J.* 2000 Dec;14(15):2380-2. *http://pmid.us/11024006.*

[191] Lionetti V et al. Hyaluronan mixed esters of butyric and retinoic acid affording myocardial survival and repair without stem cell transplantation. *J Biol Chem.* 2010 Mar 26;285(13):9949-61. *http://pmid.us/20097747.*

[192] Håkansson A et al. Blueberry husks, rye bran and multi-strain probiotics affect the severity of colitis induced by dextran sulphate sodium. *Scand J Gastroenterol.* 2009;44(10):1213-25. *http://pmid.us/19670079.*

Gut bacteria prolifically convert resistant starch to butyrate. For instance, resistant starch from sago (one of our "safe starches") generates much more butyrate than fructo-oligosaccharide (FOS) supplements.[193]

Cellulose-rich foods, such as the squashes (pumpkin, zucchini, acorn squash, butternut squash) and stalk vegetables like celery or bok choy, may also generate beneficial amounts of butyrate.

Pectin, gums, and mucilage – commonly called water-soluble fiber or viscous fiber – are probably beneficial. These fibers, common in fruit and vegetables like apples or tomatoes, appear to protect against atherosclerosis.[194]

Fermented Foods

Another seemingly healthful strategy is to let bacteria pre-digest vegetables outside the gut, and eat the fermented foods. Fermented foods include the many varieties of Korean kimchi, sauerkraut, yogurt, and pickles.

Presumably, traditional methods of food fermentation have selected foods and fermentation methods that yield probiotic, not pathogenic, bacteria. (If kimchi made Koreans sick, it would not be so popular.)

There May Be Benefits to Limiting Fiber

Although gut bacteria generate healthful short-chain fats, they also generate harmful "endotoxins" – toxic bacterial proteins that excite an immune response.

THE HUMAN BODY REGULATES BACTERIAL POPULATIONS AND ENDOTOXIN LEVELS

Endotoxins are fat-soluble proteins and they are carried into the body with dietary fats. The immune system monitors endotoxin levels and tries to keep them – and the bacterial population that produces them – at an appropriate level:

- When endotoxin levels are high, the immune system attacks gut bacteria to reduce their population.

- When endotoxin levels are low, the immune system relaxes to let gut bacteria proliferate.

It turns out the reason antibiotics often lead to pathogenic infections is that, by killing off probiotic bacteria, antibiotics reduce endotoxin levels and cause immune cells to let down their guard. This allows pathogens to invade the body.[195]

---

[193] Siew-Wai L et al. Fermentation of Metroxylon sagu Resistant Starch Type III by Lactobacillus sp. and Bifidobacterium bifidum. *J Agric Food Chem.* 2010 Feb 24;58(4):2274-8. *http://pmid.us/20121195.*

[194] Wu H et al. Dietary fiber and progression of atherosclerosis: the Los Angeles Atherosclerosis Study. *Am J Clin Nutr.* 2003 Dec;78(6):1085-91. *http://pmid.us/14668268.*

HIGH FIBER INTAKE MAY BE COUNTERPRODUCTIVE

High fiber intake increases gut bacterial population, but it will also increase immune activity in order to keep the gut bacterial population down to the body's preferred level.

This means that with high fiber intake, the gut will be exposed to more bacterial endotoxins and also to inflammation generated by immune activity.

Toxins and inflammation aren't healthy for anyone, but they are especially problematic for people with damaged "leaky" guts.

Leaky guts allow toxic or allergenic bacterial proteins, and pathogens themselves, to enter the body. With a leaky gut, the harms from toxin and pathogen entry to the body may far outweigh the benefits from bacteria-produced short-chain fats.

A SMALL BUT WELL-NOURISHED BACTERIAL POPULATION MAY BE OPTIMAL

A few lines of evidence suggest that low or moderate fiber intake may be healthful.

Bacteria not only need carbohydrates for food, they need phospholipids for their membranes and amino acids for their proteins. And well-nourished gut bacteria may be more likely to cooperate probiotically with their host.

This may be a reason that tree nuts are healthful. Almond fats, for instance, have been shown to help probiotic bacteria flourish. The benefits of almonds are lost when the fat content is removed.[196]

If gut bacteria need fats, and if providing fats makes the gut healthier, then high-carb low-fat diets may sabotage the gut by creating a scarcity of nourishing fats for gut bacteria. A low-carb, high-fat diet will create a smaller but healthier – and friendlier – population of gut bacteria.

FIBER MAY NOT BE ESSENTIAL

Human breast milk has no fiber, and in traditional societies infants often suckled for 2-3 years before weaning. Recent work has shown that probiotic strains that flourish in infants, such as *B. bifidum*, are able to digest human mucus.[197] This

---

[195] Brandl K et al. Vancomycin-resistant enterococci exploit antibiotic-induced innate immune deficits. *Nature*. 2008 Oct 9;455(7214):804-7. *http://pmid.us/18724361*. Hat tip Peter Dobromylskyj, *http://high-fat-nutrition.blogspot.com/2009/02/fats-absorbing-endotoxin.html*.

[196] Mandalari G et al. Potential prebiotic properties of almond (Amygdalus communis L.) seeds. *Appl Environ Microbiol*. 2008 Jul;74(14):4264-70. *http://pmid.us/18502914*.

[197] Ruas-Madiedo P et al. Mucin degradation by Bifidobacterium strains isolated from the human intestinal microbiota. *Appl Environ Microbiol*. 2008 Mar;74(6):1936-40. *http://pmid.us/18223105*.

raises the intriguing possibility that we may not need fiber at all to maintain probiotic gut flora.

Mucin, the main component of mucus, is a glycoprotein, composed of a protein bonded to sugars. It may be that gut mucus, like human breast milk, is designed to feed friendly species of bacteria, enabling them to outcompete pathogenic strains in the mucus layer which is adjacent to human cells. Biofilms of probiotic bacteria heavily colonize the intestinal mucus layer.[198]

Conclusion: Stick to Paleo Fiber

Research into gut bacteria, fiber, and their influence upon health is still in early stages. Any specific prescription might be overturned by future research.

However, a few tentative conclusions seem warranted:

- *Foods that have been in the human diet for hundreds of thousands of years – fruits, vegetables, and starchy tubers – are the healthiest sources of fiber.* Neolithic foods, like cereal grains, supply harmful fiber. We can't guarantee that science won't in time identify harmful effects of fiber from some Paleo foods, or beneficial effects of fiber from some Neolithic plants. But for now, it appears that the Paleo principle holds: eat what our Paleo ancestors ate, and avoid the rest.

- *In people with healthy guts* that keep bacteria and their toxins from entering the body, *fiber from food is generally healthful.* However, there's no need to go out of one's way to get additional fiber. Supplemental fiber may be ill-advised.

- *In people with damaged guts, the case for fiber is much less clear.* People with bowel disorders may benefit from obtaining short-chain fats from coconut oil and butter, and limiting fiber to keep down the gut's bacterial population and endotoxin production.

The Perfect Health Diet, containing one to two pounds of daily plant matter from fiber-rich starches like sweet potato or taro, fruit such as a bowl of berries and a banana, and vegetables to taste as an accompaniment to meat dishes, should provide sufficient fiber for excellent gut health.

---

[198] Macfarlane S et al. Colonization of mucin by human intestinal bacteria and establishment of biofilm communities in a two-stage continuous culture system. *Appl Environ Microbiol.* 2005 Nov;71(11):7483-92. *http://pmid.us/16269790.*

Summary: Perfect Macronutrients

We've covered a lot of ground and it deserves a summing up. The Perfect Health Diet prescription is:

- About 400 carb calories per day, derived mainly from "safe starches" like sweet potatoes, yams, taro, white rice, sago, tapioca, and potatoes. Fruits and berries, and other fructose-containing carbs, should constitute a minority of carb calories. The plateau range for carbs is 200 to 600 calories.

- The plateau range for protein is also 200 to 600 calories. However, carb and protein together should add up to at least 600 calories.

- Some factors influencing carb and protein intake:

  - Athletes may wish to occupy the high end of the protein and carb plateau ranges. A suitable intake for elite athletes might be: carb calories, 500 plus 50 to 100 per hour of intense training; protein calories, 500 to 600 with half from sources like whey which are rich in ketogenic and branched-chain amino acids.

  - For longevity, the low end of the plateau ranges may be desirable. This would be 600 total calories of carb and protein.

- Omega-6 fatty acids should be limited to less than 4% of calories. To get down to this level, do not eat any vegetable seed oils; do eat low-omega-6 oils like butter and coconut oil and low-omega-6 meats like beef, lamb, and fish.

- Long-chain omega-3 fats from cold-water fish like salmon, sardines, and anchovies should be eaten to balance tissue omega-6s. Up to a pound of oily fish per week is likely to be healthful.

- Saturated and monounsaturated fats are the safest calorie source – indeed the only calorie source that is non-toxic in very high doses – and should provide the bulk of calories. Eat as much as you like. Meats, fish, and eggs are excellent sources. So are dairy fats like butter and cream.

- At least two tablespoons (30 ml) of coconut oil should be taken daily to provide short-chain fats to protect the health of the gut, liver, nerves, brain, and cardiovascular system.

- More short-chain fats are generated in the gut by eating fiber. Fiber should be obtained from "Paleo" foods: the safe starches, fruits and berries, and vegetables to taste. These are the fiber sources which generate the healthiest portfolio of gut bacteria and the most abundant colonic production of beneficial short-chain fats.

Ideas For Macronutritious Eating

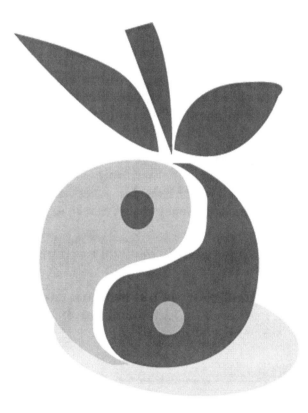

Two Simple Rules to Optimize Macronutrients

Now that we know the optimal macronutrient ratios, we have to learn a way of eating that provides them.

We favor a few very simple and easy-to-apply rules of thumb, which we'll describe. A few illustrations will help give you an idea of proportions.

> *If you wish to be more scientific, consider buying a kitchen scale and tracking your food for a few days until you are familiar with quantities and proportions. To do this, simply weigh your food before preparation and use* http://nutritiondata.com, http://fitday.com, *or similar sites to look up composition.*

Getting the Right Amount of Fat

The simplest way to get fat-protein-carb ratios right is to combine every carb or protein food with fats in a 1 calorie to 2 calorie proportion:

1. When preparing a starch, always **combine the starch with fats** in a calorie ratio of **one-third carbs to two-thirds fat**. Fruits and berries can also be beneficially combined with fat sources such as ice cream, yogurt, or heavy cream.

2. When eating meat (or other protein sources), make sure it is **fatty and moist**, not lean and dry. This will naturally provide a calorie ratio of about **one-third protein to two-thirds fat**. Lean meats should be combined with a fat source – chicken breast with avocado or olive oil or coconut milk, for instance.

Just following these simple practices will assure a macronutrient ratio that is close to the optimum – about 65% fat.

Remember to include **omega-3 sources like salmon, sardines, and anchovies**, and to favor **low-omega-6 meats like beef, lamb, and seafood** and **low-omega-6 oils like butter and coconut oil**.

The Carb to Protein Ratio

Since meats are more calorie-dense than most plants, you will get a good carb-to-protein ratio (we recommend about 20% of calories from carbs, 15% from protein) by eating **two to three times as much plant foods by weight as you eat meat**. We typically eat ½ pound meat and 1.5 pounds of plant foods per day.

Vegetables can be eaten to taste. Since supermarket salad dressings are generally made with high-omega-6 fats like soybean oil and canola oil, **we recommend making your own salad dressings with coconut oil, butter, or olive oil**.

Macronutritious Plant Foods

We favor eating three groups of plant foods each day: safe starches, fruits and berries, and vegetables.

Safe Starches

Most carb calories – about 300 per day for us – should be obtained from safe starches. As the safe starches lack fructose, omega-6 fats, and natural toxins, and provide potassium and other nutrients as well as fiber, they are among the most healthful plant foods, and the best source of glucose calories.

TARO

Taro, the starchy corm that is the raw material for poi, is a very healthy safe starch. Taro provides 600 calories of glucose per pound: thus, the daily target of 300 calories would require a half pound, or 4 corms, of taro.

We boil taro corms for about 20 minutes, then cut them in half, spread cream cheese on top, and squeeze the inedible hairy skin to release the edible starch.

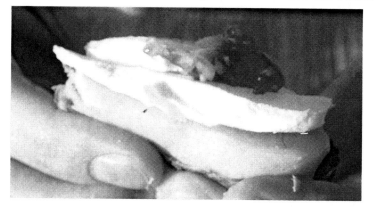

A half taro corm with cream cheese and a fig spread. We are here squeezing the cooked corm out of its brown skin.

SWEET POTATOES, YAMS, AND POTATOES

Sweet potatoes, yams, and potatoes provide 300 calories of glucose per pound, so one pound (454 g) will provide our daily target of safe starches.

We are fond of a chestnut-flavored yellow-colored variety of sweet potato sold in our local Asian supermarket, and often make mashed sweet potatoes with butter and coconut oil.

WHITE RICE

If you have a rice cooker, there's no easier starch to cook than rice – or more adaptable to a wide range of foods. We prefer white rice, as there may be toxins in rice bran. The sticky variant, mochi rice, is also excellent.

Rice has about 1300 calories per pound: thus, a quarter pound (100 g), or about 3/4 cup (180 ml) of cooked rice, will provide the daily 300-400 calories.

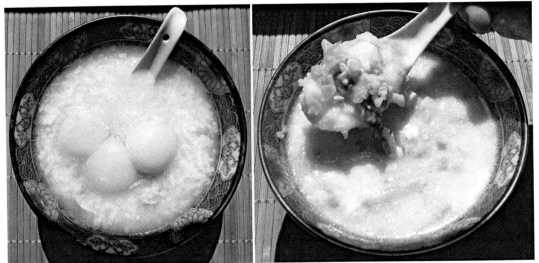

One of our favorite ways to eat rice is in a chicken soup. We boil a whole chicken with 20 garlic cloves, then remove it and add uncooked rice to the broth. Later we'll return shredded chicken meat to the soup. Left: adding egg yolks to rice soup to get our 1 calorie carb to 2 calorie fat ratio. Right: finished meal.

If you like cheese and crackers, or pasta, go ahead – just use rice noodles and rice crackers, not wheat products. Most supermarkets carry crackers and noodles made from rice. Asian supermarkets in particular have a wide variety of rice products.

AVOID PREPARED FOODS

Potato products like French fries are healthy if they are cooked in healthy oils – that is, SaFA and MUFA rich oils like coconut oil or beef tallow.

Unfortunately, most commercial foods are now prepared with omega-6 rich oils like soybean oil, corn oil or canola oil. McDonald's for decades made its French fries with 93% beef tallow; Ray Kroc, McDonald's founder, declared in his autobiography that this excellent French fry "was almost sacrosanct to me." Unfortunately such a healthy French fry could not survive the lipid hypothesis, and in 1990 McDonald's switched to vegetable oils. In general, we recommend avoiding commercial foods, even if they are made with safe starches, until food producers adopt healthier cooking oils.

Fruits and Berries

Because many fruits contain as much fructose as glucose, we don't wish to get most of our carb calories from fruits. Fortunately, they don't have a lot of calories. We normally eat 2-3 portions or ½ lb of fruit and berries per day, averaging 30-40 calories of fructose.

THE COMPOSITION OF FRUITS AND BERRIES

In the table below we present the nutritional content of various fruits and berries:

- **Glucose** and **fructose** are given as the number of calories per pound. For most fruits and berries one serving (about one cup) weighs about a third of a pound, so divide by three to get the calories per serving. The healthiest fruits and berries have low levels of fructose.

- The last column, the **Potassium to Fructose ratio**, is a measure of nutritional value. Potassium may be the most important nutrient in fruits and berries; fructose is the major toxin. So, a high potassium to fructose ratio indicates a healthy fruit or berry.

The table lists the fruits and berries from healthiest to least healthy based on their potassium to fructose ratio.

Table: Nutritional content of fruits and berries

Fruit or berry	Glucose (cal/lb)	Fructose (cal/lb)	Potassium:Fructose (mg/g)
Raspberries	36	44	62
Papaya	77	77	60
Banana	210	110	59
Strawberries	40	49	57
Peach	79	71	49
Plum	106	70	41
Orange	75	80	38
Pomegranate	124	124	35
Watermelon	40	72	28
Grapes	132	149	23
Pineapple	86	93	21
Mango	134	134	21
Pear	57	120	18
Apple	64	126	15
Blueberries	90	91	15

Berries are healthy: they tend not to have a lot of fructose – less than 50 fructose calories per pound for raspberries and strawberries, or about 15 fructose calories per one-cup (half-pint) serving – and most have high potassium-fructose ratios. Blueberries appear low in the table due to low potassium levels, but their fiber may be notably beneficial.

Among the fruits, there is great variation in nutritional value. Bananas have twice as much glucose as fructose, and plums 50% more; while pears and apples have twice as much fructose as glucose. Potassium levels also vary widely: papayas, bananas, and peaches are great sources of potassium, while pears and apples are poor sources.

We don't oppose eating pears and apples; but we would recommend looking for ancestral varieties. The modern, bred-for-sweetness (and high fructose!) varieties are the least nutritious of the fruits and berries.

EATING STRATEGY

Since fructose is a highly reactive compound that easily "fructates" and damages polyunsaturated fats, fructose should **not** be eaten with PUFA. We therefore recommend eating fruits and berries between meals or with foods that contain little PUFA, such as yogurt or cream.

Vegetables and Spices

Vegetables are too low in calories to be concerned about their macronutrient composition. For instance, spinach has 3 calories of fructose per pound. Vegetables are mainly a source of fiber and flavor. They are food for gut bacteria, and they add variety and taste to meals.

Eat as many or as few vegetables as you like: but strive to include some seaweed. Seaweed is an important source of minerals, especially iodine, that cannot easily be obtained from other sources. Seaweed is readily available at Asian supermarkets; Korean seasoned seaweed makes a great snack with a bit of rice.

SPICES

Spices are great ways to vary the flavor of meals. Most spices were discovered by our Paleolithic ancestors and handed down as traditional foods because they are good for the health. Some spices, like the Indian spice turmeric, have been scientifically studied for their health benefits.

Very hot peppers, like chilis and jalapenos, should be eaten in moderation, since capsaicin and related compounds are toxins and the "dose makes the poison." Too much can damage your digestive tract.

One spice deserves special mention: **salt**. Salt has been vilified, since excess sodium with low potassium can aggravate high blood pressure. However, some salt is essential: sodium is an essential electrolyte for the blood, and chlorine is necessary for stomach acid production. A quarter teaspoon per day is adequate if carbs are plentiful, but more is needed if carbs are restricted. Trust your taste buds: when salt tastes good, you need it.

EATING STRATEGY

We generally cook our vegetables together with our meats. It's a good idea to combine vegetables with meats: some of the beneficial nutrients in vegetables can only be absorbed by the digestive tract if they are eaten with fats; and antioxidants in vegetables can help protect meats from oxidation.

Summary: Plant Foods

The total amount of daily plant foods on the Perfect Health Diet can vary, but for us it is usually around 1.5 pounds:

- About a half pound of safe starches. For instance, 300 calories of taro, or 300 calories split evenly between rice and sweet potatoes, both weigh about half a pound.

- About a half pound of fruits and berries. A banana and a half-pint of strawberries weigh just over half a pound.

- About a half pound of vegetables. How many vegetables to eat is a matter of taste. We flavor all meat dishes with vegetables.

Although animal foods provide most of the calories, plant foods provide most of the matter. So although the Perfect Health Diet could be considered a low-carb diet, it is not a low-plant diet.

Macronutritious Animal Foods

To optimize the macronutrients in animal foods, we have four guidelines:

- **Eat ½ to 1 pound meat per day.** Lower meat consumption is good for longevity, higher meat consumption may help build muscles. Do not exceed 1 pound per day, as this risks protein toxicity.

- **Eat meat that is moist, not dry.** This assures a good fat-to-protein ratio. If meat is protein-rich and dry, like chicken breast or some fish, add a source of fat (such as coconut oil, butter, or an avocado).

- **Limit omega-6 fats.** At least four days a week, eat low-omega-6 meats like beef, lamb, and seafood. When you cook high-omega-6 meats, like duck, discard the liquid fat that drains from the duck during cooking, but keep the solid fats that stay with the meat. (Omega-6 fats have a low melting point.)

- **Eat about a pound per week of cold water fish for omega-3 fats.** Salmon, herring, and anchovies are great choices. Fish that are at the top of the ocean food chain, like tuna and swordfish, have higher risk of mercury and heavy metal toxicity and shouldn't be major sources of omega-3 fats.

Here's a table showing the macronutrient profile of common animal foods.

Table: Macronutrient profile of meats, seafoods, and eggs

Food	Calories per pound	Fat/Protein, by calories	Omega-6 as % of fat	Omega-3 as % of fat
Ribeye steak	1202	59% / 41%	3%	1%
Ground beef (85%)	1164	55% / 45%	2%	0%
Prime rib	1321	64% / 36%	3%	1%
Chicken leg	866	41% / 59%	19%	2%
Chicken breast, meat and skin	837	38% / 62%	18%	1%
Chicken breast, skinless	749	21% / 79%	17%	2%
Chicken liver	781	36% / 64%	1%	0%
Duck, roasted	1531	77% / 23%	12%	1%

Pork, country ribs	1490	71% / 29%	7%	0%
Ham	807	47% / 53%	13%	3%
Bacon	2420	70% / 30%	10%	0%
Salmon, Atlantic (farmed)	936	56% / 44%	5%	18%
Salmon, Atlantic (wild)	825	42% / 58%	3%	32%
Herring	921	53% / 47%	1%	19%
Cod	477	8% / 92%	1%	21%
Tilapia	581	19% / 81%	11%	9%
Shrimp	449	10% / 90%	2%	33%
Eggs	704	65% / 35%	11%	1%

EAT ½ LB TO 1 LB OF ANIMAL FOODS PER DAY

As the table shows, the fat content of meats can vary widely – hardly any in white fish, lots in duck, pork ribs, or bacon. However, protein content is fairly consistent. Most meats have about 500 calories per pound of protein.

We recommend two basic strategies for meat consumption:

- Low protein for longevity: eat ½ pound meat per day for 250 calories.
- High protein for muscle-building: eat 1 pound meat per day for 500 calories.

We follow the low-protein strategy of about ½ pound per day. Note that if you are on the low-protein strategy, you should make sure to eat at least 400 carb calories per day, to reach the minimum of 600 carb plus protein calories.

Do not eat more than 1 pound meat per day, to avoid protein toxicity.

EAT MOIST FATTY MEATS, NOT DRY LEAN MEATS

When we recommend that meat be "moist," or fatty, we mean that a good composition is 60% to 70% fat, 30% to 40% protein. Eating fatty meat helps optimize macronutrient ratios, and has two other advantages:

- **Fatty meat tastes better**. Taste is not merely a matter of pleasure. The unappetizing taste of lean meat is your body's way of telling you that too much protein is toxic, while fat is good for you.

- **Fatty meat provides more micronutrients**. Fat-soluble vitamins like vitamin K2 and phospholipid components like choline and inositol are more abundant in fatty meats than in oils and lean meats.

Lean meats provide too little fat to help us reach the optimal macronutrient ratios. Lean meats like skinless chicken breast (157 fat calories per pound) or cod (38 fat calories per pound) are very low in fat, but quickly provide the daily protein target.

If lean meats are eaten, they should be accompanied by sources of fat. These could include fatty plants like avocado or oils like coconut oil, olive oil, or butter. French and Thai cookbooks have a good selection of fatty sauces. Don't be afraid to use those sauces, even on moist meats!

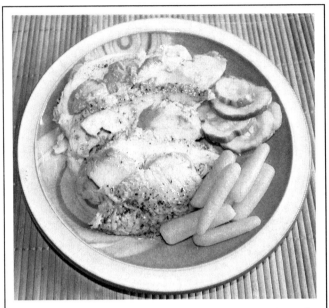

Lean meats like chicken should be combined with a fat source, such as avocado or olive oil.

LIMIT OMEGA-6 CONTENT

Overall, we want omega-6 fats to be 2% to 4% of *total* calories, or 3% to 6% of *fat* calories. Since meats provide half or more of dietary fats, we need our *meats to average less than 5% of fat calories as omega-6*.

Beef, lamb, and fish are naturally low in omega-6 fats; these should constitute half or more of each week's meat, fish, and egg intake.

Chicken, duck, pork, and eggs tend to have moderate omega-6 levels. These are healthy foods, but should provide half or less of the weekly meat intake.

Several steps can be taken to minimize omega-6 intake from chicken, duck, pork, eggs, and fish:

- If possible, buy meat and eggs from chickens that were free to roam, not caged, and that ate naturally – vegetables and insects, not cereal grains. Such naturally raised chickens have much lower omega-6 and higher omega-3 levels.

- Similarly, wild ducks and fish will have lower omega-6 levels than most domesticated ducks and farm-raised fish. We've included both farmed and wild Atlantic salmon in the table to illustrate the wild advantage: wild salmon have an omega-3 to omega-6 ratio of 10:1, farmed salmon less than 4:1.

- Omega-6 fats have a low melting point and when roasting duck or cooking bacon, much of the omega-6 fats will turn liquid and drip off the meat. Discarding most of these drippings can significantly lower the omega-6 content of these foods.

EAT COLD WATER FISH REGULARLY

Salmon, herring, and anchovies are excellent sources of omega-3 fats. We recommend eating a pound per week of these.

As the table shows, wild salmon can have nearly twice as much omega-3 per pound as farmed salmon. Nevertheless, farmed salmon has a healthy macronutrient composition. We eat farmed salmon regularly.

Summary: Animal Foods

Animal foods should be selected for their fat content: they should be fatty and moist, low in omega-6 fats, and at least some should be high in omega-3.

The meat content of the diet should be between ½ pound and 1 pound per day. Less risks protein deficiency; more risks protein toxicity.

We eat ½ pound meat per day. A typical week's animal foods include:

- a pound of salmon, providing two days of meat and meeting our omega-3 requirement;

- a pound of beef, usually ribeye steak, providing another two days of low-omega-6 meat; and

- on the other 3 days, some combination of eggs, pork (usually either ribs or pork bellies / bacon), chicken, duck, organ meats like beef liver, or shellfish like crabs or mussels.

Macronutritious Oils and Fatty Snacks

So far, we've obtained about 400 carb calories from roughly 1.5 pounds of plant foods; and 250 to 500 protein and 500 to 1000 fat calories from ½ to 1 pound of meat.

We're aiming for about 400 glucose calories, 300 protein calories, and – assuming 2,200 calories per day – 1400 fat calories. This means we still need another 600 calories or so of fat that should come from protein-free foods – that is, not meat.

What are these foods? There are three main sources: oils, desserts, and snacks.

Oils

Each tablespoon of oil provides about 130 calories, so 4-5 tablespoons of oil per day would optimize the diet's fat-to-carb-and-protein ratio.

To optimize fatty acid ratios, oils should be predominantly composed of saturated and monounsaturated fats, and have low levels of omega-6 fats.

ANIMAL AND DAIRY FATS

Animal fats are among the healthiest fats, partly because of their healthy fatty acid proportions and partly because the supply important nutrients like choline and fat-soluble vitamins. Here is a list of animal and dairy fats, ordered from low to high in omega-6:

Fat	% SaFA	% MUFA	% Omega-6	% Omega-3
Salmon oil	19.9%	29.0%	1.5%	35.3%
Tallow (beef)	49.8%	41.8%	3.1%	0.6%
Butter	63.6%	25.9%	3.4%	0.4%
Salmon (farmed) fat	22.6%	28.2%	7.3%	18.7%
Lard (pork)	39.2%	45.1%	10.2%	1.0%
Duck fat	33.2%	49.3%	12.0%	1.0%
Egg yolks	37.5%	46.0%	15.5%	1.0%
Chicken fat	29.8%	44.7%	19.5%	1.0%

We've included both farmed salmon fat and wild salmon oil to illustrate the point that wild animals and cage-free, naturally fed animals generally have lower levels of omega-6 and higher levels of omega-3 fats than their caged, grain-and-soybean fed relatives. Thus, farm-raised Atlantic salmon have roughly 5-fold more omega-

6 and half as much omega-3 as their wild relatives. Similarly, chickens and their eggs, when raised in cages and fed grain, are high in omega-6 and low in omega-3 compared to chickens allowed to roam and feed on grass and insects.

The PUFA fraction is partly determined by the temperature of an animal's environment. Cold-water fish, like salmon or herring, need high omega-3 levels so that fats will not solidify and become rigid in their bodies.

Animal fats may be used in cooking. Good cooking fats are low in both omega-6 and omega-3 fats, because these polyunsaturated fats are easily damaged by heat. Beef tallow (only 3.7% PUFA) and lamb/mutton fat (4% PUFA) make excellent cooking fats, lard (11.2% PUFA) an acceptable one.

Butter would make an excellent cooking oil but for its milk sugars and proteins which can burn at high heat and cause leftover food to go bad in a few days. Fortunately, the sugars and protein can be removed by *clarifying* the butter to make clarified butter or ghee (the Indian name).

The classic way to clarify butter is to cook it at low heat, keeping it a low simmer, until all the water evaporates and the sugars and proteins separate into solid particles which can be removed by straining through a cheesecloth.

A quick but imperfect method is to melt butter in a microwave oven, allow the yellow fat to separate from the watery portion containing most sugars and proteins, and skim off the fat. Adding water and repeating for several cycles will remove most water-soluble sugars and proteins.

Egg yolks are a highly nutritious fat, rich in folate, vitamin A, and selenium. We eat about 3 egg yolks per day – not more because of their moderately high omega-6 content. The egg whites are almost entirely made of protein; we discard them to keep protein levels down.

HEALTHY VEGETABLE OILS

Plants, like animals, tend to be low in PUFA if they come from tropical climes and high in PUFA if they come from cold climates. Thus, the healthiest plant fats are from tropical plants like the coconut, palm, and cocoa trees, or near-tropical plants like the olive and avocado.

Oil	*% sat*	*% monounsat*	*% omega-6*	*% omega-3*
Palm kernel oil	81.7%	11.4%	1.6%	0.0%
Coconut oil	86.7%	5.8%	1.8%	0.0%
Cocoa butter	59.6%	32.9%	2.8%	0.1%
Palm oil	49.1%	37.0%	9.1%	0.2%
Olive oil	13.8%	73.1%	9.8%	0.8%

Avocado oil	11.6%	70.6%	12.5%	1.0%
Cashew butter	20.3%	59.5%	16.5%	0.3%
Almond butter	9.5%	64.8%	20.1%	0.7%

Palm kernel oil, coconut oil, cocoa butter, nutmeg butter, macadamia nut butter, and ucuhuba butter have the lowest omega-6 levels among the vegetable oils and make great cooking and general-use oils.

We particularly recommend coconut oil, as its valuable short-chain fats are difficult to obtain elsewhere. We recommend eating at least 2 tbsp per day coconut oil to obtain our recommended 6.5% of energy as short-chain fats.

Cocoa butter is a very healthy fat. Chocolates made with cocoa butter are very healthy treats, as long as they don't have much sugar.

Palm oil, olive oil, avocado oil, and most tree nut butters are healthy in moderation. They are a little high in omega-6 fats, with levels similar to those in duck and chicken fat. They are best used as flavoring agents and sauces or dressings, rather than as primary cooking oils.

TOXIC VEGETABLE OILS

And here, for comparison only, is a similar table of oils you should NOT eat due to high omega-6 levels and possible natural or industrial toxins:

Oil	*% sat*	*% monounsat*	*% omega-6*	*% omega-3*
Canola oil	7.4%	63.3%	18.6%	9.1%
Peanut oil	16.9%	46.2%	32.0%	0.0%
Soybean oil	15.6%	22.8%	50.4%	6.8%
Corn oil	12.9%	27.6%	53.5%	1.2%
Wheat germ oil	18.8%	15.1%	54.8%	6.9%
Safflower oil	6.2%	14.4%	74.6%	0.0%

Note that canola oil is excluded, for two reasons:

- Its PUFA content, at 27.7%, is quite a bit higher than our most PUFA-rich healthy fats, almond butter at 20.8% and chicken fat at 20.5%.

- As we'll see in Step Two, canola oil may contain additional toxins from its industrial preparation process.

Fatty Snacks

Our recommended between-meal snack foods are nuts, fruit, cheeses, and fatty plant foods like avocado and olive. Fatty foods taste great and, as long as they are low in omega-6 fats, are extremely healthy.

Tree Nuts

Nuts, along with fruit and cheese, make an excellent snack.

Nuts do have a few toxins. Some nut toxins have been removed by breeding: for instance, wild almonds have a toxin, amygdalin, that makes them inedible, but modern almonds have been bred to remove the amygdalin gene. Most of the toxins that remain in raw nuts can be removed by overnight soaking, though this is necessary only if large quantities are to be eaten. The principal nutritional defect of tree nuts is a moderately high omega-6 fat content.

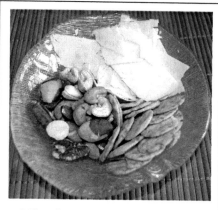

Mixed nuts, cheese, and rice crackers.

Table: Nuts with their toxin loads

Food	Calories per pound	Fructose (% calories)	Omega-6 (% calories)
Macadamia Nuts	3260	1.3%	1.6%
Cashews	2511	2.1%	12.7%
Almonds	2611	1.3%	18.9%
Pistachio	2528	2.6%	21.3%
Pecans	3137	1.2%	26.9%
Walnuts	2968	0.8%	52.4%

The table lists some popular nuts, ordered from low to high in omega-6:

- Macadamia nuts are probably the healthiest nuts, due to their low omega-6 levels, and can be eaten in unlimited quantities.

- Cashews, almonds, and pistachios have omega-6 levels similar to the more omega-6-rich meats, like pork, duck, and chicken. They should be eaten in moderation.

- Walnuts are best avoided, due to their high omega-6 content.

Brazil nuts are a special case: they are high in selenium, which is an important and desirable mineral essential for thyroid hormone and glutathione peroxidase production, but is toxic in high doses. We often eat 2 to 3 Brazil nuts in a day, but never more than 4.

Remember also that peanuts are legumes, not tree nuts, and best avoided.

CHEESES AND FATTY PLANT FOODS

Cheeses make excellent snack foods. They are very low in fructose and omega-6 fats. Paté – fatty duck or goose liver – and fish roe also make good cracker toppings.

Avocado and olives are our two favorite "fatty plant" snacks. We call them fatty plants because most calories come from fats, and like them as snacks because their omega-6 levels are fairly low. But they are not very fatty – they have only one-third as many calories per pound as cheese, and one-fifth as many as nuts.

Table: Fructose and Omega-6 Levels of Cheeses and Fatty Plants

Food	Calories per pound	Fructose (% calories)	Omega-6 (% calories)
Cheese, Cheddar	1830	0.3%	1.3%
Cheese, Brie	1517	0.3%	1.4%
Avocado	545	0.8%	11.8%
Olives	522	0.0%	6.6%

Conclusion

You can easily obtain near-perfect macronutrient ratios with a few simple rules:

Eat three kinds of plant foods: 300 calories safe starches PLUS ½ lb fruit or berries PLUS vegetables including seaweed.

Combine starches with fats or oils.

Eat meats fatty enough to be moist.

Eat red meat and salmon for low omega-6 and high omega-3.

Eat fatty desserts and snacks.

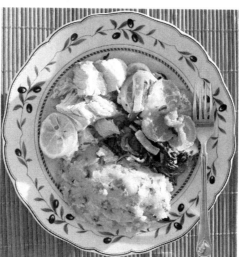

A representative meal: Salmon, vegetables, and sweet potatoes mashed with butter and coconut oil.

Step Two to Perfect Health: Eat Paleo, Not Toxic

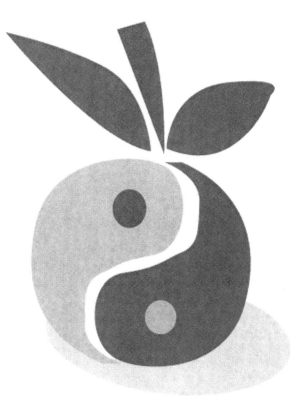

About Food Toxins

In the Introduction, we introduced the "marginal benefit curve" for nutrients. Most nutrients eventually become toxic; nutrients should be eaten in their "plateau range," between the points where benefits end and toxicity begins.

But what about foods that don't have ANY benefits, compared to alternative foods? And what if they have toxins that can damage health, even in small doses? The "marginal benefit curve" would look like this:

Figure: Marginal Benefit Curve for Toxins

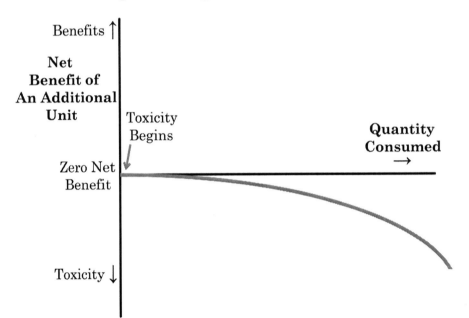

This is the profile of a poisonous food. Our advice: don't eat such foods.

Seems like a simple rule, doesn't it? But identifying which foods are poisonous is not easy: The ill effects may not show up for many years. In some foods, toxins are combined with beneficial nutrients. Finally, some poisons can be good for you in small doses – even as large doses seriously damage your health.

Four Principles of Food Toxicology

Four principles are the key to understanding food toxins.

Animal foods are generally non-toxic.

In general, animals receive no benefit from harboring in their flesh compounds toxic to humans. Animal biology is very similar to human biology. Any compounds that are poisonous to humans are also poisonous to animals. Even snake venom can be eaten – it is undigested venom that poisons.

Animal food toxins usually come from bacteria – for instance, every once in a while there's a report of ground beef contamination with subtilase cytotoxin from *E. coli* bacteria. But most meats have very low toxin levels.

All plants make pesticidal toxins.

Plants, on the other hand, have a very different biology.   They can make compounds toxic to us but safe for them, or disable their toxins at critical times such as germination.[199]   Plants make toxins because they are in danger of being eaten – and *they can't run away.* Becoming poisonous to insects, fungi, and herbivores is their best defense.

All plants, therefore, generate toxins. Bruce Ames and Lois Gold estimate that Americans eat 5,000 different natural plant pesticides, many of them carcinogens, averaging 1.5 grams of plant toxins per day.[200]

> The disabling of plant toxins by special enzymes during germination is why some plants that are normally quite toxic, like beans, have non-toxic sprouts that may safely be eaten.

The toxicologists' rule: "The dose makes the poison."

The harm done by most toxins depends on the amount. In small amounts, the body removes the poison before it does lasting harm, and there is full recovery. In large doses, however, cells are killed or irretrievably damaged before the toxin can be removed, and the effects can be serious.

This means that the danger of plant toxins is not great so long as no plant is eaten in large amounts. It is much safer to eat small quantities from a wide variety of plants, than large quantities of a single species.

> The toxicologists' rule was first formulated by Paracelsus, the "father of toxicology": *http://en.wikipedia.org/wiki/Paracelsus.*

Hormesis: Small doses of some toxins can be beneficial

Hormesis is a beneficial response of the body to small doses of a toxin. Some examples: fasting may improve health, but starvation kills; exercise improves health, but running the first marathon killed Pheidippides; moderate alcohol may

---

[199] Enzymatic detoxification of gluten by germinating wheat proteases: implications for new treatment of celiac disease. *Ann Med.* 2009;41(5):390-400. *http://pmid.us/19353359.*

[200] Ames BN, Gold LS. Paracelsus to parascience: the environmental cancer distraction. *Mutation Research* 2000 Jan 17; 447(1):3-13. *http://pmid.us/10686303.*

have health benefits, but alcoholism is devastating; various poisons, such as botulinum toxin[201], are used as medicines in small doses.

Hormesis may or may not occur from any given food toxin – a review found that only 1% of scientific articles showing a dose-response function reported hormesis[202] – but it is thought that low doses of some toxins may stimulate the body's repair mechanisms, which then proceed to repair other defects.

A Practical Application of Hormesis

The most famous experimenter with hormesis may have been Mithridates VI, king of Pontus from 119 to 63 BC.

Mithridates, one of the most successful leaders ever to oppose the Romans (in the three Mithridatic Wars), made himself resistant to poisons by regularly consuming small doses.

When, in his 70s, he was finally defeated by the Romans, he tried to commit suicide by poison, but failed because of the immunity he had built up. He prevailed upon a friend to kill him with a sword.

Together, these principles suggest that eating a large amount of any one plant is likely to be dangerous, but that occasional small amounts will only be harmful if the plant is especially toxic.

The Four Most Dangerous Foods

Since "the dose makes the poison," the most damaging foods in Western diets are also among the most common. They are:

1. **Cereal grains**,

2. **Legumes**,

3. **Vegetable oils**, and

4. **Fructose** sugar.

Let's look at the scientific evidence of toxicity from each of those foods.

---

201 Erbguth FJ. From poison to remedy: the chequered history of botulinum toxin. J Neural Transm. 2008;115(4):559-65. *http://pmid.us/17458494.*

202 Calabrese EJ, Baldwin LA (Aug 2001). "The frequency of U-shaped dose responses in the toxicological literature". Toxicol Sci. 62 (2): 330–8. *http://pmid.us/11452146.*

The Most Toxic Food: Cereal Grains

The cereal grains – wheat, corn, rice, barley, sorghum, oats, rye, and millet – are the seeds of grasses. They are the staple crops of the modern human diet. Wheat, corn, rice, and barley together account for nearly 70% by weight of the world's agricultural crops – 76% with sorghum, oats, rye, and millet. These eight cereal grains provide 56% of the food calories and 50% of the protein consumed by humanity.[203]

Grasses evolved in concert with grazing mammals: both originated at the same time and they became common together. Grasses, unlike other plants, grow their leaves from the base rather than the tip, and so are less damaged by grazing. Grasses are killed by shade, but grazers trample and eat saplings, so that land cleared by fire can remain savannah, steppe, or prairie.

> Grasses and herbivorous mammals originated about 65-55 million years ago and really began to flourish c. 20 million years ago, when grasslands populated by herds of grazing mammals took over 30% of the earth's land area.
>
> For a discussion of the co-evolution and mutual adaptations of grasses and herbivorous mammals, see Wikipedia, *http://en.wikipedia.org/wiki/Poaceae*.

To reproduce successfully despite being regularly eaten, grasses evolved two innovations. First, they generate a multitude of seeds per plant – tens of thousands annually – so that many seeds can be eaten, as long as a few scatter and take root. This fecundity is what makes the grains so attractive for agriculture: much of the harvest can be consumed as food while still retaining plentiful seed for next year's crop.

The second innovation was a set of toxic compounds specifically designed to sabotage the digestive tracts of mammals. The plant's strategy is to pass its seeds intact through the digestive tract of grazing animals so that they emerge (with manure!) to take root in a new location.

> The ability of grains to sabotage digestion is well illustrated by this fact:
>
> > For every gram of wheat bran eaten, fecal weight increases by 5.7 grams.[1]
>
> Eating wheat causes large amounts of food to be excreted instead of digested!
>
> [1] Cummings JH. The effect of dietary fibre on fecal weight and composition. In: Spiller GA, ed. *Handbook of dietary fibre in human nutrition*. 2nd ed. Boca Raton, FL: CRC Press, 1993. Pp 547–73.

---

[203] Cordain, Loren (1999) "Cereal Grains: Humanity's Double-Edged Sword," in Simopoulos AP (ed): Evolutionary Aspects of Nutrition and Health. Diet, Exercise, Genetics and Chronic Disease. *World Rev Nutr Diet*. Basel, Karger, 1999, vol 84, pp 19–73. Refs. 1 & 3.

Grazing mammals have evolved defenses for these toxins – for instance, digestive organs like rumens that allow the brunt of the toxins to be taken by bacteria. Humans, lacking such organs, are comparatively defenseless.

Alcohol as a less toxic grain

We can detoxify grains the way cows do: by replacing rumens with vats, and fermenting grains into alcohol. In the Middle Ages, alcoholic beverages like mead and ale made up about half of calories – similar to the modern percentage taken by the grains. We would never recommend obtaining half your calories from alcoholic beverages, but we suspect the medieval practice was healthier than today's!

Grain toxins are proteins and are most abundant in the bran, but present in all parts of kernels. White wheat flour is about 10% protein by weight, while crude wheat bran is about 16% protein by weight.[204]

We'll focus on wheat, which seems to be the most dangerous of the grains (with corn a close second), and on three wheat toxins in particular:

- **Gluten**, a compound protein that triggers autoimmune disease and promotes cancer, heart disease, and neuropathy.

- **Opioids**, which make wheat addictive and trigger schizophrenia.

- **Wheat germ agglutinin**, a protein that damages the intestine and interferes with vitamin D action, thus sabotaging the immune system and promoting chronic infections.

These are not the only toxins in cereal grains, but we hope they'll be enough to scare you!

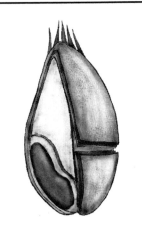

Figure: A wheat kernel. The bran, or outer shell, makes up 14% and is included in "whole" grains; the starchy endosperm makes up 83% of the kernel and provides most of the calories; and the germ makes up about 3% of the kernel.

Glutinous rice has no gluten

Anyone who is fond of *glutinous rice* (also known as *sticky rice* or *mochi rice*) can rest easy: glutinous (meaning "glue-like") rice is sticky because of the structure of its starch. Glutinous rice contains no *gluten* or other toxic proteins and is a healthy part of the Perfect Health Diet.

---

[204] *http://nutritiondata.com.*

Gluten Sensitivity and Celiac Disease

Gluten makes up 80% of the protein in wheat, rye and barley grains. Wheat gluten is compounded of two protein types: the more-toxic alcohol-soluble gliadins, and the less-toxic alcohol-insoluble glutenins.[205]

Gluten is toxic to human cells

Gluten is directly toxic to intestinal cells: it inhibits cell proliferation, increases cellular oxidation products, and changes membrane structure.[1] In the body, gluten changes the structure of the intestine: it reduces the height of villi, decreases the depth of crypts, and decreases enterocyte surface.[2]

[1] Rivabene R et al. In vitro cytotoxic effect of wheat gliadin-derived peptides on the Caco-2 intestinal cell line is associated with intracellular oxidative imbalance: implications for coeliac disease. *Biochim Biophys Acta.* 1999 Jan 6;1453(1):152-60. *http://pmid.us/9989255*; Elli L et al. Gliadin cytotoxicity and in vitro cell cultures. *Toxicol Lett.* 2003 Dec 15;146(1):1-8. *http://pmid.us/14615062.*

[2] Ciclitira PJ, Ellis HJ. In vivo gluten ingestion in coeliac disease. *Dig Dis.* 1998 Nov-Dec;16(6):337-40. *http://pmid.us/10207218.*

Gluten sabotages the gut, reducing its surface area and impairing digestion.

As all toxins do, gluten inspires an immune response. This immune response helps to clear the gluten from the intestine, preventing a build-up of toxins; however, in the process it makes the intestine inflamed.

This is a little known but important point:

Wheat triggers gut inflammation in nearly everyone.

This immune response **kills intestinal cells** and **makes the gut leaky.**[206]

There appear to be four levels of immune response to wheat:

1. About 83% of the population develops observable gut inflammation after eating wheat gluten.[207]

---

[205] Gluten composition: *http://en.wikipedia.org/wiki/Gluten.* Howdle PD. Gliadin, glutenin or both? The search for the Holy Grail in coeliac disease. *Eur J Gastroenterol Hepatol.* 2006 Jul;18(7):703-6. *http://pmid.us/16772825.*

[206] Bernardo D et al. Is gliadin really safe for non-coeliac individuals? Production of interleukin 15 in biopsy culture from non-coeliac individuals challenged with gliadin peptides. *Gut* 2007 Jun;56(6):889-90. *http://pmid.us/17519496.* Hat tip: Stephan Guyenet, *http://high-fat-nutrition.blogspot.com/2008/05/gluten-links-from-bloggeier.html.*

[207] Bernardo D et al. Is gliadin really safe for non-coeliac individuals? Production of interleukin 15 in biopsy culture from non-coeliac individuals challenged with gliadin peptides. *Gut* 2007 Jun;56(6):889-90. *http://pmid.us/17519496.*

2. About 30% of the population develops anti-wheat-gluten antibodies locally in the intestine.[208]

3. About 11% of the population develops systemic (circulating throughout the body) antibodies to wheat gluten.

4. About 0.4% of the population develops systemic antibodies that attack human cells in the intestine, thyroid, pancreas, and elsewhere.

This last group is diagnosed with celiac disease. With the immune system attacking and killing gut cells, the intestine can be damaged to the point that sufferers have difficulty absorbing needed nutrients. [209]

What determines the severity of the response to wheat?

The innate immune system provides a nonspecific, first-line reaction to toxins and microbes. Nearly everyone has an innate immune response to wheat: 83% of people tested experienced an innate immune response to wheat gluten, as shown by elevated levels of the immune signaling molecule interleukin-15. Gluten "induces epithelial stress and reprograms intraepithelial lymphocytes into natural killer (NK)-like cells leading to enterocyte apoptosis and an increase in epithelium permeability."

These are the same effects – the death of intestinal cells and gut leakiness – that occur in patients with full-blown celiac disease, only the celiac disease response is more severe.[1]

In people who tolerate wheat relatively well, only the innate immune response is triggered by wheat gluten. This immune response helps to clear wheat toxins and results in transient inflammation of the gut. Of course, if wheat is eaten regularly, the gut may be continually inflamed.

In many people, however, the innate immune response causes gliadin to be presented to the adaptive immune system leading to antibody generation and a powerful immune reaction.[2]

Genetic variations in the HLA-DQ gene seem to control how likely it is that antibodies will develop. HLA (human leukocyte antigen) molecules present other molecules, usually toxins or microbe proteins, to the adaptive immune system. People with HLA haplotypes DQ2 or DQ8 are especially prone to developing anti-wheat antibodies: these haplotypes are held by about 42% of the population, and 95% of celiac patients have one of these alleles. Only haplotype DQ4 is not known to present gliadin to the immune system. Only 0.4% of the population has both HLA-DQ alleles of type DQ4. So 99.6% of the population can develop antibodies to wheat.

How common are antibodies to wheat gluten? This depends on which antibodies are measured and how they are measured.

---

[208] Stephan Guyenet, *http://high-fat-nutrition.blogspot.com/2008/05/gluten-links-from-bloggeier.html*, quoting Dr. Kenneth Fine of EnteroLab; see the transcript of Dr. Fine's talk at *https://www.enterolab.com/StaticPages/EarlyDiagnosis.htm*.

[209] Sollid LM, Jabri B. Is celiac disease an autoimmune disorder? *Curr Opin Immunol.* 2005 Dec;17(6):595-600. *http://pmid.us/16214317*.

What determines the severity of the response to wheat? (cont.)

We can identify a spectrum of disease states, based on which antibody types are generated:

- IgA antibodies are generated by gut mucosal cells, and are the most likely to be produced. All celiac disease sufferers and 29% of apparently healthy controls show anti-wheat IgA antibodies in their stool. In some people these IgA antibodies leak into the blood, so that 76% of celiac patients and 12% of healthy controls have anti-wheat IgA antibodies in blood. These antibodies help to clear wheat toxins from the gut.

- IgG antibodies are the slowest part of the immune response to develop. They develop after long exposure to wheat toxins within the body. Up to 11% of the population may have anti-gliadin IgG antibodies. This makes for a powerful inflammatory response to wheat proteins.

- Gliadin molecules in the body often become permanently cross-linked with human molecules, such as the enzyme tissue transglutaminase (tTg). As a result, these human molecules can be presented to the immune system along with gliadin. Anti-tTg antibodies trigger autoimmune attacks against tissues in which tTg is abundant, especially the thyroid. Thus, wheat is a common cause of hypothyroidism, and all celiac disease sufferers become hypothyroid.[3] About 0.4% of Americans reach this disease stage, according to tests for anti-endomysial antibodies (EmA).[4]

Anti-endomysial antibodies are by no means a foolproof test for celiac disease. Severe damage can be done to the gut without such antibodies. As one paper notes, "EmA-negative coeliac disease is common. Reliance on EmA testing to select patients for biopsy will result in significant underdiagnosis."[5]

Whatever the level of the immune response, removal of wheat from the diet leads to a complete recovery. Restoration of wheat brings back the disease.

Those who don't have an adequate immune response to wheat are less effective in clearing wheat toxins and may ultimately suffer more, not less, damage from wheat toxicity. For instance, a deficiency in IgA antibodies, reducing the rate of wheat clearance in the intestine, increases the risk of full-blown celiac disease tenfold.[6]

[1] Bernardo D et al. Higher constitutive IL15R alpha expression and lower IL-15 response threshold in coeliac disease patients. *Clin Exp Immunol.* 2008 Oct;154(1):64-73. *http://pmid.us/18821940.*

[2] Stephan Guyenet, "Gluten sensitivity and celiac disease," *http://wholehealthsource.blogspot.com/2008/12/gluten-sensitivity-celiac-disease-is.html.* Silano M et al. Toxic, immunostimulatory and antagonist gluten peptides in celiac disease. *Curr Med Chem.* 2009;16(12):1489-98. *http://pmid.us/19355902.*

[3] *http://en.wikipedia.org/wiki/Celiac_disease.*

[4] Not T et al. Celiac disease risk in the USA: high prevalence of antiendomysium antibodies in healthy blood donors. *Scand J Gastroenterol.* 1998 May;33(5):494-8. *http://pmid.us/9648988.*

[5] Dickey W et al. Reliance on serum endomysial antibody testing underestimates the true prevalence of coeliac disease by one fifth. *Scand J Gastroenterol.* 2000 Feb;35(2):181-3. *http://pmid.us/10720117.*

[6] *http://en.wikipedia.org/wiki/Celiac_disease.*

In summary, (1) nearly everyone has an immune response to wheat, (2) the immune response can result in damage throughout the body, but usually most severely to the gut and thyroid, (3) the response to wheat varies across persons, but (4) at any time, antibodies against wheat may be acquired, making wheat damage more severe. Finally, (5) the only way to avoid wheat-generated health problems is to remove wheat from the diet.

Consequences of Gluten Sensitivity

The immune attack against wheat not only damages the gut, but other tissues too. Wheat can trigger autoimmune disease, heart disease, neuropathy, or cancer.

AUTOIMMUNE DISEASES

We mentioned that wheat consumption often triggers autoimmune attacks against the thyroid, leading to hypothyroidism.[210] Wheat can also trigger autoimmune attacks against pancreatic islet cells, inducing Type I diabetes in both rats and humans. The cause has been tracked down to a wheat protein we haven't discussed, globulin 1.[211]

Fortunately, both diabetes-related and hypothyroid-related auto-antibodies tend to disappear after wheat is removed from the diet.[212]

Wheat can even destroy the heart. Heart transplant patients usually have celiac disease, and when scientists investigated they found that antibodies against wheat gliadin also attack the heart, leading to destruction of heart tissue.[213]

Wheat can also promote autoimmune disease by other mechanisms. Wheat makes the intestine more leaky, allowing intestinal bacteria and their proteins to enter

---

[210] Ch'ng CL et al. Celiac disease and autoimmune thyroid disease. *Clin Med Res.* 2007 October; 5(3): 184–192. *http://pmid.us/18056028.* Naiyer AJ et al. Tissue transglutaminase antibodies in individuals with celiac disease bind to thyroid follicles and extracellular matrix and may contribute to thyroid dysfunction. *Thyroid.* 2008 Nov;18(11):1171-8. *http://pmid.us/19014325.*

[211] MacFarlane AJ et al. A type 1 diabetes-related protein from wheat (Triticum aestivum). cDNA clone of a wheat storage globulin, Glb1, linked to islet damage. J Biol Chem. 2003 Jan 3; 278(1): 54-63. *http://pmid.us/12409286.*

[212] Ventura A et al. Diabetes-related and hypothyroid-related autoantibodies tend to disappear when wheat is removed from the diet: Ventura A et al. Gluten-dependent diabetes-related and thyroid-related autoantibodies in patients with celiac disease. *J Pediatr* 2000;137:263–265. *http://pmid.us/10931424.*

[213] Sategna-Guidetti C et al. Binding by serum IgA antibodies from patients with coeliac disease to monkey heart tissue. *Scand J Gastroenterol.* 2004 Jun;39(6):540-3. *http://pmid.us/15223677.*

the body.[214] Some bacterial proteins are "molecular mimics" of human proteins, and production of antibodies against these bacterial proteins is thought to lead to autoimmune diseases such as lupus, rheumatoid arthritis, and type I diabetes.

Probably due to their leaky guts, celiac disease sufferers acquire autoimmune disorders – including multiple sclerosis, lupus, type I diabetes, Sjogren syndrome, and Hashimoto's thyroiditis – at a high rate. One paper says, "The comorbidity between celiac disease and other autoimmune disorders has been clearly established.... [T]he loss of the intestinal barrier function typical of celiac disease could be responsible for the onset of other autoimmune disease."[215]

CANCER

There is an association between cancer and gluten sensitivity. People diagnosed with celiac disease have a higher overall risk of cancer, but mostly in the first year after diagnosis.[216] This suggests that wheat consumption was causing or promoting the cancer, and the removal of wheat from the diet after diagnosis ends the cancer promotion.

The cancer association is most dramatic for lymphomas. People with gluten sensitivity have a 40 to 100 fold higher incidence of lymphomas.[217]

NEUROPATHY

Gluten can cause neuropathy even in the absence of intestinal distress, and in neuropathy patients with circulating antigliadin antibodies a gluten-free diet continued for one year significantly improves neurophysiology.[218]

---

[214] Lammers KM et al. Gliadin Induces an Increase in Intestinal Permeability and Zonulin Release by Binding to the Chemokine Receptor CXCR3. *Gastroenterology*. 2008 Jul;135(1):194-204.e3. *http://pmid.us/18485912*. Drago S et al. Gliadin, zonulin and gut permeability: Effects on celiac and non-celiac intestinal mucosa and intestinal cell lines. *Scand J Gastroenterol*. 2006 Apr;41(4):408-19. *http://pmid.us/16635908*.

[215] Fasano A. Systemic autoimmune disorders in celiac disease. *Curr Opin Gastroenterol*. 2006 Nov;22(6):674-9. *http://pmid.us/17053448*. See also: Sapone A et al. Zonulin upregulation is associated with increased gut permeability in subjects with type 1 diabetes and their relatives. *Diabetes*. 2006 May;55(5):1443-9. *http://pmid.us/16664703*.

[216] Askling J et al. Cancer incidence in a population-based cohort of individuals hospitalized with celiac disease or dermatitis herpetiformis. *Gastroenterology*. 2002 Nov;123(5):1428-35. *http://pmid.us/12404215*. West J et al. Malignancy and mortality in people with coeliac disease: population based cohort study. *BMJ*. 2004 Sep 25;329(7468):716-9. *http://pmid.us/15269095*. Hat tip: Stephan Guyenet, *http://wholehealthsource.blogspot.com/2008/06/more-fat-soluble-vitamin-musing-ii.html*.

[217] Hoggan R. Considering wheat, rye, and barley proteins as aids to carcinogens. *Med Hypotheses*. 1997 Sep;49(3):285-8. *http://pmid.us/9293475*.

INCREASED MORTALITY

People with gluten sensitivity die earlier.[219]

Epidemiological evidence suggests that *nearly everyone* who eats wheat dies earlier. The China Study was a huge undertaking: beginning in 1976 the Chinese government interviewed hundreds of millions of Chinese about their diet, gathered millions of blood and urine samples, and correlated diet with disease rates. We've blogged about how remarkably well the China Study correlations support the Perfect Health Diet.[220] Perhaps the most remarkable correlations in the China Study are those involving grains.

Different areas of China eat different staple grains, so the China Study correlations give a good measure of the impact of different grains on health. The correlations were:

- Wheat had a **+67%** correlation with heart disease mortality;
- Rice had a **-58%** correlation with heart disease mortality;
- Other grains had a **+39%** correlation with heart disease mortality.

Wheat was by far the most toxic food found in the China Study. The relative safety of rice fits with our classification of rice among our "safe starches."

Opioid Peptides, Wheat Addiction, and Schizophrenia

Many people have subclinical gluten sensitivity, characterized by acid reflux and bowel inflammation, and yet continue to eat wheat.

One reason they don't quit is that *wheat is addictive.* Wheat contains opioid peptides which have the same pleasure-stimulating effects as morphine.

OPIOIDS AND SCHIZOPHRENIA

The discovery of opioid peptides in wheat was first reported by Dr. Christine Zioudrou and colleagues at the National Institutes of Mental Health in 1979.[221]

---

[218] Hadjivassiliou M et al. Dietary treatment of gluten neuropathy. *Muscle & Nerve* 2006 Dec; 34(6): 762-6. *http://pmid.us/17013890*.

[219] Dickey W et al. Reliance on serum endomysial antibody testing underestimates the true prevalence of coeliac disease by one fifth. *Scand J Gastroenterol.* 2000 Feb;35(2):181-3. *http://pmid.us/10720117*.

[220] "The China Study: Evidence for the Perfect Health Diet," July 9, 2010, *http://perfecthealthdiet.com/?p=166*. Hat tip Denise Minger, *http://rawfoodsos.com/2010/07/07/the-china-study-fact-or-fallac/*.

[221] Zioudrou C et al. Opioid peptides derived from food proteins: The exorphins. *J Biol Chem.* 1979 Apr 10;254(7):2446-9. *http://pmid.us/372181*. Huebner FR et al. Demonstration of high opioid-like activity in isolated peptides from wheat gluten

They looked into the matter because of the strong association between wheat and schizophrenia.[222] A brief summary of this association:

> "Schizophrenics maintained on a cereal grain-free and milk-free diet and receiving optimal treatment with neuroleptics showed an interruption or reversal of their therapeutic progress during a period of "blind" wheat gluten challenge. The exacerbation of the disease process was not due to variations in neuroleptic doses. After termination of the gluten challenge, the course of improvement was reinstated. The observed effects seemed to be due to a primary schizophrenia-promoting effect of wheat gluten."[223]

One scientist suggests that schizophrenia is rare if grain is rare: "Epidemiologic studies demonstrated a strong, dose-dependent relationship between grain intake and the occurrence of schizophrenia."[224] In one case, longstanding schizophrenia was cured by a low-carb diet. Wheat removal may have been key to the cure.[225]

Since these early studies, evidence has continued to finger opioid peptides as wheat toxins which specifically promote schizophrenia.[226]

OPIOIDS, CANCER, AND HORMONES

In test tubes, wheat opioids cause tumor cells to multiply. This suggests that wheat opioids may stimulate cancer growth and may be partly responsible for the association between wheat and cancer.[227]

Wheat opioids may also feminize male bodies by promoting unusual hormones. "Man-boobs" may result from prolactin secretion stimulated by wheat opioids.[228]

---

hydrolysates. *Peptides.* 1984 Nov-Dec;5(6):1139-47. *http://pmid.us/6099562.* Fukudome S, Yoshikawa M. Opioid peptides derived from wheat gluten: their isolation and characterization. *FEBS Lett.* 1992 Jan 13;296(1):107-11. *http://pmid.us/1309704.*

[222] Kalaydjian AE et al. The gluten connection: the association between schizophrenia and celiac disease. *Acta Psychiatr Scand.* 2006 Feb;113(2):82-90. *http://pmid.us/16423158.*

[223] Singh MM et al Wheat gluten as a pathogenic factor in schizophrenia. *Science.* 1976 Jan 30;191(4225):401-2. *http://pmid.us/1246624.*

[224] Dohan FC et al 1984 Is schizophrenia rare if grain is rare? *Biol Psychiatry.* 1984 Mar;19(3):385-99. *http://pmid.us/6609726.*

[225] Kraft BD, Westman EC. Schizophrenia, gluten, and low-carbohydrate, ketogenic diets: a case report and review of the literature. *Nutr Metab (Lond).* 2009 Feb 26;6:10. *http://pmid.us/19245705.*

[226] Ross-Smith P, Jenner FA. Diet (gluten) and schizophrenia. *J Hum Nutr.* 1980 Apr;34(2):107-12. *http://pmid.us/6989901.*

[227] Zagon IS et al. Opioid growth factor-opioid growth factor receptor axis is a physiological determinant of cell proliferation in diverse human cancers. *Am J Physiol Regul Integr Comp Physiol.* 2009 Oct;297(4):R1154-61. *http://pmid.us/19675283.*

Opioid peptides can be generated from other foods besides wheat. Incomplete digestion of milk proteins, rice albumin, and other food proteins can create peptides with opioid activity.[229]

Wheat Germ Agglutinin

Wheat germ agglutinin (WGA) is a lectin, a protein that bonds strongly to certain sugars. Whole wheat flour has about 30-50 mg WGA per kg; many Americans consume 10 mg of WGA per day. WGA specifically bonds to certain glycoproteins found in the human gastrointestinal tract, immune system, blood vessels, and nerves. Similar lectins are found in other grains and legumes.

WGA IN THE GUT

WGA is toxic to intestinal cells. It damages the integrity of the gut lining and makes it permeable, allowing gut bacteria, partially digested food fragments, and bacterial waste to enter the body. At extremely low concentrations, only a few parts in a billion, WGA stimulates immune cells in the gut to release inflammatory cytokines, further loosening the gut barrier.[230]

WGA causes shedding of the intestinal brush border and shrinkage in the surface area of the intestine.[231] In addition to promoting the shedding of mature gut cells, WGA increases the rate of cell division in the cells lining the intestine, leaving the intestinal lining in an immature state that doesn't digest food well. After ingestion of WGA, rats develop celiac disease.[232]

WGA IN THE BODY

A large part of dietary WGA is transported across the gut wall into the blood, where it is deposited onto immune cells, vessel walls and later into nerves.

---

[228] Fanciulli G et al. Gluten exorphin B5 stimulates prolactin secretion through opioid receptors located outside the blood-brain barrier. *Life Sci.* 2005 Feb 25;76(15):1713-9. *http://pmid.us/15698850.* (Hat tip Dr. BG: *http://drbganimalpharm.blogspot.com/2008/05/wheat-would-you-give-your-kids-crack.html.*)

[229] Teschemacher H. Opioid receptor ligands derived from food proteins. *Curr Pharm Des.* 2003;9(16):1331-44. *http://pmid.us/12769741.*

[230] Dalla Pellegrina C et al. Effects of wheat germ agglutinin on human gastrointestinal epithelium: insights from an experimental model of immune/epithelial cell interaction. *Toxicol Appl Pharmacol.* 2009 Jun 1; 237(2): 146-53. *http://pmid.us/19332085.*

[231] Lorenzsonn V, Olsen WA. In vivo responses of rat intestinal epithelium to intraluminal dietary lectins. *Gastroenterology.* 1982 May;82(5 Pt 1):838-48. *http://pmid.us/6895878.*

[232] Sjölander A et al. Morphological changes of rat small intestine after short-time exposure to concanavalin A or wheat germ agglutinin. *Cell Struct Funct.* 1986 Sep;11(3):285-93. *http://pmid.us/3768964.*

In the body, WGA shrinks various organs, notably the thymus.[233]

WGA in the brain may trigger leptin resistance[234], which could lead to **obesity**.[235] (Leptin is a hormone released by fat cells which quickens metabolism. We know that obese people are leptin resistant while thin people are not; and that mice with mutated leptin – equivalent to complete leptin resistance – become extremely obese.)

WGA binds to insulin receptors, triggering an insulin-like effect. It is as effective as insulin at pushing glucose into cells and stopping the release of fat from fat cells. This means that eating wheat may block weight loss and promote weight gain, regardless of how many calories are eaten overall.[236]

WGA helps to trigger **autoimmune disease** by acting as an adjuvant to other molecules. In other words, WGA binds to proteins and causes the body to generate antibodies against them, even though the body would not form antibodies against that protein in isolation. For instance, one study found that antibodies against the egg protein ovalbumin are generated if it is accompanied by WGA.[237]

WGA is inflammatory[238], promotes clotting, and induces the release of proteins called matrix metallopeptidases that cause clots to break free[239] – all features that increase the likelihood of a **heart attack**.

---

[233] Lochner N et al. Wheat germ agglutinin binds to the epidermal growth factor receptor of artificial Caco-2 membranes as detected by silver nanoparticle enhanced fluorescence. *Pharm Res.* 2003 May;20(5):833-9. *http://pmid.us/12751642*. Pusztai A et al. Antinutritive effects of wheat-germ agglutinin and other N-acetylglucosamine-specific lectins. *Br J Nutr.* 1993 Jul;70(1):313-21. *http://pmid.us/8399111*. Pusztai A et al. Specific uptake of dietary lectins into the systemic circulation of rats. *Biochemical Society Transactions.* 1989;17, 527-528.

[234] Jönsson T et al. Agrarian diet and diseases of affluence--do evolutionary novel dietary lectins cause leptin resistance? *BMC Endocr Disord.* 2005 Dec 10;5:10. *http://pmid.us/16336696*.

[235] Scarpace PJ, Zhang Y. Leptin resistance: a prediposing factor for diet-induced obesity. *Am J Physiol Regul Integr Comp Physiol.* 2009 Mar; 296(3): R493-500. *http://pmid.us/19091915*.

[236] Cuatrecasas P, Tell GP. Insulin-Like Activity of Concanavalin A and Wheat Germ Agglutinin—Direct Interactions with Insulin Receptors. *Proc Natl Acad Sci U S A.* 1973 February; 70(2): 485–489. *http://pmid.us/4510292*.

[237] Lavelle EC et al. The identification of plant lectins with mucosal adjuvant activity. *Immunology.* 2001 Jan;102(1):77-86. *http://pmid.us/11168640*.

[238] Sodhi A, Kesherwani V. Production of TNF-alpha, IL-1beta, IL-12 and IFN-gamma in murine peritoneal macrophages on treatment with wheat germ agglutinin in vitro: involvement of tyrosine kinase pathways. *Glycoconj J.* 2007 Dec; 24(9): 573-82. *http://pmid.us/17668318*.

WGA promotes **kidney disease** by binding IgA, triggering IgA nephropathy.[240]

WGA in the body

WGA's movement through the body is well understood, because, bonded to a fluorescent marker to form a compound called WGA-HRP, it has been used for medical imaging.

Within 5 minutes, WGA coats blood vessels throughout the body, including the brain. Within a few hours, WGA is absorbed into endothelial cells lining the vessels through a process called endocytosis, and coats various intracellular organelles. Most toxins absorbed by endocytosis are destroyed in lysosomes, but WGA is able to evade destruction and exit the cell via transcytosis. This allows it to cross the blood-brain barrier and enter the brain and cerebrospinal fluid. Twelve hours after injection, WGA is found within nerve cells neighboring blood vessels.[1]

[1] Broadwell RD et al. Transcytotic Pathway for Blood-Borne Protein through the Blood-Brain Barrier. *Proc Natl Acad Sci USA.* 1988 Jan;85(2):632-6. *http://pmid.us/2448779.* Balin BJ, Broadwell RD. Transcytosis of protein through the mammalian cerebral epithelium and endothelium. I. Choroid plexus and the blood-cerebrospinal fluid barrier. *J Neurocytol.* 1988 Dec;17(6):809-26. *http://pmid.us/3230399.* Villegas JC, Broadwell RD. Transcytosis of protein through the mammalian cerebral epithelium and endothelium. II. Adsorptive transcytosis of WGA-HRP and the blood-brain and brain-blood barriers. *J Neurocytol.* 1993 Feb; 22(2):67-80. *http://pmid.us/7680372.*

WGA, as well as other grain and legume lectins such as kidney bean phytohaemagglutinin, have been shown to denude the small intestine of mucus, stimulate stomach acid production, and promote overgrowth of bacteria including H. Pylori. These are conditions that lead to **acid reflux** and **stomach ulcers**.[241]

Interference with Vitamin D

Rickets is a softening of the bones in children leading to fractures and deformity. In the early 20th century, rickets was common, and was associated with mortality. Ninety percent of children who died before the age of 4 had rickets, and the death rate among children was 3 to 10 fold higher where rickets was prevalent than in areas where it was rare.

WHEAT CAUSES VITAMIN D DEFICIENCY DISEASE

Rickets is said to be a vitamin D deficiency disease, yet rickets has always been associated with grain consumption. In Edward Mellanby's pioneering

---

[239] Dubois B et al. Regulation of gelatinase B (MMP-9) in leukocytes by plant lectins. *FEBS Lett.* 1998 May 8; 427(2): 275-8. *http://pmid.us/9607327.*

[240] Freed DL. Do dietary lectins cause disease? *BMJ.* 1999 Apr 17;318(7190):1023-4. *http://pmid.us/10205084.*

[241] Freed DL. Do dietary lectins cause disease? *BMJ.* 1999 Apr 17;318(7190):1023-4. *http://pmid.us/10205084.*

experiments, he induced the disease by feeding dogs a diet of oats or wheat bread, and then cured it by adding cod liver oil (which contains vitamin D). Either dietary fats or sunlight cured rickets; a cereal-based diet combined with confinement indoors caused rickets.[242]

However, it seems that rickets can be caused by cereal grains even when sun exposure is high. Today, rickets is mainly found in sunny countries such as Nigeria, South Africa, and Bangladesh, where it is the result of "cereal-based diets with limited variety and little access to dairy products," and is cured by the addition of dairy foods, not vitamin D.[243]

Rickets With Normal Vitamin D

Blood tests confirm that rickets can coincide with normal vitamin D levels, as in the case of this Bedouin woman:

> Vitamin D was present in normal amounts in the plasma of our patient so this excludes the premise that she was deprived of vitamin D. Bedouin women are sunburned over the anterior half of their head and forearms. They go about their tasks at home unveiled. Vitamin D levels would be expected to be normal from the area of skin available for irradiation and the intensity of sunlight in this area.[1]

A study of rickets in Nigeria concludes, "Vitamin D deficiency appears unlikely to be the primary etiologic factor of rickets in African children. Moreover, low dietary calcium intake alone does not account for rickets. Insufficient dietary calcium probably interacts with genetic, hormonal, and other nutritional factors to cause rickets in susceptible children."[2]

[1] Berlyne GM et al. Bedouin osteomalacia due to calcium deprivation caused by high phytic acid content of unleavened bread. *Am J Clin Nutr.* 1973 Sep;26(9):910-1. *http://pmid.us/4727748.*

[2] Thacher TD et al. Case-control study of factors associated with nutritional rickets in Nigerian children. *J Pediatr.* 2000 Sep;137(3):367-73. *http://pmid.us/10969262.*

In animals, rickets is known to occur with adequate vitamin D and calcium due to food toxins. One study of rickets in farm turkeys concluded: "Because the feed contained adequate vitamin D, calcium, and phosphorus, the cause of this outbreak of field rickets is thought to be a toxic feed contaminant."[244]

---

[242] Mellanby E. (March 15 1919) An experimental investigation on rickets. *The Lancet* 193(4985):407-412. Reprinted in *Nutrition.* 1989 Mar-Apr; 5(2): 81-6; discussion 87. *http://pmid.us/2520279.*

[243] Pettifor JM. Nutritional rickets: deficiency of vitamin D, calcium, or both? *Am J Clin Nutr.* 2004 Dec;80(6 Suppl):1725S-9S. *http://pmid.us/15585795.*

[244] Huff WE et al. Research on the probable cause of an outbreak of field rickets in turkeys. *Poult Sci.* 1999 Dec;78(12):1699-702. *http://pmid.us/10626644.*

Another link with wheat is that rickets patients frequently have celiac disease. Possibly the immune response to gluten contributes to rickets.[245]

Feeding wheat bran to infants creates mineral deficiencies, a shift in gut flora to protein-digesting species, and early signs of rickets.[246] The likely explanation for the mineral deficiencies is phytic acid in wheat, which binds minerals like calcium and can deplete them from the digestive tract and body.[247] The resulting calcium deficiency might contribute to rickets.

WHEAT INTERFERES WITH VITAMIN D

There are two known ways in which wheat interferes with vitamin D:

1. By an unknown mechanism, wheat causes people to burn through their vitamin D stores. One study found that eating just 20 g (0.7 ounces) per day of wheat bran caused vitamin D to be depleted 43% faster.[248]

2. Japanese researchers found that WGA can prevent the vitamin D receptor (VDR) from entering the cell nucleus.[249] This would prevent the VDR from fulfilling its function as a transcription factor for genes involved in the innate immune response.

The Japanese result suggests that those who eat wheat may be particularly vulnerable to infectious disease. Bacteria and viruses probably block or downregulate the VDR in order to protect themselves from the immune system. If wheat also does this, then it must obstruct immune function.

Wheat depletes vitamin D and blocks its function ... thus impairing immune defense against bacteria and viruses.

---

[245] Thapa BR. Celiac disease in India. *Indian J Pediatr*. 1999;66(1 Suppl):S16-20. *http://pmid.us/11132463*. See also Rawashdeh MO et al. Celiac disease in Arabs. *J Pediatr Gastroenterol Nutr*. 1996 Nov; 23(4):415-8. *http://pmid.us/8956178*.

[246] Zoppi G et al. Potential complications in the use of wheat bran for constipation in infancy. *J Pediatr Gastroenterol Nutr*. 1982; 1(1): 91-5. *http://pmid.us/6310074*.

[247] Berlyne, GM et al. Bedouin osteomalacia due to calcium deprivation caused by high phytic acid content of unleavened bread. *Am J Clin Nutr*. 1973 Sep;26(9):910-1. *http://pmid.us/4727748*. Harinarayan, CV et al. High prevalence of low dietary calcium, high phytate consumption, and vitamin D deficiency in healthy south Indians. *Am J Clin Nutr*. 2007 Apr;85(4):1062-7. *http://pmid.us/17413106*.

[248] Batchelor AJ, Compston JE. Reduced plasma half-life of radio-labelled 25-hydroxyvitamin D3 in subjects receiving a high-fibre diet. *Br J Nutr*. 1983 Mar;49(2):213-6. *http://pmid.us/6299329*. Hat tip Stephan Guyenet, *http://wholehealthsource.blogspot.com/2008/06/more-fat-soluble-vitamin-musing-ii.html*.

[249] Miyauchi Y et al. Importin 4 Is Responsible for Ligand-independent Nuclear Translocation of Vitamin D Receptor. *J Biol Chem*. 2005 Dec 9;280(49):40901-8. *http://pmid.us/16207705*.

Wheat may therefore make the body more prone to chronic infectious diseases. Chronic infections have been implicated in aging, autoimmunity, atherosclerosis, Alzheimer's and multiple sclerosis.

Cumulatively, the evidence suggests wheat eaters have impaired vitamin D function and higher vitamin D needs than those who don't eat wheat.

Other Grains

We have focused on wheat in this section. However, all of the grasses share similar toxins. Peculiar toxic effects are found from many grains.

Just to give one example, corn (maize), the domesticated form of the grass teosinte, is able to induce pellagra by mechanisms that are not understood. Pellagra was unknown until the introduction of maize into Europe from the New World.[250] Much as vitamin D supplementation cures wheat-induced rickets, niacin supplementation cures corn-induced pellagra.[251]

Finally, some people are starch-sensitive, possibly due to toxins produced by pathogenic gut bacteria as they digest starches. Grains seem to be particularly good at provoking this reaction, and association of starch sensitivity with ancestral gene alleles suggests that the provoking foods have only recently entered the human diet (see green box, "Is Ankylosing Spondylitis Caused by Starches?").

---

[250] Lanska DJ. Chapter 30 Historical aspects of the major neurological vitamin deficiency disorders: the water-soluble B vitamins. *Handb Clin Neurol.* 2009;95:445-76. *http://pmid.us/19892133.*

[251] Carpenter KJ, Lewin WJ. A critical review: A reexamination of the composition of diets associated with pellagra. *J Nutr* 1985 May;115(5):543–552. *http://pmid.us/3998856.*

Is Ankylosing Spondylitis Caused By Starches?

A starch branching structure which is abundant in legume and grain starches and indigestible by humans is digested by the pullulanase enzyme of the bacteria *Klebsiella*. Pullulanase from *Klebsiella* resembles human collagen and, in people with the ancestral form of the gene HLA-B27, stimulates an autoimmune response.[1] (Recently evolved forms of this gene are more tolerant of pullulanase than the ancestral HLA-B*2705 haplotype[2]; probably adoption of agriculture initiated selection for grain-tolerant haplotypes.) This response may cause ankylosing spondylitis.[3]

[1] Rashid T et al. Role of Klebsiella and collagens in Crohn's disease: a new prospect in the use of low-starch diet. *Eur J Gastroenterol Hepatol.* 2009 Aug;21(8):843-9. *http://pmid.us/19352192.*

[2] Mathieu A et al. The interplay between the geographic distribution of HLA-B27 alleles and their role in infectious and autoimmune diseases: a unifying hypothesis. *Autoimmun Rev.* 2009 Mar;8(5):420-5. *http://pmid.us/19185064.*

[3] Ebringer A et al. A possible link between Crohn's disease and ankylosing spondylitis via Klebsiella infections. *Clin Rheumatol.* 2007 Mar;26(3):289-97. *http://pmid.us/16941202.* Fielder M et al. Molecular mimicry and ankylosing spondylitis: possible role of a novel sequence in pullulanase of Klebsiella pneumoniae. *FEBS Lett.* 1995 Aug 7;369(2-3):243-8. *http://pmid.us/7649265.* See also Carol Sinclair's book *The IBS Low-Starch Diet: Why Starchy Food May Be Hazardous to Your Health.* Hat tip Peter Dobromylskyj, *http://high-fat-nutrition.blogspot.com/2006/11/food-pyramids-food-and-pyramids.html.*

Conclusion

Cereal grains damage the intestine and impair digestion. They impair the innate immune response and make people vulnerable to chronic infections. They are addictive and cause or worsen schizophrenia and other mental illnesses. They trigger autoimmune disease. They promote cancer growth. They measurably increase mortality in gluten-sensitive and diseased populations. They are the food most strongly associated with mortality in the China Study.

It's fair to infer that health is likely to improve, maybe substantially, with elimination of grains from the diet.

We know how hard it is to give up bread. Yet there may be no single step which can do more to improve health.

Almost-Grains: Legumes

Common food legumes include soybeans, the fifth largest global agricultural product and the largest non-grain crop; kidney beans; lentils; and peanuts.

Legumes are toxicologically similar to grains. Like grains, they are eaten by herbivores and have developed toxins against mammals, including humans. Important legume toxins include lectins (similar in function to grain lectins like WGA) and alpha-amylase inhibitors (which are also found in grains).

Here is a sample of known toxicity effects from legumes:

- **Leaky gut, bad digestion, diarrhea, bloating.** Kidney beans make rat intestines leaky, allowing bacteria and toxins to enter the body.[252] The kidney bean lectin phytohaemagglutinin (PHA) blocks production of stomach acid. This prevents proper digestion, especially of proteins.[253] PHA induces overpopulation of the gut with immature cells that do not digest food well. Immature gut cells are easily exploited by diarrhea-inducing bacteria like E. coli. Thus, PHA ingestion "was accompanied by a reversible and PHA dose-dependent overgrowth with E. coli."[254] High doses of PHA disturb the mucus and shorten villi.[255] Feeding rats the alpha-amylase inhibitor found in kidney beans leads to extreme gut bloating:

  > "As starch digestion ... was negligible ... the cecum was practically blocked by solidified digesta.... [A]s the distension was not always sufficient, **the [intestine] was occasionally ruptured** and the rats had to be killed."[256]

- **Retarded body growth and shrinkage of organs.** Rats fed legume alpha-amylase inhibitors show impaired digestion and retarded growth.[257]

---

[252] Greer F, Pusztai A. Toxicity of kidney bean (Phaseolus vulgaris) in rats: changes in intestinal permeability. *Digestion.* 1985;32(1):42-6. *http://pmid.us/4018443.*

[253] Kordás K et al. Phytohaemagglutinin inhibits gastric acid but not pepsin secretion in conscious rats. *J Physiol Paris.* 2001 Jan-Dec;95(1-6):309-14. *http://pmid.us/11595455.*

[254] Pusztai A et al. Kidney bean lectin-induced Escherichia coli overgrowth in the small intestine is blocked by GNA, a mannose-specific lectin. *J Appl Bacteriol.* 1993 Oct;75(4):360-8. *http://pmid.us/8226393.*

[255] Prykhod'ko O et al. Precocious gut maturation and immune cell expansion by single dose feeding the lectin phytohaemagglutinin to suckling rats. *Br J Nutr.* 2009 Mar;101(5):735-42. *http://pmid.us/18644165.*

[256] Pusztai A et al. Inhibition of starch digestion by alpha-amylase inhibitor reduces the efficiency of utilization of dietary proteins and lipids and retards the growth of rats. *J Nutr.* 1995 Jun;125(6):1554-62. *http://pmid.us/7782910.*

[257] Ibid.

Feeding soybeans to rats alters organs: the "pancreas was significantly heavier while the liver was lighter in soyabean-fed rats."[258] Kidney bean lectin (PHA) given to human volunteers caused their gallbladders to contract to 2/3 normal size.[259]

- **Heart disease and tendon damage.** The human body has two enzymes called sterolins devoted to removing plant phytosterols from the body by pumping them back into the gut. People with mutations in their sterolin genes that allow phytosterols to enter the body have a disease called phytosterolemia, which results in premature atherosclerosis, early death from heart attacks, and tendon and liver damage. Soy and other legumes have high levels of phytosterols.[260]

Typical legume toxicity effects include acid reflux and gut bloating, but poorly cooked batches of legumes can trigger more severe reactions. A British hospital in 1988 offered a "healthy eating day" in its staff cafeteria and served a dish of red kidney beans. Within a few hours, eleven staff had suffered profuse vomiting, some with diarrhea. A surgical registrar vomited in the operating room. The trouble was traced to high levels of PHA.[261]

Legume Allergies

Peanut and soybean allergies are among the most common allergies.

Legume allergies can be quite serious. People with celiac disease who aren't healed by removal of wheat often turn out to have antibodies to soybeans or other legumes, and need to remove legumes from their diet as well:

> "Circulating antibodies to soya-derived protein antigens have been measured in patients with duodenitis, Crohn's disease, ulcerative colitis and coeliac disease. Significantly raised antibody titres were

---

[258] Pusztai A et al. Novel dietary strategy for overcoming the antinutritional effects of soyabean whey of high agglutinin content. *Br J Nutr.* 1997 Jun;77(6):933-45. *http://pmid.us/9227190.*

[259] Purhonen AK et al. Duodenal phytohaemagglutinin (red kidney bean lectin) stimulates gallbladder contraction in humans. *Acta Physiol (Oxf).* 2008 Jul;193(3):241-7. *http://pmid.us/18248661.*

[260] Wikipedia, *http://en.wikipedia.org/wiki/Sitosterolemia.* Stephan Guyenet, *http://wholehealthsource.blogspot.com/2009/03/margarine-and-phytosterolemia.html.*

[261] Freed DL. Do dietary lectins cause disease? *BMJ.* 1999 Apr 17;318(7190):1023-4. *http://pmid.us/10205084.*

found frequently in the coeliac group, particularly those patients showing a suboptimal response to a gluten-free diet ..."[262]

Another Issue: Industrial Processing of Legumes

Legumes are so toxic in their raw state – raw kidney beans at 1% of diet can kill rats in two weeks – that they need processing to reduce toxin levels. Traditional methods of reducing toxin levels are soaking, sprouting, boiling, and fermentation.

Modern factories rely on fast, mechanized methods to turn legumes into edible foods. Some question whether such methods are safe. Dr. John Briffa describes how soy foods are created:

> [A] slurry of soy beans is treated with acid and alkali solutions to get the protein to precipitate out. In this process the product can be tainted with the metal aluminum (aluminum exposure has been linked with an increased risk of degeneration of the nervous system and Alzheimer's disease). The resultant protein-rich 'curd' is spray dried at high temperature to produce a powder ... [and] heated and extruded under pressure to make a foodstuff known as textured vegetable protein (TVP).... TVP will often have monosodium glutamate (MSG) added to it to impart a 'meaty' flavour before it is fashioned into products such as vegetarian burgers, sausages and mince.[263]

Whether or not these industrial processing methods are safe, we prefer foods that don't need such processing.

Conclusion

Legumes are dangerous, and the dangers are not yet fully understood. Since human carbohydrate needs can easily be met with other more nutritious and healthy foods, there seems little reward to eating these plants.

---

[262] Haeney MR et al. Soya protein antibodies in man: their occurrence and possible relevance in coeliac disease. *J Clin Pathol.* 1982 Mar; 35(3):319-22. *http://pmid.us/7040491.*

[263] Dr. John Briffa, "It's not just the salt that makes many meat-substitute foods a thoroughly unhealthy option," *http://www.drbriffa.com/blog/2008/05/19/its-not-just-the-salt-that-makes-many-meat-substitute-foods-a-thoroughly-unhealthy-option/*

Liquid Devils: Vegetable Oils

Beginning in the 1950s, and especially after promotion of vegetable oil by the US government in the 1970s, many scientists embraced the idea that omega-6-rich vegetable oils would be healthy because of their cholesterol-lowering effect.

This turned out to be a fateful mistake. Dr. William E. Lands wrote,

> "We had been looking at essential ... fatty acids as 'angels' but **in excessive amounts they turn into devils.**"[264]

Vegetable oils are conveniently cheap. Unfortunately, they are toxic:

- Vegetable oils are loaded with **omega-6 fatty acids**, which are toxic in high doses. The omega-6 content of soybean oil is 55%; corn oil, 54%; safflower oil, 75%; canola oil, 18%.[265]

- Vegetable oils, especially grain and legume oils like soybean oil, peanut oil, corn oil, and wheat germ oil, also contain **plant toxins**.

The Problem of Excess Omega-6

We've already presented evidence that omega-6 fats become toxic above about 4% of calories. We won't repeat all the evidence, just two key facts:

1. Most Americans get about 10% of dietary calories from omega-6 fats, triple the safe level. This omega-6 excess is causally linked to a host of health problems, including cardiovascular disease, cancer, mental illness, and obesity, as well as to increased mortality.

2. The omega-6 excess is primarily caused by excessive intake of vegetable oils.

A casual look at the items on supermarket shelves will show how prevalent the use of vegetable oils is in industrially prepared foods. From salad dressings to cookies, soybean oil appears high on the list of ingredients.

Plant Toxins in Omega-6-Rich Vegetable Oils

Nearly all plants which contain abundant omega-6 are also full of toxins. Given our earlier discussion of grain and legume toxicity, you may not be surprised to hear that grain and legume oils are some of the most dangerous.

---

[264] Lands WE. Dietary fat and health: the evidence and the politics of prevention: careful use of dietary fats can improve life and prevent disease. *Ann N Y Acad Sci.* 2005 Dec;1055:179-92. *http://pmid.us/16387724.*

[265] Fatty acid content of vegetable oils can be found at *http://nutritiondata.com.*

PEANUT OIL AND CARDIOVASCULAR DISEASE

Giving rhesus monkeys 40% of fat calories from peanut oil induces atherosclerosis in all monkeys, and heart attacks in one-third, in 16 months. The culprit appears to be either the lectin peanut agglutinin (PNA) or toxic triglycerides that have a particular combination of a peanut phospholipid with omega-6 fats.[266]

Tree-nut oils and cocoa butter do not have this effect. Therefore, we recommend replacement of peanut butter with tree nut butters.

CORN OIL AND CARDIOVASCULAR DISEASE

Corn oil, another oil that probably contains plant toxins, is about as atherogenic as peanut oil.[267] Corn oil could be the most lethal intervention ever tested on humans in a randomized trial. In the Rose Corn Oil Trial, the death rate was 364% higher in the group eating corn oil compared to the control group eating animal and dairy fats.[268]

SOYBEAN OIL AND LIVER DAMAGE

Some babies are born with "short bowel syndrome" and need to be given "parenteral" nutrition, or nutrition delivered intravenously directly to the blood, until their digestive tracts grow and heal.

Since 1961, parenteral nutrition has used soybean oil as its source of fat.[269] And for decades, babies on parenteral nutrition have suffered devastating liver and brain damage. The death rate on soybean oil is 30% by age four.

Finally, doctors at Boston's Children's Hospital investigated whether the liver and brain damage might be due to vegetable oils. After studies in mice showed that the liver damage was due to soybean oil, they tried substituting a fish oil based formula. The results were "freaking amazing," according to a Children's Hospital doctor; parents called it "a miracle." [270]

---

[266] Kritchevsky D et al. Lectin may contribute to the atherogenicity of peanut oil. *Lipids* 1998 Aug; 33(8): 821-3. *http://pmid.us/9727614.*

[267] Kritchevsky D et al. Influence of native and randomized peanut oil on lipid metabolism and aortic sudanophilia in the vervet monkey. *Atherosclerosis.* 1982 Mar;42(1):53-8. *http://pmid.us/7082418.*

[268] Rose GA et al. Corn oil in the treatment of ischaemic heart disease. *Br Med J.* 1965 Jun 12;1(5449):1531-3. *http://pmid.us/14288105.*

[269] Waitzberg DL et al. New parenteral lipid emulsions for clinical use. *JPEN J Parenter Enteral Nutr.* 2006 Jul-Aug;30(4):351-67. *http://pmid.us/16804134.*

[270] "Old-fashioned lifeline," Boston Globe, Jan. 9, 2009, *http://www.boston.com/news/local/massachusetts/articles/2009/01/09/old_fashioned_lifeline/.*

Of 42 babies given the fish oil in a clinical trial, 3 died and 1 required a liver transplant; of 49 babies given soybean oil, 12 died and 6 required a liver transplant.[271] The death-or-liver-transplant rate was reduced from 37% with soybean oil to 9% with fish oil.

The Slow Pace of Medical Progress

Why did it take 43 years to figure out that soybean oil was killing these babies? An explanation was offered by Dr. Mark Puder of Children's Hospital:

> In trying to figure out what was causing PN [parenteral nutrition] to damage the liver, some researchers, like Children's Judah Folkman, MD, and Robert Shamberger, MD, hypothesized that the injury was due to a missing nutrient that is present in regular food. Others thought that individual components of the solutions themselves might be to blame. Over the years, each theory was ruled out …

> Fortunately for Puder, he's not an expert on PN, or he might have ruled out the lipid as the problem from the beginning…. "One of the things I didn't do was read the literature to find out what everyone else was already thinking."

> In fact, Puder didn't realize what everyone else was thinking until he began telling people about his observations, and they, in turn, began telling him he was wrong.

> "When researchers took the lipid out of PN, and it still caused liver injury, they probably assumed that some other part of the PN preparation was the culprit," he says. "They never thought to question the type of lipid they were using."[1]

Basically, supplying all calories as carbohydrates causes fatty liver disease through sugar poisoning. Replacing some of the carbs with soybean oil maintains fatty liver disease, this time due to a mix of sugar and omega-6 toxicity. The solution was to reduce carbs AND omega-6 fats, but this was never tried.

[1]   "Fishing for the right solution," Children's Hospital Boston, *http://childrenshospital.org/dream/dream_fall06/fishing_for_the_right_solution.html*

Other studies in parenteral nutrition have found that soybean oil kills immune cells. To reduce this destruction of lymphocytes, researchers are considering switching from a 100% soybean oil formula to one with 80% olive oil, 20% soybean oil. The new formula still kills immune cells, but less prodigiously.[272]

---

[271] Puder M et al. Parenteral fish oil improves outcomes in patients with parenteral nutrition-associated liver injury. *Ann Surg.* 2009 Sep;250(3):395-402. *http://pmid.us/19661785.* Gura KM et al. Reversal of parenteral nutrition-associated liver disease in two infants with short bowel syndrome using parenteral fish oil: implications for future management. *Pediatrics.* 2006 Jul;118(1):e197-201. *http://pmid.us/16818533.*

[272] Cury-Boaventura MF et al. Effect of olive oil-based emulsion on human lymphocyte and neutrophil death. *JPEN J Parenter Enteral Nutr.* 2008 Jan-Feb;32(1):81-7. *http://pmid.us/18165452.*

Toxins Introduced By Industrial Processing

Many vegetable oils undergo extensive processing to make them palatable. Canola oil (an oil invented in the 1970s and named for "Canadian Oilseed, Low-Acid"), for instance, is rapeseed oil bred and processed to remove erucic acid and glucosinolates. During processing, the oil is treated with the solvent hexane and very high temperatures; the oil may also be subject to caustic refinement, bleaching, and degumming.[273] Soybean oil, corn oil, peanut oil, safflower oil, and other vegetable oils undergo similar processing to remove toxins and odors and improve taste.

Unfortunately such processing can introduce artificial toxins. First, heating, either during the oil's original manufacture or later when foods are prepared, can hydrogenate the oil to create toxic trans-fats. Grains and legumes naturally contain omega-6 fats, and vegetable oils like soybean oil are added to many prepared foods. In baking and storage, many of these omega-6 fats convert to trans-fats. Supermarket breads, cakes, cookies, crackers, potato or corn chips, French fries, and pizza crusts often contain 10% to 40% of fat calories as trans-fats.[274] Commercial liquid canola oil can have trans-fat levels as high as 4.6%.[275] Shelf storage and cooking at home will also generate toxic trans-fats from vegetable oils.

In many prepared foods, oils are intentionally hydrogenated to extend the shelf life. Such processing not only creates unhealthy trans-fats, it also alters compounds dissolved in the oil.

For instance, the plant form of vitamin K is hydrogenated into dihydrophylloquinone in soybean and canola oil based foods. Dihydrophylloquinone is a sort of anti-vitamin: it competes with vitamin K in the body but is incapable of activating vitamin-K dependent proteins. Dihydrophylloquinone intake was associated in the Framingham Offspring Study with lower bone mineral density.[276]

---

[273] Sally Fallon & Mary Enig, "The Great Con-ola," *http://www.westonaprice.org/The-Great-Con-ola.html.*

[274] Ratnayake WM et al. Fatty acids in some common food items in Canada. *J Am Coll Nutr.* 1993 Dec;12(6):651-60. *http://pmid.us/8294720.*

[275] O'Keefe S et al. Levels of Trans Geometrical Isomers of Essential Fatty Acids in Some Unhydrogenated US Vegetable Oils. *Journal of Food Lipids* Sept 1994; 1(3):165-176. *http://www3.interscience.wiley.com/journal/119973548/abstract.*

[276] Booth SL et al. Effects of a hydrogenated form of vitamin K on bone formation and resorption. *Am J Clin Nutr.* 2001 Dec; 74(6):783-90. *http://pmid.us/11722960.* Troy LM et al. Dihydrophylloquinone intake is associated with low bone mineral density in men and women. *Am J Clin Nutr.* 2007 Aug;86(2):504-8. *http://pmid.us/17684225.*

Conclusion

Americans eat at least three times more omega-6 fats than is safe, and have a tissue omega-6 to omega-3 ratio about 10 times the optimum. The foods primarily responsible for excess omega-6 intake, vegetable seed oils, also contain natural plant toxins and artificial toxins introduced during industrial processing. Vegetable oil consumption is associated with heart disease mortality, depression, violence, cancer mortality, bowel disease, and liver damage.

Vegetable oils should be replaced in the diet by healthy fats and oils: animal fats like lard and tallow, dairy fats like butter and cream, and low-omega-6 plant oils like coconut oil, palm oil, cocoa butter, nutmeg butter, tree nut butters, olive oil, and avocado.

The Sweet Toxin: Fructose

Table sugar is composed of two sugars, glucose and fructose. Glucose, the "good" sugar, is healthy in moderation. Fructose is more dangerous.

Fructose in the diet comes from two main sources:

- **Fruit, berries, and some vegetables** (e.g. carrots).

- **Sweeteners**, like sugar and high fructose corn syrup, and sweetened products, like candies and colas.

> Sweeteners are a major product of global agriculture. Table sugar is obtained from the cane sugar plant, the world's sixth largest crop with 3.3% of agricultural production, and from beets, the twelfth largest crop with 1.7% of agricultural production. High fructose corn syrup is manufactured from corn, the world's second largest crop with 21.6% of agricultural production.

How Much Fructose Can Be Eaten, and When?

Fructose is a poison, but in small doses the liver can rapidly dispose of it, so it does no harm. The liver has two pathways for fructose disposal:

1. **Conversion to liver glycogen.** This only works when the liver's glycogen stores have space available. The liver can store a total of 70-100 g of glycogen, but never allows this reservoir to become empty.

2. **Conversion to fat.** This is a slower pathway along which most fructose toxicity occurs.

On the American diet, liver glycogen stores are probably nearly always full. After an overnight fast, there may be room to convert 15 g or so of fructose to glycogen; this is about the amount in two bananas. Breakfast, therefore, may be the safest time to consume fruit.

One benefit of a diet like the Perfect Health Diet that provides a little less glucose than the body needs is that it keeps liver glycogen a little depleted. This makes the body more tolerant of the modest amounts of fructose in fruits, berries, and vegetables.

Sugar and high fructose corn syrup are best avoided. They just add up too quickly. A large cola contains about 45 g of fructose – far beyond the liver's capacity for glycogen conversion. One cup (8 fluid ounces) of soda contains six times more fructose than a cup of raspberries.

There is another danger with fructose. Fructose reacts with polyunsaturated fats to create toxic products. Therefore, fruits and sweets are best eaten on an empty stomach, between meals; and should be combined only with cream or coconut oil, which are very low in polyunsaturated fats, not omega-6 or omega-3 containing fats.

Fructose Is a Poison

In an excellent talk which the University of California has posted on Youtube[277], Dr. Robert H. Lustig explains that fructose has all the characteristics of poison: It damages the body, provides no benefit, and is shunted directly to the liver for disposal in order to keep it away from the rest of the body.

This sharply contrasts to the way glucose is handled. Glucose from food is allowed to bypass the liver and proceed into the bloodstream.

"High Fructose Corn Syrup and sucrose ... are both dangerous.... It goes way beyond empty calories.... [F]ructose is a poison. It's not about the calories, has nothing to do with the calories. It's a poison by itself." (Dr. Robert H. Lustig, at 21:00)

One of the primary mechanisms by which fructose poisons is by reacting with proteins to form "advanced glycation endproducts" (AGEs) that disrupt normal functions. Fructose is seven times more likely than glucose to cross-link with proteins to form AGEs.[278] AGEs cross-link collagen for stiff joints and aged skin, damage DNA, hasten aging[279], stiffen vessels to cause high blood pressure, and cause kidney disease.[280]

Fructose Poisons the Liver And Ruins Blood Lipids

The liver detoxifies excess fructose by converting it to fat. As more fructose is eaten, the liver is poisoned and becomes fatty, a condition known as non-alcoholic fatty liver disease or NAFLD. Since the liver processes fructose the same way it processes alcohol, fructose generates almost the same litany of problems as alcohol abuse: high blood pressure, bad lipid profiles, heart attacks, pancreatitis, obesity, cirrhosis, and fetal insulin resistance.[281]

Liver damage deranges the metabolism, creating *metabolic syndrome*, the first step toward diabetes and obesity, and a blood lipid profile characteristic of high risk for cardiovascular disease. For instance, shifting 25% of dietary calories from

---

[277] Lustig RH, *http://www.youtube.com/watch?v=dBnniua6-oMl*.

[278] Gaby, AR, Adverse effects of dietary fructose. *Alt Med Rev.* 2005 Dec; 10(4): 294-306. *http://pmid.us/16366738*; Schalkwijk, CG et al. Fructose-mediated non-enzymatic glycation: sweet coupling or bad modification. *Diabetes Metab Res Rev.* 2004 Sep-Oct;20(5):369-82. *http://pmid.us/15343583*.

[279] Hipkiss, AR. Dietary restriction, glycolysis, hormesis and ageing. *Biogerontology.* 2007 Apr;8(2):221-4. *http://pmid.us/16969712*.

[280] Gaby, AR, Adverse effects of dietary fructose. *Alt Med Rev.* 2005 Dec; 10(4): 294-306. *http://pmid.us/16366738*.

[281] Lustig RH, *http://www.youtube.com/watch?v=dBnniua6-oMl*.

glucose to fructose raises small dense LDL, the worst blood lipid, by 45%; increases post-meal triglycerides 100%; and increases abdominal fat 4-fold faster than glucose.[282]

A study compared rats fed a diet of 60% fructose with rats fed conventional chow.[283] After 5 weeks, the fructose-fed rats had 15% higher blood pressure, 198% higher blood triglycerides, and 90% higher blood cholesterol. In humans, when overweight women were fed 25% of calories in the form of fructose for ten weeks, there was a 140% increase in circulating triglyceride levels.[284]

Fructose Causes Gout and Kidney Disease

The first step in fructose detoxification is its conversion to fructose-1-phospate. The phosphate is drawn from the energy molecule ATP (adenosine triphosphate), creating a shortage of phosphate and excess of adenosine. The adenosine is disposed of by conversion to uric acid which is released to the blood. High levels of fructose consumption beget high levels of uric acid.

This is problematic because humans, along with dogs and apes, are the only species lacking the enzyme uricase which breaks down uric acid. Fructose consumption therefore leads to an accumulation of uric acid crystals in the joints, causing intense pain, a condition called gout.[285] People with impaired fructose metabolism get gout at a high rate.[286]

---

[282] Stanhope KL et al. Consuming fructose-sweetened, not glucose-sweetened, beverages increases visceral adiposity and lipids and decreases insulin sensitivity in overweight/obese humans. *J Clin Invest* 2009 May;119(5):1322-34. *http://pmid.us/19381015.* Teff KL et al. Dietary fructose reduces circulating insulin and leptin, attenuates postprandial suppression of ghrelin, and increases triglycerides in women. *J Clin Endocrinol Metab.* 2004 Jun;89(6):2963-72. *http://pmid.us/15181085.*

[283] Ackerman Z et al. Fructose-induced fatty liver disease: hepatic effects of blood pressure and plasma triglyceride reduction. *Hypertension.* 2005 May;45(5):1012-8. *http://pmid.us/15824194.*

[284] Stanhope KL, Havel PJ. Endocrine and metabolic effects of consuming beverages sweetened with fructose, glucose, sucrose, or high-fructose corn syrup. *Am J Clin Nutr.* 2008 Dec; 88(6): 1733S-1737S. *http://pmid.us/19064538.* Stanhope KL et al. Consuming fructose-sweetened, not glucose-sweetened, beverages increases visceral adiposity and lipids and decreases insulin sensitivity in overweight/obese humans. *J Clin Invest* 2009 May;119(5):1322-34. *http://pmid.us/19381015.*

[285] Underwood M. Sugary drinks, fruit, and increased risk of gout. *BMJ* 2008 Feb 9;336(7639):285-286. *http://pmid.us/18258933.*

[286] Seegmiller JE et al. Fructose-induced aberration of metabolism in familial gout identified by 31P magnetic resonance spectroscopy. *Proc Natl Acad Sci U S A.* 1990 Nov;87(21):8326-30. *http://pmid.us/2236043.*

Fructose, by way of uric acid, may be a major cause of kidney disease.[287]

Fructose Causes Metabolic Syndrome and Diabetes

Partly through its elevation of uric acid and partly through liver poisoning, fructose causes high blood pressure and metabolic syndrome.[288] Since metabolic syndrome is the first and crucial step toward diabetes, fructose may be a leading cause of diabetes.

Indeed, fructose intake is proportional to diabetes rates in countries worldwide[289], and the 8.7-fold rise in diabetes incidence since 1935 coincided with a 6-fold to 20-fold rise in fructose consumption.[290]

Fructose Causes Obesity

The "glycemic index," a measure of how much a food raises blood sugar, is a rough indicator of how much a food fattens. However, it doesn't account for the intensely fattening nature of fructose, which contributes little to blood sugar because it is shunted to the liver and converted directly to fat.

Yet fructose is extremely effective at inducing obesity. Each additional daily soft drink increases the rate of obesity by 60%[291], and reduction of soft drink consumption in British schoolchildren by only one-fifth of a glass (50 ml) per day reduced the number of overweight and obese children by 7.5%.[292] A review of 88

---

[287] Johnson RJ et al. Potential role of sugar (fructose) in the epidemic of hypertension, obesity and the metabolic syndrome, diabetes, kidney disease, and cardiovascular disease. *Am J Clin Nutr.* 2007 Oct;86(4):899-906. *http://pmid.us/17921363.*

[288] Perez-Poso et al. Excessive fructose intake induces the features of metabolic syndrome in healthy adult men: role of uric acid in the hypertensive response. *Int J Obes (Lond).* 2010 Mar;34(3):454-61. *http://pmid.us/20029377.* Nakagawa T et al. A causal role for uric acid in fructose-induced metabolic syndrome. *Am J Physiol Renal Physiol.* 2006 Mar;290(3):F625-31. *http://pmid.us/16234313.*

[289] Johnson RJ et al. Hypothesis: could excessive fructose intake and uric acid cause type 2 diabetes? *Endocr Rev.* 2009 Feb;30(1):96-116. *http://pmid.us/19151107.*

[290] 20-fold: Gross, LS et al: Increased consumption of refined carbohydrates and the epidemic of type 2 diabetes in the United States: an ecologic assessment. *Am J Clin Nutr* 2004;79: 774–9. *http://pmid.us/15113714.* 6-fold: Bray GA. How bad is fructose? *Am J Clin Nutr.* 2007 Oct;86(4):895-6. *http://pmid.us/17921361.*

[291] Ludwig DS et al. Relation between consumption of sugar-sweetened drinks and childhood obesity: a prospective, observational analysis. *Lancet.* 2001 Feb 17;357(9255):505-8. *http://pmid.us/11229668.*

[292] James J et al. Preventing childhood obesity by reducing consumption of carbonated drinks: cluster randomised controlled trial. *BMJ.* 2004 May 22;328(7450):1237. *http://pmid.us/15107313.*

studies found that higher intakes of soft drinks was associated with greater caloric consumption, higher body weight, lower intake of other nutrients and worse indicators of health.[293]

A possible mechanism was discovered when it was shown that fructose causes leptin resistance. Leptin is a hormone that normally causes fat reduction, quickened metabolism, and weight loss, but leptin-resistant people don't respond to leptin and tend to become obese.[294]

For the benefit of those seeking to lose weight, some have recommended replacing the glycemic index with a new "fructose index":

> "[S]tarch-based foods don't cause weight gain like sugar-based foods and don't cause the metabolic syndrome like sugar-based foods," said Dr. Richard Johnson…. "Potatoes, pasta, rice may be relatively safe compared to table sugar. A fructose index may be a better way to assess the risk of carbohydrates related to obesity."[295]

Fructose Poisons the Body and the Brain

When ingested in large quantities, fructose spills out of the liver and poisons the whole body, a problem that is especially severe in diabetics. The brain is impacted: A high fructose diet impairs memory in rats.[296] Fructose also increases the blood pressure and shortens the lifespan of rats.[297]

Fructose poisoning is most damaging in diabetics. Organ damage in diabetes comes from glycation of proteins, creating "advanced glycation endproducts" that trigger oxidation of other proteins and can render tissues dysfunctional. But

---

[293] Vartanian LR, et al. Effects of soft drink consumption on nutrition and health: a systematic review and meta-analysis. *Am J Public Health.* 2007 Apr;97(4):667-75. *http://pmid.us/17329656.*

[294] Shapiro A et al. Fructose-induced leptin resistance exacerbates weight gain in response to subsequent high-fat feeding. *Am J Physiol Regul Integr Comp Physiol.* 2008 Nov;295(5):R1370-5. *http://pmid.us/18703413.*

[295] "Too Much Fructose Could Leave Dieters Sugar Shocked," *ScienceDaily,* *http://www.sciencedaily.com/releases/2007/12/071212201311.htm.* Segal MS et al. Is the fructose index more relevant with regards to cardiovascular disease than the glycemic index? *Eur J Nutr.* 2007 Oct;46(7):406-17. *http://pmid.us/17763967.*

[296] Ross AP et al. A high fructose diet impairs spatial memory in male rats. *Neurobiol Learn Mem.* 2009 Oct;92(3):410-6. *http://pmid.us/19500683.*

[297] Preuss HG. Effects of diets containing different proportions of macronutrients on longevity of normotensive Wistar rats. *Geriatr Nephrol Urol.* 1997;7(2):81-6. *http://pmid.us/9422703.*

fructose is far more likely to glycate and oxidize proteins than glucose.[298] Fructose consumption by diabetics is particularly associated with retinopathy – a major cause of blindness.[299]

Fructose Feeds Bacteria

Fructose also promotes bacterial infections. Human cells are not generally able to use fructose, but bacteria can and do metabolize it. Fructose consumption is therefore a risk factor for overgrowth of bad gut bacteria and for chronic bacterial infections within the liver and body generally.

Intriguing evidence for the possibility that fructose, but not glucose, consumption leads to bacterial infection of the liver comes from a recent study. In mice, as in humans, fructose causes fatty liver disease while glucose does not. Intriguingly, blood endotoxin levels, a bacterial waste product, were higher in mice consuming fructose than in all other groups, and "treatment of fructose fed mice with antibiotics ... markedly reduced hepatic lipid accumulation."[300] This suggests the possibility that fatty liver disease stems from bacterial infection, either in the liver or in the gut with the liver damage mediated by endotoxins that travel from the gut to the blood. If that is so, then fructose avoidance would cure a fatty liver.

Chronic infections have been linked to a host of diseases. Any dietary factor which feeds infections is likely to degrade health.

Conclusion

Fructose in small quantities – say, the amount in a few pieces of fruit per day – is nothing to be concerned about. We believe 50 calories of fructose per day is a reasonable upper limit.

But "the dose makes the poison," and the large quantities of sugar and high-fructose corn syrup that most Americans eat are highly toxic. Fructose-induced liver damage, aggravated by excess omega-6 vegetable oils, may be at the root of the current epidemic of metabolic syndrome, obesity, and diabetes. Fructose also promotes chronic infections which may be behind many diseases of aging, such as dementia.

---

[298] Takagi Y. Significance of fructose-induced protein oxidation and formation of advanced glycation end product. *J Diabetes Complications* 1995 Apr-Jun; 9(2): 87-91, *http://pmid.us/7599353.*

[299] Kawasaki T et al. Postprandial plasma fructose level is associated with retinopathy in patients with type 2 diabetes. *Metabolism* 2004 May; 53(5): 583-8, *http://pmid.us/15131761.*

[300] Bergheim I et al. Antibiotics protect against fructose-induced hepatic lipid accumulation in mice: role of endotoxin. *J Hepatol.* 2008 Jun; 48(6): 983-92. *http://pmid.us/18395289.*

Other Sources of Food Toxicity

Removing the four major toxic foods – grains, legumes, sugars, and vegetable oils – will remove the bulk of the food toxins in most diets. A few further steps can reduce toxin levels even more.

Avoid Sugar-Cured Meats

All meats are safe to eat in their natural state, fresh from the animal. However, meats may become dangerous after industrial processing.

There is evidence for health dangers from industrially processed meats. An epidemiological study reports that while beef, pork, and lamb do not increase disease rates, a daily hot dog, or equivalent weight of processed deli meat, raises the risk of heart disease by 42% and risk of diabetes by 19%. The lead author notes that "processed meats contained, on average, 4 times more sodium and 50% more nitrate preservatives.... [D]ifferences in salt and preservatives ... might explain the higher risk of heart disease and diabetes seen with processed meats, but not with unprocessed red meats."[301] If nitrates are responsible, then supplemental vitamin C would help prevent toxicity, since vitamin C inhibits nitrosation.[302]

Other authorities argue that nitrates, which are abundant in leafy green vegetables, are beneficial, and that a more likely culprit is the sugar used in curing to impart flavor and color. Toxic sugar compounds known as advanced glycation endproducts (AGEs) are abundant in processed meats.[303]

We recommend limiting processed meat intake. Fresh meats are preferable. We eat uncured bacon and smoked salmon, but do not eat meats cured with sugar.

Nightshades

Nightshades – eggplant, tomato, peppers, and potato – have high toxin levels in leaves, but toxin levels in eggplant, tomato, and pepper fruits and potato tubers are low and do not seem to cause problems for most people.

---

[301] Micha R et al. Red and Processed Meat Consumption and Risk of Incident Coronary Heart Disease, Stroke, and Diabetes Mellitus. A Systematic Review and Meta-Analysis. *Circulation.* 2010 May 17. [Epub ahead of print] *http://pmid.us/20479151.* "Eating processed meats, but not unprocessed red meats, may raise risk of heart disease and diabetes, study finds." *ScienceDaily.* June 6, 2010, *http://www.sciencedaily.com/releases/2010/05/100517161130.htm.*

[302] Ward MH. Too much of a good thing? Nitrate from nitrogen fertilizers and cancer. *Rev Environ Health.* 2009 Oct-Dec;24(4):357-63. *http://pmid.us/20384045.*

[303] Stephan Guyenet, "Nitrate: A Protective Factor in Leafy Greens," June 10, 2010, *http://wholehealthsource.blogspot.com/2010/06/nitrate-protective-factor-in-leafy.html.*

The medical literature does not contain reports of nightshade poisoning, but anecdotally some people report sensitivity to these foods. A writer for the Weston A. Price Foundation suggests that nightshade toxins promote calcification of soft tissues and arthritic symptoms, and recommends that anyone with arthritis, sclerodoma, or muscle and bone pain test for nightshade sensitivity by removing nightshades from the diet entirely for six weeks, followed by a "nightshade party day" – salsa and eggs for breakfast, tomato and eggplant for lunch, potatoes for dinner. If symptoms improve on the nightshade free diet and return with the party, this indicates nightshade sensitivity.[304]

Keep Safe Starches Safe

Starchy foods, attractive to insects and herbivores due to their calorie content, often generate toxins. However, some – the ones we call "safe starches" – become nearly toxin-free with proper preparation.

Our "safe starches" include taro, white rice, sweet potatoes, yams, well-handled potatoes, sago, and tapioca. Safe starches are a nutritious and important part of the Perfect Health Diet. They provide glucose without fructose; resistant starch which improves gut health; and useful minerals like potassium.

Cooking can eliminate toxins by rendering proteins digestible. Starchy plants that are rendered safe by cooking include:

- **Taro.**[305]

- **Cassava.** Cassava contains toxic cyanogenic glucosides and improper preparation causes a disease called *konzo*. Cooking destroys most cassava toxins. **Tapioca** is made from cassava.

- **White rice.** "Antinutrition factors in the rice grain … include phytin (phytate), trypsin inhibitor, oryzacystatin and haemagglutinin-lectin…. All the antinutrition factors are proteins and all except phytin (phytate) are subject to heat denaturation. Phytin … is responsible for the observed poorer mineral balance of subjects fed brown rice diets in comparison to that of subjects fed milled rice diets."[306]

---

[304] Garrett Smith, "Nightshades," *Wise Traditions in Food, Farming and the Healing Arts*, Spring 2010, *http://www.westonaprice.org/Nightshades.html*.

[305] Seo YJ, et al. (1990) "The effect of lectin from Taro tuber (Colocasia antiquorum) given by force-feeding on the growth of mice." *J Nutr Sci Vitaminol (Tokyo)*, vol. 36, no. 3 (Jun.), pp. 277-285. *http://pmid.us/2292730*.

[306] Bienvenido O. Juliano (1993) *Rice in Human Nutrition*, Rome, Italy: Food and Agriculture Organization of the United Nations, *http://www.fao.org/inpho/content/documents//vlibrary/t0567e/T0567E0g.htm*

We recommend avoiding brown rice because of the phytin, mentioned above, and because rice protein – found primarily in the bran – has been found to provoke an immune response, implying toxicity. No antibodies to rice proteins have ever been identified, however, so it appears that rice toxicity cannot progress to severe disease in the way wheat toxicity can.[307]

Other plants can be kept safe with proper handling. **Potato** toxins solanine and chaconine are generated under exposure to heat and light. At low doses, these toxins are efficiently cleared from the body. Thus, potatoes kept continuously in cool dark conditions are safe. Discolored potatoes should be discarded.

Possibly Safe Starches

Some other starch sources, such as quinoa, buckwheat, and amaranth, may be safe, but lack of widespread human consumption and lack of investigation by scientists makes us reluctant to give them an unqualified endorsement.

A discussion with reader contributions may be found on our blog.[308]

Cook for Low Toxicity

High temperature can modify polyunsaturated fats and proteins, creating toxic compounds. The black chemicals on the surface of meat grilled at very high temperatures are toxic, for instance. It is safest to cook meats at lower temperatures.

Be Wary of Genetically Modified Foods

Breeding has made some plants less toxic. Wild almonds contain amygdalin, a chemical that turns into cyanide in the body. Eating only a few wild almonds may be lethal. However, breeding has eliminated amygdalin from domesticated almonds, making them relatively safe.[309]

Genetic engineering holds the promise to improve upon breeding as a means for removing plant toxins. Removal of lectins, alpha-amylase inhibitors, opioids, and modification of gliadin to reduce its immunogenicity may eventually make wheat into a safe starch.

---

[307] Mehr SS et al. Rice: a common and severe cause of food protein-induced enterocolitis syndrome. *Arch Dis Child.* 2009 Mar;94(3):220-3. *http://pmid.us/18957470.*

[308] "The Oldest Profession: Quinoa, Millett, and Emmer and Einkorn Wheat," September 20, 2010, *http://perfecthealthdiet.com/?p=582.*

[309] Mark Rieger, *Introduction to Fruit Crops* (New York: Food Products Press, 2006). Cited by Gregory Cochran & Henry Harpending, *The 10,000 Year Explosion: How Civilization Accelerated Human Evolution* (New York: Basic Books, 2009), p 17.

Unfortunately, to date genetic modifications of agricultural crops have not been made for the purpose of increasing their safety to humans, but rather to *increase their toxicity to insects*. Such modifications may increase crop yields, but are not likely to improve human health.

There are valid concerns that genetically modified cereal grains may be more toxic to humans than their (already toxic) wild ancestors. (See text box for more.)

The Uncertain Safety of Genetically Modified Foods

One strategy in genetic modification efforts has been to protect crop plants from insects by incorporating pesticides from other plant species into crop plant genomes.

Most genetically modified crops have been tested in animals for only **90 days**, which may be too little time to detect negative health effects.

Such is the complexity of biology that seemingly innocuous genetic alterations can have far-reaching effects. A good example of this is provided by the "Pusztai affair."

In the 1990s an English biotechnology company developed a genetically modified potato by adding the gene for a lectin from the snowdrop plant. Snowdrop lectin is highly toxic to insects but, by itself, safe for mammals.

Árpád Pusztai, a leading expert on plant lectins, tested the new genetically modified potatoes. Rats fed ordinary potatoes mixed with snowdrop lectin remained healthy, but rats fed the genetically modified potatoes developed damage to their intestines and immune systems. The damage was not due to snowdrop lectins, but to derangement of potato biology from alterations to gene expression. The modification had triggered much higher expression of native potato toxins.

No biologist would be shocked at this result: gene networks are intricately connected, and seemingly minor changes to regulatory sequences can have far-reaching effects.

What was shocking, however, was the response to Pusztai's findings. Pusztai and his research team lost their jobs at a British government research institute. A House of Commons committee attacked Pusztai. Pusztai was blocked from publishing his work, though after new data was collected the results appeared in the *Lancet* after an extraordinary review process. Pusztai found employment in the United States, his collaborator Stanley Ewen was pushed to retirement, and the *Lancet* editor was threatened. Allegedly, pressure had been applied from Prime Minister Tony Blair and US President Bill Clinton to suppress the findings on behalf of the genetically modified food industry. The biotech company went out of business.

Wikipedia, "Arpad Pusztai," *http://en.wikipedia.org/wiki/%C3%81rp%C3%A1d_Pusztai*. Ewen, SW. Pusztai, A. Effect of diets containing genetically modified potatoes expressing Galanthus nivalis lectin on rat small intestine. *Lancet*. 1999 Oct 16; 354(9187): 1353-4. *http://pmid.us/10533866*.

What's the best way to detoxify genetically modified grains? Let animals eat them first. In Ohio before the steamboat, when it was prohibitively expensive to carry corn to market, pigs were called "walking corn" since they could profitably be driven to market. We could with equal justice say that bacon is "healthy corn."

"Paleo"-Style Eating For Low Toxicity

"Paleo" style eating, which avoids "Neolithic" foods like cereal grains and vegetable oils, has been recommended on the basis that most of our evolutionary past was spent eating the Paleolithic way. But how do Paleolithic diets stack up in terms of toxicity?

Our Paleolithic Ancestors and Toxic Foods

Paleolithic hunter-gatherers did sometimes eat toxic foods. Clear evidence for the grinding of cereal grains has been found at a site in Israel dating to 21,500 BC[310], and sorghum grain residues have also been found on stone tools at a site in Mozambique, Africa dating to 103,000 BC.[311] Middle Stone Age Africans used sorghum grasses for bedding, kindling, and (possibly) baskets, and may occasionally have prepared and cooked sorghum grains, though there is no direct evidence of this.

However, Paleolithic diets were much less toxic than modern diets, for several reasons:

1. Plant foods were generally less than 35% of the diet by calories, compared to 55% in the western diet.

2. Paleolithic hunter-gatherers ate a much wider variety of plant foods – hundreds of species[312], rather than a handful as in western diets – so the quantity of any one toxin was far lower. Since "the dose makes the poison," this reduces the toxicity of the diet dramatically.

3. The most toxic foods in the modern diet were not available:

   a. Grains and legumes were only eaten seasonally, not stored for year-round consumption. Nor were they eaten in quantity even when in season: since grains require laborious processing and cooking, they were probably backup or "starvation" foods.

---

[310] Piperno DR et al. Processing of wild cereal grains in the Upper Palaeolithic revealed by starch grain analysis. *Nature.* 2004 Aug 5; 430(7000): 670-3. *http://pmid.us/15295598.*

[311] Mercader J. Mozambican grass seed consumption during the Middle Stone Age. *Science* 2009 Dec 18; 326:1680-1683. *http://pmid.us/20019285.* See also: *http://sciencenow.sciencemag.org/cgi/content/full/sciencenow;2009/1217/2.*

[312] Gordon Hillman found archaeological residues from 157 plant species at the village of the Paleolithic hunter-gatherers at Abu Hureyra, Syria, and believed that at least another hundred species must have been eaten that left no residues. Source: Hillman, G.C. 2000. The plant food economy of Abu Huraya 1 and 2. In *Village on the Euphrates* (ed. A.M.T. Moore, G.C. Hillman & A.J. Legge), pp 327-99. Oxford: Oxford University Press.

b. Aside from honey and fruits, there were no available sources of fructose. The discovery of how to crystallize sugar cane was not made until 350 AD, and as late as 1500 AD imports of sugar into Europe were only a few tons.[313]

c. High-omega-6 vegetable oils did not enter the human diet until industrial processing methods were available to remove toxins and concentrate the oils. For instance, canola oil was not invented until the 1970s. Paleolithic fats were overwhelmingly from animals, though some plant oils – palm oil, coconut oil, tree nut oils, olive oil – were probably extracted. For instance, Mesolithic American Indians extracted hickory nut oil.[314]

4. Paleolithic hunter-gatherers, like modern hunter-gatherers, probably prepared plant foods in ways that reduced the toxin load. For instance, seeds may have been soaked in water overnight to start the germination process, or fermented. Modern industrial food processing, on the other hand, tends to be optimized for speed rather than health.

Eating Paleo-style – excluding grains, legumes, vegetable oils, and sugars; and eating a diverse array of plant foods – naturally generates a diet very low in food toxins.

Health Benefits of Paleo-Style Eating

So Paleolithic diets had a very low toxin load. If we are right that reducing the level of food toxins is important for modern health, then:

- Paleolithic humans should have been notably healthy, while Neolithic humans who adopted grains and legumes as staples should have experienced impaired health.

- Modern humans who eat Paleo-style should experience improved health.

Evidence from both sources is consistent with the idea that adoption of low-toxicity diets can yield dramatic, unexpected gains in health.

Paleolithic Health, Neolithic Decline

Paleoanthropologists have always commented on the tall stature and healthy bones of Paleolithic skeletons.

Most skeletal evidence comes from the Upper Paleolithic, the period after humans expanded from East Africa and the Near East into Eurasia about 50,000 years ago.

---

[313] Bairoch, P. (1995) *Economics and World History: Myths and Paradoxes*, Chicago: University of Chicago Press, p 93. *http://books.google.com/books?id=LaF_cCknJScC.*
[314] *http://www.stonepages.com/news/archives/001708.html.*

The Upper Paleolithic is divided into two stages:

- The early stage (the "EUP") lasted from about 40,000 BC to the Last Glacial Maximum (LGM) about 18,000 BC.

- The late stage (the "LUP") lasted from the LGM at 18,000 BC to the global warming that ended the Paleolithic about 9,600 BC.

Paleolithic Health: Evidence from Stature

EUP humans were tall and slender. EUP men averaged 174.1 cm (5'9") in height, women 161.8 cm (5'4").[1] Another review gives heights about an inch taller.[2]

After the LGM in Europe, heights lessened and bodies became stockier; perhaps this was in part an adaptation to cold, or perhaps it was driven by higher population densities and less rich nutrition. LUP men in Europe averaged 165.3 cm (5'5") while LUP men along the Nile averaged 170.2 cm (5'7"); LUP women in Europe averaged 154.5 cm (5'1") while LUP women along the Nile averaged 162.4 cm (5'4").

At lower latitudes there was no strong trend toward shorter heights. Some Epipaleolithic (10,500 BC to 8,500 BC) Natufians were as tall as EUP Europeans.

[1] Holt BM, Formicola V. Hunters of the Ice Age: The biology of Upper Paleolithic people. *Am J Phys Anthropol.* 2008;Suppl 47:70-99. *http://pmid.us/19003886.*

[2] Formicola V, Giannecchini M. 1999. Evolutionary trends of stature in Upper Paleolithic and Mesolithic Europe. *J Hum Evol.* 1999 Mar;36(3):319-33. *http://pmid.us/10074386.*

Throughout the Upper Paleolithic, skeletons indicate that humans were notably healthy. Cavities were rare, and signs of malnutrition or stress in bones were also rare, though they became more common in the LUP:

> With few exceptions, oral health conditions remain good in the LUP.... The generally good health conditions observed in UP dentition also characterize other parts of the skeleton. Signs of infectious diseases are extremely infrequent....
>
> Enamel hypoplasias are infrequent and of low intensity in EUP material from ... Europe ...
>
> In conclusion, specific and nonspecific stress indicators emphasize the concept, evidenced by previous studies, of UP groups as healthy people, but also point to differences through time. In particular, LUP samples show an increase in frequency but not in severity of enamel hypoplasia and Harris lines, compared to EUP. Caries become less sporadic in the LUP, indicating a possible increase in consumption of vegetal food rich in carbohydrates.[315]

---

[315] Holt BM, Formicola V. Hunters of the Ice Age: The biology of Upper Paleolithic people. *Am J Phys Anthropol.* 2008;Suppl 47:70-99. *http://pmid.us/19003886.*

Holt & Formicola point out that the slight deteriorations in health and stature of the LUP were minor compared to what occurred later:

> It is important to point out, however, that differences in nutritional status during the UP in no way approximate those seen in more recent prehistoric times.[316]

The adoption of farming in the Neolithic greatly increased toxin loads. Farmers needed crops that yielded many calorie-rich seeds from each seed planted, so the harvest could feed the farmer's family for a year and supply seeds for sowing in the spring. This meant grains and legumes – the most toxic foods.

If our thesis that eliminating natural food toxins is a key to health is true, then we should see that Neolithic health deteriorated.

And it did. After the adoption of agriculture, stature lessened; smaller tendon attachments show that muscles weakened; bone and teeth pathologies, such as cavities and osteoporosis, became common; hypoplasias show that periods of malnutrition were common; and signs of infections and inflammation become common.

The evidence is scattered in journal articles, unpublished anthropology Ph.D. theses, and in books such as *Paleopathology at the Origins of Agriculture* (1984, by Mark Nathan Cohen and George J. Armelagos), *Bioarchaeology: Interpreting Behavior from the Human Skeleton* (1999, by Clark Larsen), and *The Backbone of History: Health and Nutrition in the Western Hemisphere* (2002, Richard H. Steckel and Jerome C. Rose, eds.). A large-scale systematic study, "The history of European health project," is now underway.[317] A few tidbits:

- Average height dropped, reaching bottom at about 5'3" for men, 5'0" for women around 3,000 BC – about five inches shorter than in the EUP.[318]

- Bones from the Neolithic site of Ganj Dareh in Israel, studied by the anthropologist Anagnostis Agelarakis, showed hypoplasias on the teeth, indicative of malnutrition when young; signs of ear infections and gum

---

[316] Holt & Formicola, citing Brennan, MU. *Health and disease in the Middle and Upper Paleolithic of southwestern France: A bioarchaeological study*. PhD dissertation, New York University, 1991.

[317] Steckel RH et al. The history of European health project: a history of health in Europe from the late paleolithic era to the present. *Acta Univ Carol Med Monogr*. 2009;156:19-25. *http://pmid.us/20063662*.

[318] Jared Diamond, "The Worst Mistake in the History of the Human Race," *Discover* 8, no. 5 (1987): 64-66.

inflammation; broken or fractured bones; and arthritis.   Those who survived childhood struggled to reach middle age.[319]

- Nine of sixteen Bronze Age mummies – and seven of the eight that died after age 45 – in the Museum of Egyptian Antiquities, Cairo, had atherosclerosis.[320]

Clinical Trials: Toxin Elimination is a Key to Health

Clinical trials of Paleolithic diets have only recently been undertaken. Results have been remarkable: health improvements have been unexpectedly large.

For instance, a study led by Swedish doctor Staffan Lindeberg found that "a Paleolithic diet improved glycemic control and several cardiovascular risk factors compared to a Diabetes diet in patients with type 2 diabetes."[321] A Paleo diet outperformed the standard diet recommended to diabetics.

Paleo-style eating seems to rapidly cure metabolic syndrome, induce weight loss in the obese, and improve biomarkers in diabetics. One paper concludes:

> It is difficult to refute the assertion that if modern populations returned to a hunter-gatherer state then obesity and diabetes would not be the major public health threats they now are.[322]

These early trials suggest the importance of eliminating food toxins for good health. One study, which differed substantially from the Perfect Health Diet in having lots of carbs (1000 carb calories per day) and disappointingly high levels of fructose from honey and carrot juice, is helpful because both the "Paleo" arm and the control arm ate the same macronutrient ratios. So the improved lipid profiles, glucose tolerance, and blood pressure seen in the "Paleo" arm were likely due to elimination of food toxins from grains and legumes. The improvements came quickly – in days:

---

[319] Agelarakis, Anagnostis. *The Palaeopathological Evidence: Indicators of Stress of the Shanidar Proto-Neolithic and the Ganj-Dareh Tepe Early Neolithic Human Skeletal Collections*, Ph.D. dissertation, Columbia University, 1989. Summary in Mithen, Steven (2004) *After the Ice: A Global Human History, 20,000-5000 BC*, Cambridge: Harvard University Press, p 424.

[320] Allam AH et al. Computed tomographic assessment of atherosclerosis in ancient Egyptian mummies. *JAMA.* 2009 Nov 18;302(19):2091-4. *http://pmid.us/19920233.*

[321] Jönsson T et al. Beneficial effects of a Paleolithic diet on cardiovascular risk factors in type 2 diabetes: a randomized cross-over pilot study. *Cardiovasc Diabetol.* 2009 Jul 16;8:35. *http://pmid.us/19604407.* Hat tip Stephan Guyenet, *http://wholehealthsource.blogspot.com/2009/09/paleolithic-diet-clinical-trials-part.html.*

[322] O'Rahilly S. Human genetics illuminates the paths to metabolic disease. *Nature.* 2009 Nov 19;462(7271):307-14. *http://pmid.us/19924209.*

Even short-term consumption of a paleolithic type diet improves BP and glucose tolerance, decreases insulin secretion, increases insulin sensitivity and improves lipid profiles ... in healthy sedentary humans.[323]

Another trial, comparing a Paleolithic diet with a Mediterranean diet among Type II diabetes patients, similarly found that elimination of toxic foods benefits health, even if macronutrient ratios are unchanged. The authors concluded:

The larger improvement of glucose tolerance in the Paleolithic group was independent of energy intake and macronutrient composition, which suggests that **avoiding Western foods is more important than counting calories, fat, carbohydrate or protein**. The study adds to the notion that healthy diets based on whole-grain cereals and low-fat dairy products are only the second best choice in the prevention and treatment of type 2 diabetes. (emphasis added)[324]

Note that the diet containing whole-grain cereals, though described as "healthy," was inferior to the diet that had no grains at all.

Conclusion

Science is only beginning to understand the far-reaching impact of natural food toxins on human health. However, it seems likely that almost everyone's health would greatly improve by completely excluding the four major toxic foods – grains, legumes, sugars, and vegetable oils – from the diet.

Paleolithic diets are healthier than modern diets, and lower levels of food toxins are probably the reason. We hope we've persuaded you to reduce the toxicity of your diet.

---

[323] Frassetto LA et al. Metabolic and physiologic improvements from consuming a paleolithic, hunter-gatherer type diet. *Eur J Clin Nutr.* 2009 Aug;63(8):947-55. *http://pmid.us/19209185.*

[324] Lindeberg S et al. A Palaeolithic diet improves glucose tolerance more than a Mediterranean-like diet in individuals with ischaemic heart disease. *Diabetologia.* 2007 Sep;50(9):1795-807. *http://pmid.us/17583796.* Hat tip Stephan Guyenet, *http://wholehealthsource.blogspot.com/2008/10/paleolithic-diet-clinical-trials.html* and *http://wholehealthsource.blogspot.com/2008/10/paleolithic-diet-clinical-trials-part.html.*

Ideas For Non-Toxic Eating

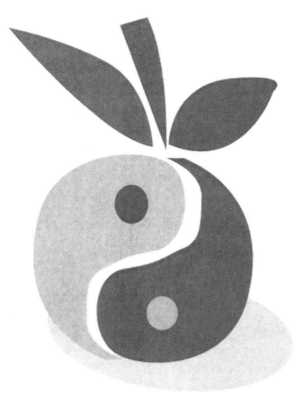

How To Replace Grains

Cereal for breakfast, sandwiches for lunch, pasta for dinner – these are all very convenient foods. When people first try to give up grains, they often find themselves at a loss for replacements.

Here are a few ideas.

Cereal-Free Breakfasts

Eggs and sweet potatoes with butter, yogurt and berries, or a banana with coffee and heavy cream are all common breakfasts in our house.

If you don't eat at home, boiled eggs are easily portable. To make them easy to peel, shock the eggs by moving them rapidly from boiling to icy cold water.

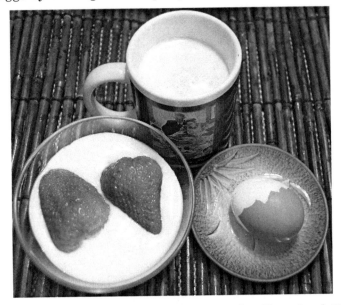

Some breakfast ideas. Paul often eats a banana and coffee mixed 50-50 with heavy cream; Shou-Ching likes whole milk yogurt and berries, sometimes a boiled egg.

Bread and Cracker Substitutes

Rice crackers are a low-toxin substitute for cookies and crackers.

For a zero-carb substitute, leafy vegetables, like romaine lettuce, can double as a sandwich wrap.

Pasta Substitutes

Rice is the savior of pasta lovers. Rice noodles are great in almost all pasta dishes. We eat spaghetti with rice noodles often, and rice noodle lasagna.

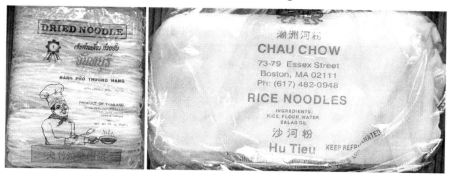

Asian supermarkets offer various styles of rice noodles. The spaghetti-style noodles on the left are pure rice. The lasagna-style noodles on the right have some flour and vegetable oil; buy pure rice noodles if you can find them.

For a zero-carb substitute, use vegetables like boiled cabbage leaves in place of lasagna noodles.

Flour-Free Baking

We don't bake, but those who do will be glad to hear there are substitutes for wheat flour.

Some companies sell gluten-free flours that are also grain-free. (Avoid gluten-free flours that contain cornstarch, corn meal, or grains like millet and sorghum.) Good flours use the "safe starches": rice flour, potato starch, potato flour, tapioca flour or tapioca starch.

The King Arthur flour company suggests making your own baking flour with 6 cups rice flour, 2 cups potato starch, and 1 cup tapioca flour or tapioca starch and a ½ teaspoon xantham gum per cup of flour, for texture.[325]

Other "Paleo" cooks recommend using almond flour or meal in "quick-bread" type recipes, like muffins, nut breads, and pancakes. Grind almonds in a blender or food processor, but not so far as to make almond butter; or buy almond meal at supermarkets. Extra eggs may be required for texture.

---

[325] *http://www.kingarthurflour.com/glutenfree/.*

How To Replace Vegetable Oils

Vegetable oils should be replaced in the diet by healthy fats and oils.

The best cooking, salad, and sauce oils are very low in omega-6 fats:

- red-meat animal fats like beef tallow or lamb (mutton) fat, and dairy fats like butter and cream.

- tropical plant oils like coconut oil, palm kernel oil, cocoa butter, nutmeg butter, macadamia nut butter, and ucuhuba butter.

When using butter as a cooking oil it's desirable to clarify it first, otherwise its sugars and proteins will cause leftover food to go bad quickly, or form toxic glycation endproducts.

Less desirable as cooking oils, because their moderate (~10%) omega-6 fats can be oxidized under heat, but healthful when added to dishes after cooking in sauces and salad dressings, are:

- animal fats like lard (pork) and egg yolks.

- plant oils like olive oil, tree nut butters, and avocado.

We use the low-omega-6 fats for cooking, include egg yolks in the daily diet for nutritional reasons, and vary the flavor of our dishes sometimes by adding olive oil, tree nut butters, or avocado to dishes **after** they have been cooked.

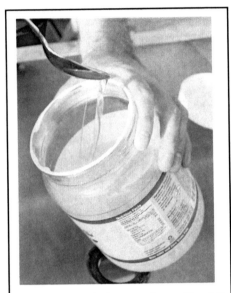

Coconut oil is a clear liquid above 76°F, a white solid below. "Extra virgin organic" brands taste best.

Make Your Own Salad Dressing

Unfortunately, commercial salad dressings are almost invariably made from unhealthy oils like soybean oil or canola oil. Until food companies remedy that, it is best for salad-lovers to make their own dressings.

Everyone is familiar with simple Italian dressings made of olive oil, balsamic vinegar, and herbs. However, this is far from the only alternative. Find a recipe for your favorite salad dressing, and substitute healthy oils for unhealthy ones.

We happen to like Thousand Island, a mayonnaise-based dressing. Mayonnaise is made by mixing an oil such as coconut oil or olive oil with egg yolks, vinegar, and lemon juice. The dressing is made by adding herbs, spices, and vegetables diced finely in a food processor. We favor pickles, onion, tomato, bell pepper, carrots, and olives in our home-made mayonnaise.

Sauces

Any sauce will be healthy as long as the oils used are healthy; and traditional recipes are usually the tastiest.

Butter and cream sauces are the delight of French cooking. Coconut milk is the secret to the wonderful sauces and curries of Thai cuisine.

Cookbooks from the days before vegetable oils may be mined for recipes. Look for old editions of *The Good Housekeeping Cookbook* or anything by Julia Child; or, if you really want to go back, to Fannie Farmer's cookbooks, first published in 1896.

Conclusion

We hope that food manufacturers will soon start creating healthier products, such as olive oil or coconut oil based salad dressings.

Until then, it is necessary to make your own sauces and dressings. This is a nuisance: There are dishes to clean, and as home-made dressings lack preservatives they may not last as long in the refrigerator. The consolation is that homemade dressings and sauces are unbeatably healthy and tasty.

How To Replace Sweets

Most people obtain fructose from drinks – for instance, soda and fruit juices – and desserts. But you don't need a lot of sugar in drinks and desserts.

Drinks

Healthy drinks have no sugar. We particularly recommend:

- Tea, especially green tea.
- Coffee.
- Water.
- Cream (better than whole milk or half-and-half).
- Wine.

We recommend heavy cream over milk because dairy proteins, especially casein, are potentially problematic. Cream has about half the protein per glass as milk. (Butter also has some protein; clarify the butter to remove its protein and sugars.)

Artificially sweetened zero-calorie beverages should be drunk only as a transitional drink while adapting to the diet. (Paul drank sucralose-sweetened fruit-flavored drinks when he first gave up sugary beverages.)

We recommend avoiding:

- Any sugary beverage.
- Fruit juices – instead, eat the fruit with a glass of water.
- Low-fat milk. Prefer fatty dairy: Stick to cream or whole milk.

Desserts

Food should always be enjoyable, so don't deprive yourself of dessert. But try to make it healthy.

Any mix of a carb with a fat makes for a tasty dessert. Choose the carb from our safe starches, fruits, and berries, and the fat from our healthy fats, and you will have a healthy dessert. Our favorites are:

- A bowl of fruit or berries with cream or coconut milk.
- Homemade ice cream – 6 egg yolks, a pint of cream, and flavorings like raspberries, cocoa powder, vanilla extract, and minimal sugar. Sometimes we include starches like tapioca, for a taste reminiscent of south Asian desserts like rice pudding or kheer.
- Dark chocolate or cocoa butter truffles made with minimal sugar.

A Traditional Pacific Islander Diet

Now that we have designed the diet, it may be helpful to summarize the differences between the Perfect Health Diet and western diets.

Americans in 2005 obtained 23% of calories from cereal grains, 3% from legumes, 23% from vegetable oils, and 17% from sugar and high-fructose corn syrup.[326] Americans get two-thirds of calories from foods the Perfect Health Diet eliminates!

To adopt the Perfect Health Diet, Americans will have to find healthy foods to replace the two-thirds of calories from grains, legumes, vegetable oils and sugars. Specific foods the Perfect Health Diet recommends eating more of include:

- **Safe starches like sweet potatoes, taro, and rice.** These should increase from about 3% in the American diet to about 15% of calories.

- **Fruits and berries.** These should increase from 2.9% to 5% of calories.

- **Sea vegetables.** Negligible in the American diet, should be common.

- **Ocean fish**, providing omega-3 fats. Less than 0.6% of the American diet, these should provide about 7% of calories.

- **Coconut oil and coconut milk**, providing short-chain fats. Negligible in the American diet, these should be over 6% of calories.

- **Meat, eggs, and other fats and oils.** These should rise from 23.6% of the American diet to about 55% of calories.

Looking over the foods that should be increased in the diet, we noticed something interesting: These are precisely the staple foods of traditional Pacific islander diets. The Perfect Health Diet is a Pacific islander diet!

Let's look at some of the traditional Pacific islander diets, and see what they did for islanders' health.

The Okinawan Diet

The traditional diet of Okinawa consists of sweet potatoes, fish, pork, eggs, and vegetables including seaweed. All parts of pigs were eaten ("tails to nails"), and lard was used ubiquitously for cooking. Gerontologist Kazuhiko Taira describes traditional Okinawan food as "very, very greasy."[327]

---

[326] USDA, "Nutrient Content of the U.S. Food Supply 2005," *http://www.cnpp.usda.gov/Publications/FoodSupply/FoodSupply2005Report.pdf.*

[327] Deborah Franklyn, "Take a Lesson from the People of Okinawa," *Health*, September 1996, pp 57-63; cited by Sally Fallon and Mary Enig, "Adventures in Macro-Nutrient Land," *http://www.westonaprice.org/Adventures-in-Macro-Nutrient-Land.html.* Sho H.

On this diet Okinawans had the longest life expectancy in the world, with numerous centenarians. The age-adjusted death rate from heart disease was 82% lower than the US, from cancer 27% lower, and from all causes 36% lower. Hormone-dependent cancers, like breast, cancer, ovarian, and colon cancer, were 50-80% less frequent in Okinawa than the US. [328]

Centenarians had the highest intake of milk, meat, fish, eggs, fat and oils.[329]

Unfortunately, during the post-World War II US occupation Okinawans began to eat vegetable oils, grains, and industrially prepared foods. Okinawans now have widespread obesity, rising rates of heart disease, cancer, and diabetes, and shortening lifespans.[330]

The Kitavan Diet

In 1989, a global search for aboriginal peoples eating in their traditional manner discovered the islanders of Kitava, off the coast of New Guinea. The residents of Kitava lived on safe starches (yam, sweet potato, taro, tapioca, cassava), fruit (banana, papaya, pineapple, mango, guava, watermelon, pumpkin), fish, coconuts, and vegetables. Lauric acid, the 12-carbon SaFA found in coconut oil, was the dominant dietary fatty acid.[331]

Despite a fair number of elderly, with ages up to 95, a research team led by Staffan Lindeberg was unable to find a single person who had ever had a heart attack based on EKG examinations. The Kitavans were entirely free of heart disease. They were also free of stroke, diabetes, and dementia. No one was overweight, no one had acne, and no one had high blood pressure. Infections – primarily malaria – and accidents – drowning and falling from coconut trees – were the leading causes of death.[332]

History and characteristics of Okinawan longevity food. *Asia Pac J Clin Nutr.* 2001;10(2):159-64. *http://pmid.us/11710358.*

[328] The Okinawa Centenarian Study, *http://www.okicent.org/.*

[329] Shibata H et al. Nutrition for the Japanese elderly. *Nutr Health.* 1992;8(2-3):165-75. *http://pmid.us/1407826.*

[330] Hokama T, Binns C. Declining longevity advantage and low birthweight in Okinawa. *Asia Pac J Public Health.* 2008 Oct;20 Suppl:95-101. *http://pmid.us/19533867.*

[331] Lindeberg S et al. Lipoprotein composition and serum cholesterol ester fatty acids in nonwesternized Melanesians. *Lipids.* 1996 Feb;31(2):153-8. *http://pmid.us/8835402.* Lindeberg S et al. Cardiovascular risk factors in a Melanesian population apparently free from stroke and ischaemic heart disease: the Kitava study. *J Intern Med.* 1994 Sep;236(3):331-40. *http://pmid.us/8077891.*

[332] Lindeberg S, Lundh B. Apparent absence of stroke and ischaemic heart disease in a traditional Melanesian island: a clinical study in Kitava. *J Intern Med.* 1993

The Hawai'ian Diet

The traditional diet of the native Hawai'ians consisted of taro (often prepared as poi), sweet potatoes, breadfruit, coconut, fish, squid, shellfish, pork, fowl including chicken, taro leaves, seaweed and *limu* (algae), and a few sweet fruits.

A famous *lu'au* offered by King Kamehameha III in 1847 served "271 hogs, 482 large calabashes of *poi*, 602 chickens, 3 whole oxen, 2 barrels salt pork, 2 barrels biscuit, 3,125 salt fish, 1,820 fresh fish, 12 barrels *lu'au* and cabbages, 4 barrels onions, 80 bunches bananas, 55 pineapples, 10 barrels potatoes, 55 ducks, 82 turkeys, 2,245 coconuts, 4,000 heads of taro, 180 squid, oranges, limes, grapes and various fruits."[333] Except for the biscuits – hardly a food that would have been available seventy years earlier – these are all foods we can highly recommend. As this menu suggests, most calories came from meat, fish, taro, and coconut.

Early European explorers remarked on the beauty, strength, good nature and excellent physical development of the native Hawai'ians.

Conclusion

We did not know when we began writing that we would be recommending a traditional Pacific islander diet. Nevertheless, we are reassured that the Perfect Health Diet, which we arrived at from our study of the scientific literature, is so similar to traditional diets known to produce superb health.

To our Hawaiian readers: *Mahalo!*

Mar;233(3):269-75. *http://pmid.us/8450295*. Lindeberg S. The Kitava Study. *http://www.staffanlindeberg.com/TheKitavaStudy.html.*

[333]*Hawaiian Annual* (1930), cited *http://www.pacificworlds.com/nuuanu/native/native5.cfm.*

Step Three to Perfect Health: Be Well Nourished

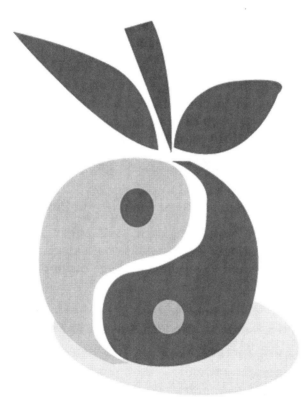

Why Moderns Are Malnourished

Good health doesn't only depend on removing toxins and getting the right macronutrients. The human body also needs micronutrients like vitamins and minerals. This raises several questions:

Are people malnourished on modern diets? How much of each nutrient is optimal? Which nutrients are toxic in excess? Should we supplement?

Six Reasons Why People are Malnourished

Modern people are malnourished compared to our Paleolithic ancestors – and Paleolithic people were not always well nourished. Here are six reasons why we should expect that most moderns are malnourished:

First: Modern living is sedentary. People don't burn as many calories, so they don't eat as much food. This reduces nutrient intake.

Our Paleolithic ancestors probably ate 3,000 calories per day or more. Modern !Kung and Ache hunter-gatherers average 49 calories per kg per day, compared to 32 calories per kg per day for modern office workers.[334] For an 80 kg man and 55 kg woman, those translate to 3900 calories for men and 2700 for women among the hunter-gatherers, versus 2560 for men and 1760 for women among moderns.

If our Paleolithic ancestors ate 50% more calories, they were probably eating at least 50% more nutrients.

Second: Modern foods are nutrient-poor compared to Paleolithic foods.

Modern plant foods like wheat, rice, corn, and sugar have around 1300-1500 calories per pound and relatively few nutrients per calorie. Paleolithic plant foods like starchy tubers, fruits, and vegetables average around 200 calories per pound and are nutrient rich.

Paleolithic humans ate the whole carcass of animals, including nutrient-rich tissues like liver and bone marrow. Modern Americans eat only skeletal muscle.

If, in addition to consuming 50% more calories, Paleolithic people were getting several times more nutrients per calorie than modern Americans, then they must have been obtaining vastly more nutrients.

Third: Agricultural food production and water treatment diminish the mineral content reaching consumers.

---

[334] Cordain L et al. Physical activity, energy expenditure, and fitness: an evolutionary perspective. *Int J Sports Med.* 1998 Jul;19(5):328-35. *http://pmid.us/9721056.*

Repeated plantings of a single crop on the same plot of land diminish the mineral content of the soil, and ultimately the mineral content of the plants, unless fertilizer adequately replaces minerals. Wikipedia notes:

> Many inorganic fertilizers do not replace trace mineral elements in the soil which become gradually depleted by crops. This depletion has been linked to studies which have shown a marked fall (up to 75%) in the quantities of such minerals present in fruit and vegetables.[335]

Mineral deprivation in pasture land leads to deficiencies in animal meats, eggs, and dairy. A study found that copper levels in UK foods have declined by 90% in dairy foods, 55% in meat and 76% in vegetables.[336]

Minerals are also lost in treatment of drinking water. Water was the largest source of magnesium in Paleolithic diets, but modern water treatment removes most dissolved minerals.

Fourth: Modern cooking methods often leave nutrients behind.

Traditional diets usually made soups or broths when cooking in water, thus retaining water-soluble nutrients in the diet. They also added inedible organic matter, like bones, to the soup, allowing minerals and other nutrients to leach into it. But modern cooks discard bones and when they boil foods, discard the cooking water and its dissolved nutrients.

Similarly, when modern foods are fried, the cooking oil is often discarded, along with fat-soluble nutrients drawn from foods.

Fifth: Modern foods contain antinutrients that lock up nutrients as well as toxins that impair intestinal absorption of micronutrients.

We've discussed elsewhere how antinutrients like phytic acid lock up minerals and prevent their absorption, and how toxins in grains and legumes impair digestion. Many of these toxins specifically target protein digestion; for instance, trypsin inhibitors prevent the breakdown of proteins into amino acids. This sabotage likely affects micronutrient intake much more than overall caloric intake, since sugars and fats can still be digested, but many micronutrients are chelated to proteins or bound in enzymes.

Sixth: Even on their low toxin and high-nutrient diets, Paleolithic humans may have been malnourished.

---

[335] "Fertilizer," Wikipedia, *http://en.wikipedia.org/wiki/Fertilizer.*

[336] Thomas D. The mineral depletion of foods available to us as a nation (1940-2002)--a review of the 6th Edition of McCance and Widdowson. *Nutr Health.* 2007;19(1-2):21-55. *http://pmid.us/18309763.* Hat tip Robert Andrew Brown, *http://wholehealthsource.blogspot.com/2010/04/copper-and-cardiovascular-disease.html.*

Anthropologists have detected occasional signs of malnourishment, such as tooth hypoplasia, in Paleolithic skeletons.

Moreover, on theoretical grounds we should not expect Paleolithic nutrition to have been optimal for individual health. Though Paleolithic diets were undoubtedly largely non-toxic, Malthusian population growth would likely have increased the population above the level optimal for individual human health. Widespread slight malnourishment was probably the norm, especially after the Last Glacial Maximum.

Cumulatively, these factors suggest that micronutrient deficiencies are widespread today. But how harmful are they?

Malnourishment Is Perilous

Although we have a good understanding of acute diseases arising from severe nutrient deficiencies, such as scurvy, rickets, beri beri, and pellagra, little is known about the long-term effects of chronic deficiencies. Long-term effects may be insidious and hard to trace.

A plausible theory, proposed by Bruce Ames of the University of California at Berkeley and called "triage theory," holds that when nutrients are scarce, the body prioritizes functions needed for reproduction and short-term survival – such as the ability to hunt – while short-changing maintenance functions that sustain a long, healthy life.[337] Triage theory predicts that the chronically malnourished will die younger and be less healthy in their older years.

Support for this idea comes from studies of the long-term effects of youthful malnourishment. Famines such as the Dutch World War II famine and the Chinese Great Leap Forward famine have provided natural laboratories in which we know a certain birth cohort suffered malnourishment.

Remarkably, although experiencing a famine at any time increases rates of chronic disease later in life, *the worst health may belong to people whose mothers experienced famine shortly before they were conceived.*

For instance, maternal exposure to the Dutch famine *prior to conception* doubled the risk of adult depression in the offspring, but maternal exposure to the famine *during pregnancy* had no effect. [338]

---

[337] Ames BN. Low micronutrient intake may accelerate the degenerative diseases of aging through allocation of scarce micronutrients by triage. *Proc Natl Acad Sci U S A.* 2006 Nov 21;103(47):17589-94. *http://pmid.us/17101959.*

[338] Maternal exposure to the Dutch famine before conception and during pregnancy: quality of life and depressive symptoms in adult offspring. *Epidemiology.* 2009 Nov;20(6):909-15. *http://pmid.us/19752733.*

Similarly, in rural China as a result of the Great Leap Forward Famine, "the post-famine cohort had the highest risk of developing schizophrenia, and there was virtually no difference in schizophrenia risk between the pre-famine and the famine cohort."[339]

This is not to suggest that malnourishment during pregnancy is harmless. Those who were malnourished in the womb go on to experience high rates of chronic disease, including obesity and diabetes. The same effects occur in animals.[340]

The Enduring Effects of Malnutrition

Two remarkable sets of data imply that malnutrition not only damages one's own health, but is also, to borrow a Biblical phrase, visited upon the sons to the third and fourth generation.

POTTENGER'S CATS

Dr. Francis Marion Pottenger, Jr. was a veterinarian who worked in a lab producing adrenal hormones for medical use. At the time there was no good way to evaluate the strength of manufactured hormone, so the evaluation was done in cats with surgically removed adrenal glands.

Pottenger's cats had a high death rate, but he noticed that when the offal portion of the diet – liver, tripe, sweetbreads, brains, and heart – was fed raw rather than cooked, the health of the cats improved tremendously.

This observation led him to conduct a remarkable experiment from 1932 to 1942. The experiment evaluated five diets over four generations, and included 900 cats. The work was described in his book, *Pottenger's Cats*.

Cats fed raw milk and raw meat and offal maintained remarkable health through four generations.

However, cats fed cooked meat and pasteurized, evaporated or condensed milk experienced steadily deteriorating health:

- First generation cats developed degenerative diseases late in life.

- Second generation cats developed degenerative diseases in mid-life.

- Third generation cats developed diseases, allergies, soft bones, and succumbed to parasitic infections early in life. Most cats could not produce offspring.

---

[339] Song S et al. Famine, death, and madness: schizophrenia in early adulthood after prenatal exposure to the Chinese Great Leap Forward Famine. *Soc Sci Med.* 2009 Apr;68(7):1315-21. *http://pmid.us/19232455*.

[340] Stocker CJ et al. Fetal origins of insulin resistance and obesity. *Proc Nutr Soc.* 2005 May;64(2):143-51. *http://pmid.us/15960859*.

- Not a single fourth generation cat could reproduce. Fourth generation cats **"suffered from most of the degenerative diseases encountered in human medicine."**[341]

It's now generally accepted that the decline of Pottenger's cats was due to nutritional deficiencies induced by cooking. Cooking destroys some nutrients, like vitamin C. More significantly for cats, the taurine in cooked meat but not raw meat is degraded in the intestinal tract.[342] Taurine is an essential dietary nutrient for cats, and taurine deficiency in cats causes many of the symptoms seen in Pottenger's cats.[343]

We find two aspects of Pottenger's experiments especially fascinating:

- The effects of a malnourishing diet were passed down through generations, such that health deteriorated in every generation. *This reproduces the effects seen in famine studies, where malnourished mothers produced children prone to obesity and disease.*

- On the malnourishing diets, most human degenerative diseases were recapitulated. *This suggests that much human disease may be due to malnourishment.*

THE FLYNN EFFECT

When immigrants from poor countries came to the United States in the late 19th and early 20th centuries, their descendants' IQ increased by about 10 points per generation for three to four generations, a phenomenon known as the "Flynn effect." There has been a similar, but smaller, effect in Americans. The Flynn effect only operates in people with low IQs; people with high IQs have negligible IQ increases over generations. The Flynn effect seems to have ceased operating in the late 20th century.[344]

---

341 Wikipedia, "Francis M. Pottenger, Jr.", *http://en.wikipedia.org/wiki/Francis_M._Pottenger,_Jr.*

342 Hickman MA et al. Effect of processing on fate of dietary [14C]taurine in cats. *J Nutr.* 1990 Sep;120(9):995-1000. *http://pmid.us/2144588.* Kim SW et al. Dietary antibiotics decrease taurine loss in cats fed a canned heat-processed diet. *J Nutr.* 1996 Feb;126(2):509-15. *http://pmid.us/8632225.* Kim SW et al. Maillard reaction products in purified diets induce taurine depletion in cats which is reversed by antibiotics. *J Nutr.* 1996 Jan;126(1):195-201. *http://pmid.us/8558301.* Hat tip Jean-Louis Tu, "Is Cooked Food Poison?", *http://www.beyondveg.com/tu-j-l/raw-cooked/raw-cooked-1a.shtml.*

343 Sturman JA et al. Feline maternal taurine deficiency: effect on mother and offspring. *J Nutr.* 1986 Apr;116(4):655-67. *http://pmid.us/3754276.*

344 Wikipedia, "Flynn effect," *http://en.wikipedia.org/wiki/Flynn_effect.*

The Flynn effect has been linked to improved nutrition.[345] It appears that chronic malnourishment impairs IQ, and that improved nutrition causes IQ to return to natural levels over three to four generations.

Iodine intake could be a critical factor. Iodine deficiency is the leading global cause of mental retardation, and even a moderate iodine deficiency lowers IQ by 10 to 15 points.[346]

Conclusion

Famine studies, Pottenger's cats, and Flynn's humans all point to one conclusion: Malnourishment has long-lasting, even trans-generational, effects on health, and may be one of the primary factors in human disease.

We believe it is very important to keep the body well nourished throughout life. All nutrient deficiencies should be eradicated.

Nor is it enough to assure that *macronutrient* deficiencies are relieved. It is common for children of obese mothers to experience stunted growth.[347] The children are malnourished, but not for lack of calories. They lack micronutrients — vitamins and minerals.

We have already discussed how to optimize macronutrients — fat, carbs, and protein. Now we need to learn how to optimize micronutrients: how to eat and supplement so as to bring all micronutrients into their plateau ranges.

---

[345] Colom R, Lluis-Font JM, Andrés-Pueyo A. (2005) "The generational intelligence gains are caused by decreasing variance in the lower half of the distribution: Supporting evidence for the nutrition hypothesis," *Intelligence* **33**: 83–91.

[346] "In Raising the World's I.Q., the Secret's in the Salt," *New York Times*, December 16, 2006, *http://www.nytimes.com/2006/12/16/health/16iodine.html*.

[347] Garrett J, Ruel MT. The coexistence of child undernutrition and maternal overweight: prevalence, hypotheses, and programme and policy implications. *Matern Child Nutr.* 2005 Jul;1(3):185-96. *http://pmid.us/16881899*.

Multivitamins: Good or Bad?

Multivitamins are extremely convenient – just one pill per day. About half of Americans routinely supplement with a multivitamin.

It seems logical that if most people are malnourished, as we believe they are, then multivitamins should deliver health benefits. The health improvement from repairing some deficiencies is **huge**. Some deficiency diseases – rickets (vitamin D), scurvy (vitamin C), beri beri (vitamin B1), and pellagra (vitamin B3), plus many mineral deficiencies – can be *fatal*. Even subclinical deficiencies can have large but insidious effects on health.

Yet studies have generally been unable to detect much effect, positive or negative, from multivitamins:

- A study of 161,808 women followed over eight years as part of the Women's Health Initiative found that the 42% of women who regularly used multivitamins had no difference in rates of cancer, heart attack, stroke, or mortality from women who did not take multivitamins. The multivitamin users were 2% more likely to die, a result that was considered insignificant.[348]

- A meta-analysis of eight clinical trials conducted in the elderly found "weak and conflicting" evidence for benefits from multivitamins. Multivitamin users had the same number of infections as non-users, but got over them in about half the time, experiencing 17.5 fewer days per year with infections. The study was unable to analyze death rates, which had not been adequately reported.[349]

What are we to make of this?

Multivitamins May Contribute to Nutrient Imbalances

As we'll see when we analyze the optimal intake for various micronutrients, multivitamin formulas are not optimal. They provide

- Too little of certain nutrients, like magnesium, vitamin C, vitamin D and vitamin K2.

---

[348] Neuhouser ML et al. Multivitamin use and risk of cancer and cardiovascular disease in the Women's Health Initiative cohorts. *Arch Intern Med.* 2009 Feb 9;169(3):294-304. *http://pmid.us/19204221*. Hat tip Stuart Buck, *http://stuartbuck.blogspot.com/2009/02/dont-take-your-vitamins.html*.

[349] El-Kadiki A, Sutton AJ. Role of multivitamins and mineral supplements in preventing infections in elderly people: systematic review and meta-analysis of randomised controlled trials. *BMJ.* 2005 Apr 16;330(7496):871. *http://pmid.us/15805125*.

- Too much of some potentially toxic nutrients, notably vitamin A. Depending on the rest of the diet, multivitamins could also contribute to toxicity from niacin, calcium, iron, vitamin E, or folic acid.

Certain nutrients, such as vitamins A and D, need to be in a proper ratio to one another. We believe that the main problem with multivitamins is that, by providing about 4,000 IU of vitamin A and only 400 IU of vitamin D, they exacerbate the excessive A to D ratio that plagues most westerners due to their lack of sun exposure.

Our Take

Multivitamins, as currently formulated and used, appear to be neutral in their health effects.

This is probably due to a balance of beneficial and toxic effects. The main toxicity effect is probably an excessive ratio of vitamin A to vitamin D. This is significant because most people get too little sun exposure and are vitamin D deficient.

We believe that if vitamin D and vitamin K2 were optimized, then the A-to-D balance will be optimized even with multivitamin consumption. As a result, there will be little or no toxicity from multivitamins, the benefits will dominate, and multivitamin use will be clearly beneficial.

Therefore, **we recommend taking a multivitamin daily** as a first step toward optimizing micronutrition.

Pregnant and menstruating women should take a multivitamin with iron, others without.[350]

---

[350] "Iron," *http://lpi.oregonstate.edu/infocenter/minerals/iron/*.

Eight Highly Beneficial Nutrients

In this chapter we discuss eight micronutrients for which there is clinical evidence that *health would improve for nearly everyone* if intake were increased beyond what is contained in food and multivitamins.

We urge anyone with impaired health to obtain good levels of the following micronutrients. This need not involve supplementation; eating specific foods provides an abundance of some nutrients: seaweed provides iodine, beef liver provides copper, and Brazil nuts provide selenium. In the case of vitamin D, regular mid-day sun exposure can repair deficiency.

We discuss the micronutrients in order of their likelihood to improve health, as follows:

1. Most likely to reduce mortality and extend life: **vitamin D** and **vitamin K2**.

2. Most likely to improve well-being and important for cancer prevention: **selenium** and **iodine**.

3. Likely to prevent cardiovascular disease: **magnesium, copper,** and **chromium**.

4. Too important to risk a deficiency: **vitamin C**.

These eight nutrients also share a common feature: each one is important for immune function. As we believe chronic infections are the primary cause of aging and chronic disease, this is no surprise to us.

Vitamin D

Vitamin D is crucial for health. Vitamin D deficiencies are a causal factor in a host of diseases, including heart disease, high blood pressure, arthritis, depression, inflammatory bowel disease, obesity, premenstrual syndrome, fibromyalgia, multiple sclerosis, autoimmune disorders, autism, dementia, and cancer.

VITAMIN D BIOLOGY

Three forms of vitamin D are important:

- Cholecalciferol, or **vitamin D3**, is produced from the action of sunlight on cholesterol in the skin, or can be obtained from supplements. It is biologically inactive – a sort of raw material.

- The liver converts cholecalciferol into 25-hydroxyvitamin D. This is an active form of vitamin D that circulates throughout the body and crosses cell membranes. We'll call this form **25OHD** for short.

- All human cells can convert 25OHD into a still more active form, $1\alpha,25$-dihydroxyvitamin D. We'll call this **1,25D** for short. This form does not cross cell membranes, so every cell has its own level. 1,25D is about 500 times more potent than 25OHD.

25OHD circulates throughout the body and provides a universal "baseline" level of vitamin D activity in every cell. Cells fine-tune their level of vitamin D activity by converting more or less 25OHD into the more potent 1,25D.[351]

There are two main functions of vitamin D:

1. Calcium management. The kidney manages blood levels of calcium by introducing 1,25D into the blood. An excess of vitamin D can lead to excess calcium in the blood. However, calcium management is a routine function which rarely causes health problems.

2. Control of gene transcription. Either 25OHD or 1,25D within cells joins with a **vitamin D receptor (VDR)** on the nuclear membrane, after which the VDR is imported into the nucleus. There, it induces the manufacture of RNA and proteins from certain genes.

For many genes, the VDR needs to combine in the nucleus with a retinoic acid X-receptor (RXR) which enters the nucleus when stimulated by vitamin A. Thus, vitamin A and vitamin D are partners and need to be in balance for proper cellular function.

The two active forms of vitamin D share an equal role as VDR activators. At optimal blood levels, the 25OHD is 500-fold more abundant than 1,25D, precisely balancing 1,25D's 500-fold greater potency as a VDR activator.

OPTIMAL VITAMIN D INTAKE AND 25OHD LEVELS

One way of estimating an optimum is by total vitamin D intake.

Dr. Robert Heaney has found that healthy men need about 3,000 to 5,000 IU of vitamin D a day from all sources to maintain a 25OHD level of 30 ng/ml through a Nebraska winter.[352] Women may need a little less. More may be needed if illness or food toxicity depletes vitamin D.

It is likely that under regular sun exposure, the body limits average daily vitamin D production to about these levels. Although up to 20,000 IU can be made in a single day[353], with regular sun exposure daily vitamin D production is reduced, in part by skin tanning.

Another way of estimating an optimum is by circulating 25OHD level.

It seems fairly clear that a 25OHD level below 32-35 ng/ml indicates a deficiency, at least in people of European descent. A number of diseases become more

---

[351] Lou YR et al. 25-Hydroxyvitamin D(3) is an agonistic vitamin D receptor ligand. *J Steroid Biochem Mol Biol*. 2010 Feb 15;118(3):162-70. *http://pmid.us/19944755*.

[352] Heaney RP et al. Human serum 25-hydroxycholecalciferol response to extended oral dosing with cholecalciferol. *Am J Clin Nutr*. 2003 Jan;77(1):204-10. *http://pmid.us/12499343*.

[353] "Vitamin D Physiology," *http://vitamindcouncil.org/vitaminDPhysiology.shtml*.

prevalent when 25OHD levels fall below 32 ng/ml.[354] For instance, bone density is highest and fracture rates lowest with 25OHD levels over 32 ng/ml. Cancer rates are reduced above this level, as are rates of many other diseases.

Biokinematic studies also support establishing the lower bound of the plateau range at about 35 ng/ml. One study reports:

> One could plausibly postulate that the point at which [the liver's] 25(OH)D production becomes [saturated] constitutes the definition of the low end of normal status. This value ... is at a serum 25(OH)D concentration of 88 nmol/L (35.2 ng/mL) ... It is interesting that this estimate is very close to that produced by previous attempts to define the lower end of the normal range from the relations of serum 25(OH)D to calcium absorption and to serum parathyroid hormone concentration (ie, 75–85 nmol/L, or 30–34 ng/mL).[355]

So four independent methods agree: 25OHD levels below 35 ng/ml are inadequate, but levels above 35 ng/ml are within the optimal range.

It is more difficult to assess the 25OHD level at which vitamin D toxicity begins, because few people attain such vitamin D levels. A recent review of the literature found few contraindications for vitamin D supplementation below 10,000 IU/day, and a paucity of reports of toxicity for serum 25OHD levels below 200 ng/ml.[356] However, we believe there are strong reasons to keep serum 25OHD levels below 50 to 80 ng/ml:

- 25OHD levels after regular abundant summer sun exposure, as in lifeguards, usually peak between 45 and 80 ng/ml. For instance, outdoor workers in the tropics typically have 25OHD levels between 48 and 80 ng/ml.[357]

- Human cells begin destroying vitamin D by turning on the vitamin D degrading gene, CYP24A1, at 25OHD levels below 100 ng/ml.[358] This indicates that optimal 25OHD levels are probably well below 100 ng/ml.

---

[354] Heaney RP. Vitamin D: criteria for safety and efficacy. *Nutr Rev.* 2008 Oct;66(10 Suppl 2):S178-81. *http://pmid.us/18844846.*

[355] Heaney RP et al. 25-Hydroxylation of vitamin D3: relation to circulating vitamin D3 under various input conditions. *Am J Clin Nutr.* 2008 Jun;87(6):1738-42. *http://pmid.us/18541563.*

[356] Hathcock JN et al. Risk assessment for vitamin D. *Am J Clin Nutr.* 2007 Jan;85(1):6-18. *http://pmid.us/17209171.*

[357] Heaney RP. Vitamin D in health and disease. *Clin J Am Soc Nephrol.* 2008 Sep;3(5):1535-41. *http://pmid.us/18525006.*

[358] Lou YR et al. 25-Hydroxyvitamin D(3) is an agonistic vitamin D receptor ligand. *J Steroid Biochem Mol Biol.* 2010 Feb 15;118(3):162-70. *http://pmid.us/19944755.*

Once adequate vitamin D is provided, most people seem to reach a stable equilibrium 25OHD level around 40 to 45 ng/ml. At this level, nearly all additional vitamin D3 is placed into storage.[359]

We believe that high-dose supplementation with vitamin D3 to drive 25OHD levels above this stable level are undesirable.

A transient elevation of 25OHD – for instance, due to summer sun exposure – can usefully store vitamin D3 and 25OHD for the coming winter. But if winter is never allowed to come, then continual deposit of vitamin D into storage may build up a large reservoir. Then, if storage room runs out, or stored vitamin D is released due to weight loss, 25OHD levels could spike to toxic levels. As one study notes:

> Deposition in body fat almost certainly occurs in cases of vitamin D intoxication, and persistence of hypercalcemia for months has been attributed to sustained release of vitamin D from such body stores.[360]

Several studies also indicate potential danger from persistently elevated 25OHD levels:

- Bone mineral density peaks in the range 32 to 45 ng/ml and then falls as 25OHD rises above 45 ng/ml. For blacks, the fall in bone mineral density begins at 40 ng/ml.[361]

- Those people in the tropics who get their 25OHD level up to 80 ng/ml? They have a 3-fold higher rate of heart attack.[362]

- Lifeguards in Israel have kidney stones 20 times more often than the general population.[363]

---

[359] Heaney RP et al. 25-Hydroxylation of vitamin D3: relation to circulating vitamin D3 under various input conditions. *Am J Clin Nutr.* 2008 Jun;87(6):1738-42. *http://pmid.us/18541563.*

[360] Heaney RP et al. 25-Hydroxylation of vitamin D3: relation to circulating vitamin D3 under various input conditions. *Am J Clin Nutr.* 2008 Jun;87(6):1738-42. *http://pmid.us/18541563.*

[361] Bischoff-Ferrari HA et al. Positive association between 25-hydroxy vitamin D levels and bone mineral density: a population-based study of younger and older adults. *Am J Med.* 2004 May 1;116(9):634-9. *http://pmid.us/15093761.* Hat tip Chris Masterjohn, *http://www.westonaprice.org/blogs/are-some-people-pushing-their-vitamin-d-levels-too-high.html.*

[362] Rajasree S et al. Serum 25-hydroxyvitamin D3 levels are elevated in South Indian patients with ischemic heart disease. *Eur J Epidemiol.* 2001;17(6):567-71. *http://pmid.us/11949730.*

[363] Better OS et al. Increased incidence of nephrolithiasis (N) in lifeguards (LG) in Israel. *Adv Exp Med Biol.* 1980;128:467-72. *http://pmid.us/7424691.*

Another likely consequence of excessive vitamin D intake is premature aging.[364]

These considerations suggest that for optimal health, 25OHD should be in the vicinity of 40 ng/ml. Such levels are normally achieved with vitamin D3 intake from sun and supplements together of 3,000 to 5,000 IU per day.

DEFICIENCY IS WIDESPREAD

In modern life, with indoor work, most people get little sun exposure.

No wonder then that many Americans are deficient in vitamin D, especially at northern latitudes and in the winter. If 25OHD below 35 ng/ml is the measure of deficiency, then about 80% of Americans are deficient:

- 69% of US children have 25OHD levels below 30 ng/ml.[365]

- 77% of US adults have 25OHD levels below 30 ng/ml.[366]

SUMMARY: VITAMIN D TARGETS AND NEED FOR SUPPLEMENTATION

Cumulatively, the evidence suggests that:

- 25OHD levels between 35 and 50 ng/ml are probably optimal for healthy people of European descent. For people of African descent, the optimal range may be lower, 30 to 40 ng/ml.

- Most American adults would have to supplement with at least 2,000 IU/day, and most children with 1,000 IU per 50 pounds body weight, to bring 25OHD readings into the optimal range. Supplementation up to 5,000 IU/day might be required for large men who get minimal sun exposure, or for sufferers from certain diseases.

We do not recommend seeking 25OHD levels over 50 ng/ml or supplementing with more than 5,000 IU/day, except perhaps in patients with diseases that may be treatable by vitamin D (such as infectious disease, autoimmune disease, and cancer).

Now let's look at the benefits of getting adequate vitamin D. Since about 80% of Americans are deficient in vitamin D, while probably fewer than 1% have an excess, nearly all studies find great benefits to increasing vitamin D.

---

364 Tuohimaa P. Vitamin D and aging. *J Steroid Biochem Mol Biol.* 2009 Mar;114(1-2):78-84. *http://pmid.us/19444937.*

365 Mansbach JM et al. Serum 25-hydroxyvitamin D levels among US children aged 1 to 11 years: do children need more vitamin D? *Pediatrics.* 2009 Nov;124(5):1404-10. *http://pmid.us/19951983.*

366 Ginde AA et al. Demographic differences and trends of vitamin D insufficiency in the US population, 1988-2004. *Arch Intern Med.* 2009 Mar 23;169(6):626-32. *http://pmid.us/19307527.*

VITAMIN D AND CANCER

The farther north one lives, the more likely one is to die of cancer. This is true of a host of cancers, including breast, colon, and ovarian cancers.

Here are some maps from the National Cancer Institute illustrating the pattern.[367]

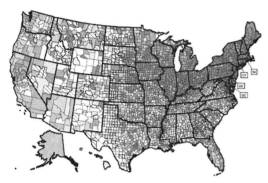 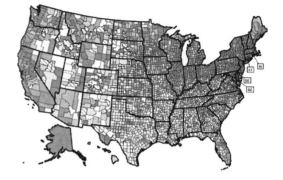

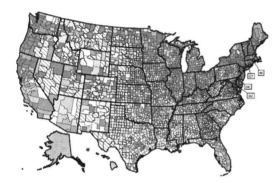

Figure: Cancer mortality in the U.S. *Top left:* Colon cancer mortality among white males. *Top right:* Breast cancer mortality among white females. *Bottom left:* Ovarian cancer mortality among white females. In all maps, darker colors represent higher mortality.

Overall, increasing 25OHD levels by 20 ng/ml can be expected to decrease breast cancer rates by up to 41%.[368] Rates for other hormone-sensitive cancers decline with increasing 25OHD in a similar fashion.

VITAMIN D AND CARDIOVASCULAR DISEASE

Levels of vitamin D predict who will die of stroke: the lower vitamin D, the more likely a fatal stroke.[369]

---

[367] National Cancer Institute, "Cancer Mortality Maps and Graphs," *http://www3.cancer.gov/atlasplus/*, based on Devesa SS et al. Atlas of cancer mortality in the United States, 1950-94. Washington, DC: US Govt Print Off; 1999 [NIH Publ No. (NIH) 99-4564].

[368] Yin L et al. Meta-analysis: Serum vitamin D and breast cancer risk. *Eur J Cancer.* 2010 Apr 22. [Epub ahead of print] *http://pmid.us/20456946*.

[369] Pilz S et al. Low vitamin d levels predict stroke in patients referred to coronary angiography. *Stroke.* 2008 Sep;39(9):2611-3. *http://pmid.us/18635847*.

Heart disease deaths in Europe are correlated with the level of solar radiation: the more sun, the fewer deaths.[370]

VITAMIN D AND MORTALITY

People with more vitamin D are less likely to die of any cause.

In one study, 25OHD levels were measured in 3258 persons and they were followed for an average of 7.7 years. Compared with patients in the highest quartile, who had a median 25OHD level of 28.4 ng/ml, those in the third quartile (median 25OHD level 13.3 ng/ml) had a 53% higher chance of dying, and those in the lowest quartile (median 25OHD level 7.6 ng/ml) had a 108% higher chance of dying.[371]

In another study, elderly in the lowest 25OHD quartile were 124% more likely to die over a 6.2-year follow-up period.[372]

VITAMIN D AND RESPIRATORY DISEASE

When rickets was rampant, victims frequently died of respiratory infections, such as pneumonia, tuberculosis, and the flu. The flu and other respiratory infections primarily strike in the winter, when vitamin D levels are low.

These associations are not coincidental. Low vitamin D levels increase the risk of tuberculosis 5-fold.[373] In a randomized trial of Japanese schoolchildren, supplementation with 1200 IU/day of vitamin D reduced the risk of influenza A by 42%.[374]

VITAMIN D AND DIABETES

Higher Vitamin D status is associated with lower rates of diabetes.[375]

---

[370] Wong A. Incident solar radiation and coronary heart disease mortality rates in Europe. *Eur J Epidemiol.* 2008;23(9):609-14. *http://pmid.us/18704704.*

[371] Dobnig H et al. Independent association of low serum 25-hydroxyvitamin d and 1,25-dihydroxyvitamin d levels with all-cause and cardiovascular mortality. *Arch Intern Med.* 2008 Jun 23;168(12):1340-9. *http://pmid.us/18574092.*

[372] Pilz S et al. Vitamin D and mortality in older men and women. *Clin Endocrinol (Oxf).* 2009 Nov;71(5):666-72. *http://pmid.us/19226272.*

[373] Talat N et al. Vitamin d deficiency and tuberculosis progression. *Emerg Infect Dis.* 2010 May;16(5):853-5. *http://pmid.us/20409383.*

[374] Urashima M et al. Randomized trial of vitamin D supplementation to prevent seasonal influenza A in schoolchildren. *Am J Clin Nutr.* 2010 May;91(5):1255-60 *http://pmid.us/20219962.*

[375] Liu E et al. Predicted 25-hydroxyvitamin D score and incident type 2 diabetes in the Framingham Offspring Study. *Am J Clin Nutr.* 2010 Jun;91(6):1627-33. *http://pmid.us/20392893.*

VITAMIN D AND INTRACELLULAR PATHOGENS

Cellular studies have shown that vitamin D is essential to the innate immune response to intracellular pathogens – viruses and cell-wall deficient bacteria. Vitamin D is essential for transcription of antimicrobial peptides such as cathelicidin, which are one of the main killing mechanisms against intracellular pathogens.[376]

Researchers are only just beginning to realize how many chronic and "autoimmune" diseases are in fact caused by persistent parasitic infections. Two such diseases are Alzheimer's and multiple sclerosis. Vitamin D appears to be effective against both.

VITAMIN D AND DEMENTIA

There is evidence that Alzheimer's may be caused by a chronic bacterial infection of the brain. The guilty bacterial species is probably *Chlamydophila pneumoniae*.[377] The bacteria steal glucose and pyruvate from neurons, starving them. The amyloid plaques that litter the brain of Alzheimer's patients may have an antibacterial function.[378]

However, a strong immune response, activated by vitamin D, may kill the bacteria or drive them into a dormant state that allows neurons to regain function.

Consistent with this idea, vitamin D is highly effective in improving cognition in Alzheimer's patients.[379]

To illustrate by one case, a Georgia doctor reported that an Alzheimer's patient who had not spoken in a year regained her ability to converse a few months after starting vitamin D at 5,000 IU/day.[380]

---

[376] Liu PT et al. Cutting edge: vitamin D-mediated human antimicrobial activity against Mycobacterium tuberculosis is dependent on the induction of cathelicidin. *J Immunol.* 2007 Aug 15;179(4):2060-3. *http://pmid.us/17675463.* White JH. Vitamin D signaling, infectious diseases, and regulation of innate immunity. *Infect Immun.* 2008 Sep;76(9):3837-43. *http://pmid.us/18505808.*

[377] Shima K et al. Chlamydia pneumoniae infection and Alzheimer's disease: a connection to remember? *Med Microbiol Immunol.* 2010 May 6. [Epub ahead of print] *http://pmid.us/20445987.*

[378] "Is Alzheimer's Caused by a Bacterial Infection of the Brain?", June 28, 2010, *http://perfecthealthdiet.com/?p=126.*

[379] Oudshoorn C et al. Higher serum vitamin D3 levels are associated with better cognitive test performance in patients with Alzheimer's disease. *Dement Geriatr Cogn Disord.* 2008;25(6):539-43. *http://pmid.us/18503256.* Llewellyn DJ et al. Serum 25-hydroxyvitamin D concentration and cognitive impairment. *J Geriatr Psychiatry Neurol.* 2009 Sep;22(3):188-95. *http://pmid.us/19073839.*

VITAMIN D AND MULTIPLE SCLEROSIS

It has long been known that multiple sclerosis (MS) has a strong latitude dependence – disease rates are much higher at northern latitudes. MS is strongly associated with low vitamin D levels.[381]

Recently, evidence has begun to accumulate that vitamin D is an effective treatment for MS. For instance, in a clinical trial giving MS patients 10,000 IU/day, "treatment group patients appeared to have fewer relapse events and a persistent reduction in T-cell proliferation compared to controls."[382]

MS is associated with simultaneous infection by the parasitic bacteria *Chlamydophila pneumoniae* and the Epstein-Barr virus (sometimes the *Varicella zoster* virus). Vitamin D's effectiveness against Epstein-Barr infections may explain the latitude dependence of MS.[383]

OUR TAKE

There are tremendous health benefits to increasing vitamin D intake, and no known toxic effects from supplementing with up to 5,000 IU/day so long as adequate vitamin K2 is obtained.

It seems prudent for everyone who obtains limited sun exposure to supplement with vitamin D, aiming for a 25OHD level around 40 ng/ml. Depending on sun exposure, it may take 2,000 to 5,000 IU/day of supplemental vitamin D3 for many adults to achieve this level.

People with some chronic diseases may find it beneficial to take higher doses. This should be done under a doctor's supervision.

Vitamin K2

Vitamin K2 is an extremely important fat-soluble nutrient that is needed to activate various proteins through a process called *carboxylation*, and has other functions as well which are poorly understood. Without vitamin K, blood doesn't clot, leading to **hemorrhage**; bones don't calcify properly, leading to **fractures**; soft tissues do calcify, leading to **atherosclerosis** and **joint disease**; and **cancer** runs rampant.

---

[380] The Vitamin D Council Newsletter, March 9, 2009.

[381] Milo R, Kahana E. Multiple sclerosis: geoepidemiology, genetics and the environment. *Autoimmun Rev.* 2010 Mar;9(5):A387-94. *http://pmid.us/19932200*.

[382] Burton JM et al. A phase I/II dose-escalation trial of vitamin D3 and calcium in multiple sclerosis. *Neurology.* 2010 Apr 28. [Epub ahead of print] *http://pmid.us/20427749*.

[383] Grant WB. Latitude and multiple sclerosis prevalence: vitamin D reduces risk of Epstein-Barr virus infection. *Mult Scler.* 2010 Mar;16(3):373; author reply 374-5. *http://pmid.us/20028708*.

Vitamin K is found in two forms: vitamin K1 (from plants) and K2 (from animals). Dietary K1 is primarily used in the liver to make clotting factors, with only a little converted to K2. So while K1 helps conserve K2, dietary K2 is essential for health.

Vitamin K2 has two principal forms, MK-4 which is the human and animal form and MK-7 which is produced by bacteria. They are functionally similar, but MK-7 may not replicate all the functions of MK-4. Most people get some MK-7 from gut bacteria and some MK-4 from foods like liver, butter, cream, cheese, and eggs.

K2 DEFICIENCY IS WIDESPREAD

Vitamin K2 deficiency seems to be common. One measure of K2 deficiency is the percentage of circulating osteocalcin that has not been activated by vitamin K2. The EPIC-Heidelberg study found that for every 10% of osteocalcin that is undercarboxylated, advanced-stage prostate cancer cases increase by 38%.[384]

If 10% osteocalcin undercarboxylation is proof of K2 deficiency, then most people are deficient. The Framingham Offspring Study found that American men average 17% undercarboxylated osteocalcin, and American women 19%. The rate of undercarboxylation was highest in postmenopausal women, and estrogen replacement improved K2 status.[385] A majority of 11- and 12-year-old Dutch girls have over 20% of their serum osteocalcin undercarboxylated.[386] In children ages 8 through 14, the range of osteocalcin undercarboxylation was 11% to 83%.[387] Another study in the Netherlands found 43% undercarboxylation in Dutch adults and 67% in Dutch children.[388] K2 deficiency is severe in children because growing bones need more K2.

Vitamin K has no significant storage pool in the body, so deficiencies develop quickly. Infants on vitamin K-free formula develop a K2 deficiency in 7-10 days.[389]

---

[384] Nimptsch K et al. Serum undercarboxylated osteocalcin as biomarker of vitamin K intake and risk of prostate cancer: a nested case-control study in the Heidelberg cohort of the European prospective investigation into cancer and nutrition. *Cancer Epidemiol Biomarkers Prev.* 2009 Jan;18(1):49-56. *http://pmid.us/19124480.*

[385] Shea MK et al. Genetic and non-genetic correlates of vitamins K and D. *Eur J Clin Nutr.* 2009 Apr;63(4):458-64. *http://pmid.us/18030310.*

[386] O'Connor E et al. Serum percentage undercarboxylated osteocalcin, a sensitive measure of vitamin K status, and its relationship to bone health indices in Danish girls. *Br J Nutr.* 2007 Apr;97(4):661-6. *http://pmid.us/17349078.*

[387] van Summeren MJ et al. Vitamin K status is associated with childhood bone mineral content. *Br J Nutr.* 2008 Oct;100(4):852-8. *http://pmid.us/18279558.*

[388] van Summeren MJ et al. Pronounced elevation of undercarboxylated osteocalcin in healthy children. *Pediatr Res.* 2007 Mar;61(3):366-70. *http://pmid.us/17314699.*

[389] Israels LG et al. The riddle of vitamin K1 deficit in the newborn. *Semin Perinatol.* 1997 Feb;21(1):90-6. *http://pmid.us/9190038.*

VITAMIN K2 PREVENTS ATHEROSCLEROSIS AND HEART DISEASE

In a healthy body, bones and teeth calcify and become hard, but no other tissues do. In many elderly, however, soft tissues improperly calcify, causing kidney stones, arthritis, cataracts, heart valve insufficiency, bone fractures, wrinkled skin, bone spurs, senility and coronary atherosclerosis.

Calcification of coronary arteries – in which the arterial walls are turned bony and stiff – is a highly accurate predictor of heart attacks and mortality.[390]

Vitamin K2 protects against all disorders of calcification, assuring that bones and teeth calcify and other tissues do not.

The Dutch Prospect arm of the EPIC study found that vitamin K2, but not K1, reduces the risk of coronary calcification[391] and heart disease[392]. Every additional 10 mcg/day of vitamin K2 reduced the rate of heart disease by 9%.

Vitamin K2 for Patients on Coumarin

In rats, blocking vitamin K2 with warfarin produces calcified arteries in only 3 weeks. However, supplemental K2 then reverses arterial calcification.[1]

As with rats, so with humans: Patients who take coumarin experience arterial calcification.[2] Such patients should supplement with vitamin K2. This will improve bone and vascular health and, with adjustment of coumarin dose, stabilize INR levels.

[1] Schurgers LJ et al. Regression of warfarin-induced medial elastocalcinosis by high intake of vitamin K in rats. *Blood.* 2007 Apr 1;109(7):2823-31. *http://pmid.us/17138823.*

[2] Rennenberg RJ et al. Chronic coumarin treatment is associated with increased extra-coronary arterial calcification in humans. *Blood.* 2010 Jun 17;115(24):5121-3. *http://pmid.us/20354170.*

VITAMIN K2 STRENGTHENS BONES

Seven clinical trials studying K2 supplementation at 45 mg/day consistently observed reduced fracture rates. On average, K2 supplementation reduced the risk of vertebral fractures by 60%, hip fractures by 77%, and non-vertebral fractures by a remarkable 81%.[393]

---

[390] Shaw LJ et al. Coronary artery calcium as a measure of biologic age. *Atherosclerosis.* 2006 Sep;188(1):112-9. *http://pmid.us/16289071.*

[391] Beulens JW et al. High dietary menaquinone intake is associated with reduced coronary calcification. *Atherosclerosis.* 2009 Apr;203(2):489-93. *http://pmid.us/18722618.*

[392] Gast GC et al. A high menaquinone intake reduces the incidence of coronary heart disease. *Nutr Metab Cardiovasc Dis.* 2009 Sep;19(7):504-10. *http://pmid.us/19179058.*

[393] Cockayne S et al. Vitamin K and the prevention of fractures: systematic review and meta-analysis of randomized controlled trials. *Arch Intern Med.* 2006 Jun 26;166(12):1256-61. *http://pmid.us/16801507.*

VITAMIN K2 SHARPLY REDUCES MORTALITY

In the Rotterdam Study, vitamin K2 intake, but not K1, was inversely proportional to mortality.[394] Over a period of 7 to 10 years, people in the upper third of vitamin K2 intake, consuming just 41 mcg/day of K2, were:

- 26% less likely to die of any cause.

- 57% less likely to die of heart disease.

- 52% less likely to suffer aortic calcification.

Perigord, France is the world capital of foie gras, or fatty goose liver, which is rich in K2. Perigord has the lowest rate of cardiovascular mortality in France.[395]

VITAMIN K2 HELPS PREVENT AND DEFEAT CANCER

It has been known for 30 years that vitamin K2 kills cancer cells, including liver, colon, lung, stomach, breast, and mouth cancers as well as leukemia and lymphoma cells. Vitamin K2 also induces leukemia cells to differentiate into more normal blood cells, and prevents cancer cells from multiplying.[396]

Observational studies show that low dietary intake of vitamin K leads to higher cancer rates. For instance, in the EPIC-Heidelberg study, being in the top quartile of dietary Vitamin K consumption produced a 24% reduction in the risk of prostate cancer and a 75% reduction in the risk of advanced-stage prostate cancer.[397]

Clinical trials show that vitamin K supplementation reduces cancer risk. The ECKO trial supplemented elderly women with 5 mg/day K1 for 2 to 4 years to see if it reduced bone loss and fractures. It did reduce fractures – there were 9 fractures among the vitamin K group and 20 among the controls – but it reduced

---

[394] Geleijnse JM et al. Dietary Intake of Menaquinone Is Associated with a Reduced Risk of Coronary Heart Disease: The Rotterdam Study. *J Nutr.* 2004 Nov;134(11):3100-5. *http://pmid.us/15514282.*

[395] Stephan Guyenet, *http://wholehealthsource.blogspot.com/2008/06/vitamin-k2-menatetrenone-mk-4.html.*

[396] Lamson DW, Plaza SM. The anticancer effects of vitamin K. *Altern Med Rev.* 2003 Aug;8(3):303-18. *http://pmid.us/12946240.* Full text: *http://www.thorne.com/altmedrev/.fulltext/8/3/303.pdf.*

[397] Nimptsch K et al. Serum undercarboxylated osteocalcin as biomarker of vitamin K intake and risk of prostate cancer: a nested case-control study in the Heidelberg cohort of the European prospective investigation into cancer and nutrition. *Cancer Epidemiol Biomarkers Prev.* 2009 Jan;18(1):49-56. *http://pmid.us/19124480.*

cancers even more: there were 3 cancers in the vitamin K group compared to 12 in the control group.[398]

Clinical trials also indicate that vitamin K can help heal cancer. In a trial of acute myeloid leukemia patients, an MK-4 dose of 45 mg/day led to regression of the cancer in 71% of patients.[399] Several clinical trials have found that vitamin K2 reduces the occurrence and recurrence of hepatocellular cancer (HCC, a form of liver cancer).[400] This disease normally results in death within 3 to 6 months.[401] A Japanese trial found that 45 mg/day K2 with a blood pressure drug "markedly inhibited the cumulative recurrence of HCC."[402] Vitamin K2 inhibits metastasis and invasion.[403] The best predictor of survival is a measure of vitamin K status.[404]

Based on this evidence, we would advise anyone with cancer to take high doses of vitamin K2 as well as vitamin D.

VITAMIN K2 PROTECTS THE NERVOUS SYSTEM

Vitamin K2 is required for embryos to develop a healthy brain and nerves. Use of the vitamin K antagonist warfarin during the first six weeks of pregnancy causes severe birth defects and, during the second and third trimesters, causes neurologic abnormalities, spasticity and seizures.[405]

---

[398] Cheung AM et al. Vitamin K supplementation in postmenopausal women with osteopenia (ECKO trial): a randomized controlled trial. *PLoS Med.* 2008 Oct 14;5(10):e196. *http://pmid.us/18922041.*

[399] Miyazawa K et al. Vitamin K2 therapy for myelodysplastic syndromes (MDS) and post-MDS acute myeloid leukemia: information through a questionnaire survey of multi-center pilot studies in Japan. *Leukemia.* 2000 Jun;14(6):1156-7. *http://pmid.us/10865985.*

[400] Azuma K et al. Vitamin K2 suppresses proliferation and motility of hepatocellular carcinoma cells by activating steroid and xenobiotic receptor. *Endocr J.* 2009;56(7):843-9. *http://pmid.us/19550077.*

[401] *http://en.wikipedia.org/wiki/Hepatocellular_carcinoma.*

[402] Yoshiji H et al. Combination of vitamin K2 and angiotensin-converting enzyme inhibitor ameliorates cumulative recurrence of hepatocellular carcinoma. *J Hepatol.* 2009 Aug;51(2):315-21. *http://pmid.us/19501932.*

[403] Murata K et al. Hypoxia-induced des-gamma-carboxy prothrombin production in hepatocellular carcinoma. *Int J Oncol.* 2010 Jan;36(1):161-70. *http://pmid.us/19956845.* Ide Y et al. Inhibition of matrix metalloproteinase expression by menatetrenone, a vitamin K2 analogue. *Oncol Rep.* 2009 Sep;22(3):599-604. *http://pmid.us/19639210.*

[404] Takahashi S et al. PIVKA-II is the best prognostic predictor in patients with hepatocellular carcinoma after radiofrequency ablation therapy. *Oncology.* 2008;75 Suppl 1:91-8. *http://pmid.us/19092277.*

[405] Tsaioun KI. Vitamin K-dependent proteins in the developing and aging nervous system. *Nutr Rev.* 1999 Aug;57(8):231-40. *http://pmid.us/10518409.*

Vitamin K2 activates enzymes that produce constituents of the brain and nerves.[406] Higher serum vitamin K2 leads directly to higher brain levels of *myelin sulfatides*, which protect against cognitive decline with age.[407] Vitamin K2 also protects cells that manufacture myelin, which sheathes nerves and is essential for their proper function.[408]

VITAMIN K2 PROTECTS AGAINST VITAMIN D TOXICITY

Large doses of supplemental vitamin D can cause improper tissue calcification and an array of symptoms including anorexia, lethargy, growth retardation, bone loss, and death.

Vitamin K2 protects against all of these effects, suggesting that vitamin K2 prevents vitamin D toxicity. Indeed, it has been argued that vitamin D is toxic *only if it induces a vitamin K2 deficiency*.[409]

It is known that vitamin D depletes vitamin K2.[410] Therefore, to avoid vitamin D toxicity and vitamin K2 deficiency, vitamin D should be co-supplemented with vitamin K2.

NO TOXICITY

There is no known toxicity from either vitamin K1 or K2. Japanese trials lasting 3 years and testing large supplemental doses of vitamin K2 – 45 mg/day, a thousand times common intake – have not detected toxicity.

Although K2 *deficiency* leads to hemorrhaging[411], high doses of K2 do not necessarily lead to excess clotting, as long as K2 dose is adjusted gradually. Because vitamin K2 activates both pro-coagulation and anti-coagulation factors in

---

[406] Denisova NA, Booth SL. Vitamin K and sphingolipid metabolism: evidence to date. *Nutr Rev.* 2005 Apr;63(4):111-21. *http://pmid.us/15869125.*

[407] Crivello NA et al. Age- and brain region-specific effects of dietary vitamin K on myelin sulfatides. *J Nutr Biochem.* 2010 Jan 19. [Epub ahead of print] *http://pmid.us/20092997.*

[408] Li J et al. Novel Role of Vitamin K in Preventing Oxidative Injury to Developing Oligodendrocytes and Neurons. *J Neurosci.* 2003 Jul 2;23(13):5816-26. *http://pmid.us/12843286.*

[409] Masterjohn C. Vitamin D toxicity redefined: vitamin K and the molecular mechanism. *Med Hypotheses.* 2007;68(5):1026-34. *http://pmid.us/17145139.*

[410] Fu X et al. 9-Cis retinoic acid reduces 1alpha,25-dihydroxycholecalciferol-induced renal calcification by altering vitamin K-dependent gamma-carboxylation of matrix gamma-carboxyglutamic acid protein in A/J male mice. *J Nutr.* 2008 Dec;138(12):2337-41. *http://pmid.us/19022954.*

[411] Dahlbäck B, Villoutreix BO. The anticoagulant protein C pathway. *FEBS Lett.* 2005 Jun 13;579(15):3310-6. *http://pmid.us/15943976.*

parallel, high serum levels of vitamin K2 are generally consistent with normal blood clotting.[412]

OUR TAKE

Vitamin K2 supplementation appears to have substantial benefits – reducing mortality by 26% in one 10-year study. It has no reported negative effects even at doses a thousand times greater than most Americans obtain. Vitamin K2 is a necessary companion to vitamin D; the two are especially effective against cancer.

We therefore recommend supplementing with at least 100 mcg per day, and perhaps several milligrams, of vitamin K2, preferably in a mix of MK-4 and MK-7 forms, plus eating plenty of vitamin K-rich foods like green leafy vegetables and pastured dairy fats.

Selenium and Iodine

Perhaps the single most important hormone for human health is the thyroid hormone triiodothyronine (T_3).

It has three major functions:

- T_3 activates the biochemical machinery of the body. T_3-activated thyroid receptors must bind to DNA in order for transcription of RNA from many genes to be activated; and T_3 itself stimulates the production of the RNA polymerases which transcribe RNA. Without T_3, essential RNA and proteins would not be produced.

- T_3 fires up the metabolism. It increases oxygen and energy consumption, increases the rate at which glucose is produced and released into the blood, increases the rate at which fats are taken up into cells for energy, and increases the heart rate and the force of heartbeats.

- T_3 is essential for development of the nervous system in embryos and infants. It stimulates production of myelin, neurotransmitters, and axon growth.

A deficiency of T_3 is called *hypothyroidism*. Hypothyroidism not only makes its sufferers fatigued and weak; it exacerbates nearly all human diseases. The body cannot heal itself if it lacks T_3.

In order to make T_3, the body needs two minerals: selenium and iodine. Thyroid hormones are composed of iodine: The precursor to T_3, thyroxine or T_4, has four iodines attached to a peptide, and T_3 is created by the action of a selenium-containing "deiodinase" enzyme that removes an iodine atom.

---

[412] Matsuzaka T et al. Relationship between vitamin K dependent coagulation factors and anticoagulants (protein C and protein S) in neonatal vitamin K deficiency. *Arch Dis Child.* 1993 Mar;68(3 Spec No):297-302. *http://pmid.us/8466266.*

IMMUNE AND ANTIOXIDANT FUNCTIONS OF SELENIUM AND IODINE

Selenium is also needed by a few dozen other enzymes. Two are *glutathione peroxidase* and *thioredoxin reductase*, which are important for maintaining the key cellular antioxidants glutathione and thioredoxin.

A deficiency in selenium strongly impacts three organs that use antioxidants heavily – the thyroid, the gut, and immune cells:

- Glutathione and thioredoxin protect the thyroid against damage from hydrogen peroxide and ROS produced during the creation of thyroid hormone. If goitrogens from toxic foods like soy are eaten, then ROS production is particularly high, and poor antioxidant function is strongly associated with thyroid damage. Thus, selenium has a double effect on thyroid function – it enables the creation of active T_3, and it protects the thyroid from harm.

- Glutathione is especially important for the gut, where most of the immune cells in the body are located and where ROS produced to control gut bacteria are common. Repairing a selenium deficiency can be extremely helpful for gut health.

- White blood cells kill pathogens by releasing reactive oxygen species (ROS); their supply of protective antioxidants, especially glutathione, determines how much ROS they can safely manufacture and release. Low selenium implies poor white cell function.

Iodine is also important for immune function. Neutrophils, a type of white blood cell, kill bacteria and fungi with a "respiratory burst" of enzymes, ROS, and acid. To make this burst, the myeloperoxidase enzyme needs a halide partner.[413] Iodide is the most effective partner.

Neutrophils draw their iodine from thyroid hormones.[414] To support neutrophil function, thyroid hormones concentrate in diseased tissue, where thyroid hormone is consumed at a rapid pace.[415] So a deficiency in thyroid hormone impairs immune defenses by depriving neutrophils of iodide; and an ordinarily adequate intake of iodine can lead to hypothyroidism during chronic infections, if thyroid

---

[413] Klebanoff SJ. Myeloperoxidase: friend and foe. *J Leukoc Biol*. 2005 May;77(5):598-625. *http://pmid.us/15689384*. Severe impairment in early host defense against Candida albicans in mice deficient in myeloperoxidase. *Infect Immun*. 1999 Apr;67(4):1828-36. *http://pmid.us/10085024*.

[414] Woeber KA, Ingbar SH. Metabolism of L-thyroxine by phagocytosing human leukocytes. *J Clin Invest*. 1973 Aug;52(8):1796-803. *http://pmid.us/4719661*.

[415] Miller JK et al. Iodine concentration in nonthyroid tissues of cows. *J Dairy Sci*. 1973 Oct;56(10):1344-6. *http://pmid.us/4742118*.

hormone is consumed by immune cells faster than it can be replenished from a limited iodine pool.

Iodine was widely prescribed for infectious diseases in the 19th century. The Nobel laureate Dr. Albert Szent Györgyi, the discoverer of vitamin C, recounted this anecdote:

> When I was a medical student, iodine in the form of KI was the universal medicine. Nobody knew what it did, but it did something and did something good. We students used to sum up the situation in this little rhyme:
>
> If ye don't know where, what, and why
>
> Prescribe ye then K and I.[416]

A standard dose of potassium iodide was 1 gram, containing 770 mg of iodine.

Since immune cells obtain iodine by stripping it from thyroid hormone using selenium-containing deiodinase enzymes, a deficiency of **either** selenium **or** iodine will impair immune function.

BENEFITS FROM INCREASED CONSUMPTION OF SELENIUM

Selenium inadequacy is associated with a number of human diseases: Keshan and Kashin-Beck disease, cancer, impaired immune function, neurodegenerative and age-related disorders, and thyroid disorders. Selenium deficiency also exacerbates conditions caused by inadequate iodine, such as cretinism.[417]

In many people, selenium may be the limiting factor in thyroid hormone production. In French women, the size of the thyroid is inversely proportional to selenium intake.[418]

Selenium supplementation improves immune function. Both healthy and immunosuppressed individuals supplemented with 200 mcg/day of selenium for eight weeks showed an enhanced immune response to foreign antigens.[419]

---

[416] Szent-Györgyi, A. (1957) *Bioenergetics*. New York: Academic Press, p. 112.

[417] Köhrle J, Gärtner R.Selenium and thyroid. *Best Pract Res Clin Endocrinol Metab.* 2009 Dec;23(6):815-27. *http://pmid.us/19942156*.

[418] Derumeaux H et al. Association of selenium with thyroid volume and echostructure in 35- to 60-year-old French adults. *Eur J Endocrinol.* 2003 Mar;148(3):309-15. *http://pmid.us/12611611*.

[419] Roy M et al. Supplementation with selenium and human immune cell functions. I. Effect on lymphocyte proliferation and interleukin 2 receptor expression. *Biol Trace Elem Res.* 1994;41(1-2):103-114. *http://pmid.us/7946898*. Kiremidjian-Schumacher L et al. Supplementation with selenium and human immune cell functions. II. Effect on cytotoxic lymphocytes and natural killer cells. *Biol Trace Elem Res.* 1994;41(1-2):115-

Selenium supplementation also seems to help prevent cancer:

- Four supplementation trials showed that "selenium showed significant beneficial effect on the incidence of gastrointestinal cancer."[420]

- More than two-thirds of over 100 published studies in 20 different animal cancers found that selenium supplementation significantly reduces tumor incidence.[421]

- An intervention trial of selenium supplementation in China in areas with high rates of liver cancer found that selenium supplementation reduced the rate of liver cancer by 35%. In a smaller subgroup of chronic hepatitis B infected patients, none of 113 selenium supplemented patients developed liver cancer, while 7 of 113 placebo supplemented patients did.[422]

- In American men with a history of skin cancer, supplementation with 200 mcg/day selenium decreased prostate cancer incidence over the following 7.4 years by 49%.[423]

BENEFITS FROM INCREASED CONSUMPTION OF IODINE

Iodine deficiency is the most common cause of preventable brain damage in the world. About 800 million people suffer from iodine deficiency disorders including hypothyroidism and mental retardation.[424]

Iodine deficiency impairs immune response and is associated with high rates of stomach cancer.[425] A mandatory program of iodine prophylaxis in Poland reduced rates of stomach cancer by 18% in men and 29% in women.[426]

---

127. http://pmid.us/7946899. Kiremidjian-Schumacher L et al. Selenium and immunocompetence in patients with head and neck cancer. *Biol Trace Elem Res.* 2000;73(2):97-111. http://pmid.us/11049203.

[420] Bjelakovic G et al. Antioxidant supplements for prevention of gastrointestinal cancers: a systematic review and meta-analysis. *Lancet.* 2004 Oct 2-8;364(9441):1219-28. http://pmid.us/15464182.

[421] Combs GF Jr, Gray WP. Chemopreventive agents: selenium. *Pharmacol Ther.* 1998 Sep;79(3):179-92. http://pmid.us/9776375.

[422] Yu SY et al. Protective role of selenium against hepatitis B virus and primary liver cancer in Qidong. *Biol Trace Elem Res.* 1997;56(1):117-124. http://pmid.us/9152515.

[423] Duffield-Lillico AJ et al. Selenium supplementation, baseline plasma selenium status and incidence of prostate cancer: an analysis of the complete treatment period of the Nutritional Prevention of Cancer Trial. *BJU Int.* 2003;91(7):608-612. http://pmid.us/12699469.

[424] Triggiani V et al. Role of iodine, selenium and other micronutrients in thyroid function and disorders. *Endocr Metab Immune Disord Drug Targets.* 2009 Sep;9(3):277-94. http://pmid.us/19594417.

Clinical trials of iodine supplementation for chronic disease are lacking, which is odd in light of the positive experiences of physicians from the 19th and early 20th centuries, as well as anecdotal accounts from many modern people who have tried high-dose iodine supplementation and seen regression of chronic diseases.

These experiences are also supported by epidemiological evidence. In general, seaweed-consuming cultures are long-lived and healthy.

The Japanese are notably long-lived, and they eat a lot of iodine-containing seaweed. Average daily iodine consumption in Japan is 1.2 mg/day.[427] People in the northern coastal region eat 50-80 mg/day.[428]

By contrast, the US RDA is only 150 mcg/day, one-eighth the consumption of a typical Japanese. The mean consumption of iodine in the US is about 240 mcg/day.[429]

IODINE IS GENERALLY NON-TOXIC

Iodine, in its inorganic form, can be among the safest of trace minerals. In humans, doses of up to 6 g/day potassium iodide, containing 4.6 g iodine – about 20,000 times the typical American's intake – have been given safely for several years.[430] The Asthma Clinic of the Free University of West Berlin treated thousands of patients with doses of 36 g/day four days per week, and found that "the unwanted effects of potassium iodide are no more important than those of many other remedies."[431]

However, high doses of iodine are not guaranteed to be benign:

[425] Venturi S et al. A new hypothesis: iodine and gastric cancer. *Eur J Cancer Prev.* 1993 Jan;2(1):17-23. *http://pmid.us/8428171.*

[426] Gołkowski F et al. Iodine prophylaxis--the protective factor against stomach cancer in iodine deficient areas. *Eur J Nutr.* 2007 Aug;46(5):251-6. *http://pmid.us/17497074.*

[427] Nagataki S. The average of dietary iodine intake due to the ingestion of seaweeds is 1.2 mg/day in Japan. *Thyroid.* 2008 Jun;18(6):667-8. *http://pmid.us/18578621.*

[428] Hetzel BS, Clugston GA. "Iodine." In: Shils M et al, eds. *Modern Nutrition in Health and Disease.* 9th ed. Baltimore: Williams & Wilkins; 1999:253-264. Hat tip Linus Pauling Institute Micronutrient Information Center, "Iodine," *http://lpi.oregonstate.edu/infocenter/minerals/iodine/.*

[429] Pennington JA. Intakes of minerals from diets and foods: is there a need for concern? *J Nutr.* 1996 Sep;126(9 Suppl):2304S-2308S. *http://pmid.us/8811790.*

[430] Bernecker C. Intermittent therapy with potassium iodide in chronic obstructive disease of the airways. A review of 10 years' experience. *Acta Allergol.* 1969 Sep;24(3):216-25. *http://pmid.us/5395878.*

[431] Bernecker C. Potassium iodide in bronchial asthma. *Br Med J.* 1969 Oct 25;4(5677):236. *http://pmid.us/5349316.*

- Iodine intake should be increased gradually to allow the thyroid time to adapt. A too rapid increase in iodine may lead to hyperthyroidism. However, if doses are altered gradually, "Normal human thyroids can adapt to excess intake of iodine by autoregulation."[432]

- In cases of pre-existing thyroid damage from thyroiditis or treatment with recombinant interferon-alpha, the thyroid may be unable to adapt to high iodine doses. In these conditions, sudden high doses of iodine can induce a hypothyroidism which fades in 2-3 weeks after iodine is stopped.[433]

- Some organic compounds containing iodine, such as the drug amiodarone, have been known to poison the thyroid and induce either hypothyroidism or hyperthyroidism.[434] This danger is generally absent from natural food sources of iodine, such as seaweed, and from inorganic iodine supplements.

- Finally, because iodine strengthens the killing ability of white blood cells, people with autoimmune disease may worsen their condition by supplementing with high doses of iodine. Ironically, the organ that is most frequently the subject of autoimmune attack is the thyroid. In people who have circulating anti-thyroid antibodies, high doses of iodine can damage the thyroid and cause hypothyroidism.[435]

We therefore recommend that high-dose iodine supplementation be avoided until several months after grains have been eliminated from the diet. Wheat is the leading cause of autoimmune attacks against the thyroid.

However, we agree with the assessment in the *New England Journal of Medicine* by Dr. Robert Utiger: "the small risks of chronic iodine excess are outweighed by the substantial hazards of iodine deficiency."[436]

SELENIUM TOXICITY

Selenium is dangerous in high doses. Fatal toxicities have occurred with accidental or suicidal ingestion of gram quantities of selenium. Clinically significant selenium toxicity was reported in 13 individuals after taking supplements that contained

---

[432] Nagataki S. The average of dietary iodine intake due to the ingestion of seaweeds is 1.2 mg/day in Japan. *Thyroid.* 2008 Jun;18(6):667-8. *http://pmid.us/18578621.*

[433] Markou K et al. Iodine-Induced hypothyroidism. *Thyroid.* 2001 May;11(5):501-10. *http://pmid.us/11396709.*

[434] Fradkin JE, Wolff J. Iodide-induced thyrotoxicosis. *Medicine (Baltimore).* 1983 Jan;62(1):1-20. *http://pmid.us/6218369.*

[435] Teng W et al. Effect of iodine intake on thyroid diseases in China. *N Engl J Med.* 2006 Jun 29;354(26):2783-93. *http://pmid.us/16807415.*

[436] Utiger RD. Iodine nutrition--more is better. *N Engl J Med.* 2006 Jun 29;354(26):2819-21. *http://pmid.us/16807421.*

27.3 mg (27,300 mcg) per tablet due to a manufacturing error. Chronic selenium toxicity may occur with smaller doses of selenium over long periods of time; the symptoms are hair and nail brittleness and loss. Other symptoms may include gastrointestinal disturbances, skin rashes, a garlic breath odor, fatigue, irritability, and nervous system abnormalities.

The Food and Nutrition Board set the tolerable upper intake level (UL) for selenium at 400 mcg/day in adults based on the prevention of hair and nail brittleness.[437]

OUR TAKE

We recommend consuming 200 mcg/day selenium in the form either of supplements or a "supplemental food" such as 3 Brazil nuts per day. Cancer patients should obtain the UL, 400 mcg/day.

Due to its non-toxicity on the Perfect Health Diet (which largely eliminates autoimmune attacks on the thyroid) and potential huge benefits for immune function, we recommend consuming at least 1 mg/day iodine via regular seaweed or kelp tablet consumption. Asian supermarkets typically have a wide selection of seaweeds. Korean seasoned seaweeds make a tasty snack by themselves; other seaweeds make excellent soups or salads.

There are additional benefits from higher doses of iodine, such as 12.5 mg/day or 50 mg/day. High-dose iodine is protective against infections and cancers. High-dose iodine from either kelp consumption or supplements (Lugol's and Iodoral are leading brands) should be begun only after elimination of grains from the diet and with a watchful eye for any autoimmune effects, monitoring of thyroid hormone levels, and slow, gradual dose increases. A good strategy is to start at 1 mg/day; wait a month; double the dose and wait three weeks or until side effects subside, whichever is longer; then double the dose and wait again, continuing this cycle until you reach your desired intake.

A Note on Hypothyroidism

Hypothyroidism is a widespread and underdiagnosed problem.

HYPOTHYROIDISM WITH "NORMAL" TSH

Most doctors diagnose hypothyroidism by measuring levels of thyroid stimulating hormone, or TSH. If the body has too little thyroid hormone, then the pituitary gland releases TSH in order to stimulate the thyroid to make more hormone.

---

[437] Food and Nutrition Board, Institute of Medicine. "Selenium." *Dietary reference intakes for vitamin C, vitamin E, selenium, and carotenoids.* Washington D.C.: National Academy Press; 2000:284-324. *http://www.nap.edu/openbook.php?record_id=9810&page=284.*

However, the "normal" levels reported on lab tests are far too wide. Most labs place the upper end of the normal TSH range around 4 mIU/L, but health worsens dramatically as TSH increases within the "normal" range:

- The HUNT study enrolled over 25,000 healthy Norwegians with normal TSH levels for 8.3 years. People with TSH in the range 1.5-2.4 were 41% more likely to die than people in the range 0.5-1.4, and people in the range 2.5-3.4 were 69% more likely to die.[438]

- An Italian study of 4123 pregnant women found that those who had a TSH between 2.5 and 5.0 mIU/L had a miscarriage rate of 6.1%, while those with TSH below 2.5 had a miscarriage rate of only 3.6%.[439]

- A Dutch study found that the likelihood of breech birth, requiring a Caesarian section, was lowest with TSH below 0.7, 5 times higher with TSH between 0.71 and 2.49, 11 times higher with TSH between 2.5 and 2.89, and 14 times higher with TSH above 2.9.[440]

So halving TSH from 2.0 to 1.0 may reduce the risk of death by a third, and a TSH of 1.0 may still indicate inadequate thyroid function!

Now consider that one-fifth of Americans have a TSH above 3.0.

If you have clinical symptoms of hypothyroidism, such as lethargy or fatigue, low body temperature, cold intolerance, weight gain, coarse dry hair or hair loss, muscle cramps and aches, constipation, depression, irritability, memory loss, or abnormal menstrual cycles, it's essential to address thyroid status. Don't let a "normal" TSH deter you.

And even if you lack hypothyroid symptoms, we would try to get TSH below 1.0.

FIXING HYPOTHYROIDISM

We believe it's best to begin with a natural approach. First, eliminate grains, legumes, and vegetable oils. Then, supplement with selenium, iodine, vitamin D, and magnesium. Vitamin A deficiency, if it exists, should also be corrected.

Iodine supplementation should start at 1 mg/day or less, and then increase gradually following a cycle of waiting three weeks or until side effects subside, and then doubling the dose. It's desirable to bring TSH close to zero.

---

[438] Asvold BO et al. Thyrotropin levels and risk of fatal coronary heart disease: the HUNT study. *Arch Intern Med.* 2008 Apr 28;168(8):855-60. *http://pmid.us/18443261*.

[439] Negro R et al. Increased Pregnancy Loss Rate in Thyroid Antibody Negative Women with TSH Levels between 2.5 and 5.0 in the First Trimester of Pregnancy. *J Clin Endocrinol Metab.* 2010 Jun 9. [Epub ahead of print] *http://pmid.us/20534758*.

[440] Kuppens SM et al. Maternal thyroid function during gestation is related to breech presentation at term. *Clin Endocrinol (Oxf).* 2010 Jun;72(6):820-4. *http://pmid.us/19832853*.

If these steps are insufficient, your doctor can prescribe thyroid hormones. Options are levothyroxine, a synthetic T4 hormone; liothyronine, a synthetic T3 hormone; and natural thyroid extracts containing a mix of T3 and T4. Most doctors prefer to start with the synthetic T4 only, but most people obtain better results from a mix of T4 and T3 than from T4 alone.[441]

Magnesium

Magnesium is a crucial mineral for health. Over 300 enzymes need it, including every enzyme associated with the energy molecule ATP and enzymes required to synthesize DNA, RNA, and proteins. Magnesium also plays a structural role in bone and in cell membranes, where it helps transport ions across the membrane.

DEFICIENCY IS WIDESPREAD

NHANES surveys have shown that most Americans are deficient in magnesium. Median magnesium intake is 326 mg/day in white men, 237 mg/day in black men, 237 mg/day in white women, and 173 mg/day in black women – in all cases far below the RDA, which is 420 mg/day for men and 320 to 400 mg/day for women.[442]

The RDA is based in part on balance studies. Under controlled dietary conditions in healthy men, intestinal absorption of magnesium begins to decrease at an intake of about 380 mg and is reduced by about 60% at twice that intake.[443]

Multivitamins are not an adequate remedy for magnesium deficiency. Magnesium is a minor component of most multivitamins due to its bulk.

CONSEQUENCES OF DEFICIENCY ARE SEVERE

Magnesium deficiency can be fatal. Symptoms of acute magnesium deficiency include muscle cramps, heart arrhythmias, tremor, headaches, and acid reflux.

Chronic magnesium deficiency causes or is associated with a host of diseases: cardiovascular disease, high blood pressure, metabolic syndrome and diabetes,

---

[441] Nygaard B et al. Effect of combination therapy with thyroxine (T4) and 3,5,3'-triiodothyronine versus T4 monotherapy in patients with hypothyroidism, a double-blind, randomised cross-over study. *Eur J Endocrinol.* 2009 Dec;161(6):895-902. *http://pmid.us/19666698.*

[442] Ford ES, Mokdad AH. Dietary magnesium intake in a national sample of US adults. *J Nutr.* 2003 Sep;133(9):2879-82. *http://pmid.us/12949381.*

[443] Food and Nutrition Board, Institute of Medicine. "Magnesium." *Dietary Reference Intakes for Calcium, Phosphorus, Magnesium, Vitamin D, and Fluoride.* Washington D.C.: National Academy Press; 1997:192. *http://www.nap.edu/openbook.php?record_id=5776&page=192.*

migraines, osteoporosis, hypothyroidism, dysmenorrhea and PMS, and asthma.[444] Actual heart attacks have been observed during magnesium-deprivation experiments.[445]

Magnesium deficiency causes mitochondrial decay and accelerated aging.[446] Magnesium is needed for proper immune function, since it is necessary to synthesize glutathione.[447]

Vitamin D function also depends on magnesium,[448] to such an extent that magnesium deficiency can induce rickets in people replete with vitamin D.[449]

Magnesium deficiency is damaging to developing babies. In one clinical trial, magnesium supplementation by pregnant mothers reduced the risk of cerebral palsy by 30%.[450]

MAGNESIUM AND MORTALITY

Epidemiologically, areas with increased water hardness (and thus higher magnesium content) have lower cardiovascular death rates.[451]

Clinical trials have shown significant mortality reduction from giving magnesium to cardiac patients. In a study of heart attack patients, magnesium therapy given

---

[444] Food and Nutrition Board, Institute of Medicine. "Magnesium." *Dietary Reference Intakes for Calcium, Phosphorus, Magnesium, Vitamin D, and Fluoride.* Washington D.C.: National Academy Press; 1997:190-249. *http://www.nap.edu/openbook.php?record_id=5776.*

[445] Ibid., p 197, *http://www.nap.edu/openbook.php?record_id=5776&page=197.*

[446] Barbagallo M, Dominguez LJ. Magnesium and aging. *Curr Pharm Des.* 2010;16(7):832-9. *http://pmid.us/20388094.*

[447] McCoy H, Kenney MA. Interactions between magnesium and vitamin D: possible implications in the immune system. *Magnes Res.* 1996 Oct;9(3):185-203. *http://pmid.us/9140864.*

[448] Carpenter TO. Disturbances of vitamin D metabolism and action during clinical and experimental magnesium deficiency. *Magnes Res.* 1988 Dec;1(3-4):131-9. *http://pmid.us/3079418.*

[449] Reddy V, Sivakumar B. Magnesium-dependent vitamin-D-resistant rickets. *Lancet.* 1974 May 18;1(7864):963-5. *http://pmid.us/4133647.*

[450] Costantine MM et al. Effects of antenatal exposure to magnesium sulfate on neuroprotection and mortality in preterm infants: a meta-analysis. *Obstet Gynecol.* 2009 Aug;114(2 Pt 1):354-64. *http://pmid.us/19622997.*

[451] Food and Nutrition Board, Institute of Medicine. "Magnesium." *Dietary Reference Intakes for Calcium, Phosphorus, Magnesium, Vitamin D, and Fluoride.* Washington D.C.: National Academy Press; 1997:198. *http://www.nap.edu/openbook.php?record_id=5776&page=198.*

before thrombolytic therapy decreased mortality by 24 percent.[452] In a Russian trial, the group given magnesium supplements was only half as likely to die.[453]

TOXICITY

Magnesium has a broad plateau range. There is no evidence that anyone has ever reached toxic levels of magnesium from food consumption.

The initial symptom of magnesium toxicity from high-dose supplementation is diarrhea. In people with healthy kidneys this is likely to be the only effect, which is why magnesium is generally safe as a laxative. An adult laxative dose of 2 g magnesium (the amount in 17 g magnesium citrate) typically produces loose stools.

Very high doses of magnesium, well above 2 g, may lead to a fall in blood pressure, which in turn induces lethargy, confusion, disturbed heart rhythm, and poor kidney function. Extremely high doses can lead to cardiac arrest.

OUR TAKE

There are tremendous health benefits from eliminating magnesium deficiency. Magnesium intake of 400 mg/day or more is needed to achieve this. Total (dietary plus supplemental) intake of 800 mg/day is unlikely to produce any toxicity. We consider 400 to 800 mg/day the "plateau range," or optimal intake range.

About half of Americans obtain less than 250 mg/day of magnesium from food, and few obtain as much as 500 mg/day. This suggests that most Americans should supplement with at least 200 mg/day to reach the plateau range.

Multivitamins rarely include much magnesium, so we recommend specific supplementation of magnesium.

Copper

Copper is another essential mineral for which deficiencies can be fatal, and many people are deficient.

DEVASTATING EFFECTS OF COPPER DEFICIENCY

Copper deficiency was first observed in animals:

- Copper deficient cattle died suddenly due to heart atrophy and scarring.[454]

---

[452] Woods KL, Fletcher S. Long-term outcome after intravenous magnesium sulphate in suspected acute myocardial infarction: the second Leicester Intravenous Magnesium Intervention Trial (LIMIT-2). *Lancet.* 1994 Apr 2;343(8901):816-9.. *http://pmid.us/7908076.*

[453] Stepura OB, Martynow AI. Magnesium orotate in severe congestive heart failure (MACH). *Int J Cardiol.* 2009 May 1;134(1):145-7. *http://pmid.us/19367681.*

- Pigs deprived of copper died of weakened and ruptured arteries and heart attacks.[455]

- Mice deprived of copper similarly died of blood clots, heart muscle degeneration, and coronary calcification.[456]

- In rats, copper deficiency shortens lifespans and can lead to sudden death by rupture of the heart. Disturbingly in light of the American diet, fructose increases their need for copper. Rats eating sugar experienced far more sudden death in response to copper restriction than rats eating starch.[457]

In a human copper restriction trial, a modest reduction of copper intake from 1.38 mg/day to 1 mg/day produced heart trouble in 4 out of 23 subjects, including one heart attack. The authors commented:

> In the history of conducting numerous human studies at the Beltsville Human Nutrition Research Center involving participation by 337 subjects, there had previously been no instances of any health problem related to heart function. During the 11 weeks of the present study in which the copper density of the diets fed the subjects was reduced … 4 out of 23 subjects were diagnosed as having heart-related abnormalities.[458]

This is a disturbing result, since the US recommended daily allowance is only 0.9 gm/day. The RDA may be much too low.

DEFICIENCY IS WIDESPREAD

According to a 2001 study, the median American copper intake is only 0.759 mg/day, well below the US RDA. A quarter of Americans got less than 0.57

---

[454] Bennetts HW et al. Studies on copper deficiency of cattle: the fatal termination ("falling disease"). *Australian Veterinary Journal* 1942 Apr; 18(2): 50-63. *http://www.interscience.wiley.com/journal/120720447/abstract*. Hat tip Stephan Guyenet, *http://wholehealthsource.blogspot.com/2010/04/copper-and-cardiovascular-disease.html*.

[455] Coulson WF, Carnes WH. Cardiovascular studies on copper-deficient swine. V. Histogenesis of the coronary artery lesions. *Am J Pathol*. 1963 Dec;43:945-54. *http://pmid.us/14099456*.

[456] Klevay LM. Atrial thrombosis, abnormal electrocardiograms and sudden death in mice due to copper deficiency. *Atherosclerosis*. 1985 Feb;54(2):213-24. *http://pmid.us/3157387*..

[457] Reiser S et al. Role of dietary fructose in the enhancement of mortality and biochemical changes associated with copper deficiency in rats. *Am J Clin Nutr*. 1983 Aug;38(2):214-22. *http://pmid.us/6881079*.

[458] Reiser S et al. Indices of copper status in humans consuming a typical American diet containing either fructose or starch. *Am J Clin Nutr*. 1985 Aug;42(2):242-51. *http://pmid.us/4025196*.

mg/day, and only a quarter got as much as 1 mg/day.[459] Considering that copper intake of 1 mg/day was sufficient in the Beltsville study to induce heart attacks, this is an alarming deficiency rate!

Widespread deficiency is no great surprise, since Americans rarely eat copper-rich foods like liver, shellfish, and nuts, and the lack of copper in most fertilizers has led to soil exhaustion. A British study estimated that since 1940 the copper content of dairy foods has declined by 90%, vegetables by 76%, and meats by 55%.[460]

Another problem is that high doses of zinc can induce a copper deficiency by preventing its absorption. For this reason, zinc intake should be limited to 40 mg/day – roughly, the level of food plus a multivitamin.

TOXICITY

Copper poisoning sometimes occurs, especially after consumption of beverages stored in copper containers. Symptoms are belly pain, nausea, vomiting, and diarrhea, all part of the body's efforts to eliminate the excess copper. Once in the body, excess copper damages the liver and kidneys.

The US Food and Nutrition Board set the tolerable upper limit for copper consumption at 10 mg/day.[461] Although many studies have reported no negative effects from copper in the range 6 to 10 mg/day, one study did observe mild negative effects from 5 months of copper at 7.8 mg/day.[462]

OUR TAKE

We estimate the plateau range of copper at 2 to 5 mg/day. The US RDA of 0.9 mg/day is too low, as significant improvements in health have been observed with an increase in copper from 1 to 1.4 mg/day.

Unfortunately, only about 5% of Americans obtain 2 mg/day of copper.

---

[459] Pang Y et al. A longitudinal investigation of aggregate oral intake of copper. *J Nutr.* 2001 Aug;131(8):2171-6. *http://pmid.us/11481413.*

[460] Thomas D. The mineral depletion of foods available to us as a nation (1940-2002)--a review of the 6th Edition of McCance and Widdowson. *Nutr Health.* 2007;19(1-2):21-55. *http://pmid.us/18309763.* Hat tip Robert Andrew Brown, *http://wholehealthsource.blogspot.com/2010/04/copper-and-cardiovascular-disease.html.*

[461] Food and Nutrition Board, Institute of Medicine. "Copper." *Dietary reference intakes for vitamin A, vitamin K, boron, chromium, copper, iodine, iron, manganese, molybdenum, nickel, silicon, vanadium, and zinc.* Washington, D.C.: National Academy Press; 2001:224-257. *http://www.nap.edu/openbook.php?record_id=10026.*

[462] Turnlund JR et al. Long-term high copper intake: effects on indexes of copper status, antioxidant status, and immune function in young men. *Am J Clin Nutr.* 2004 Jun;79(6):1037-44. *http://pmid.us/15159234.*

The most abundant dietary sources of copper are beef and lamb liver, oysters, shiitake mushrooms, cocoa or dark chocolate, sesame seeds, cashew nuts, squid, and lobster.

It is possible to buy 2 mg copper supplements, or combined zinc and copper supplements. However, we believe that "supplemental foods" like the livers of red-meat animals are the healthiest source.

We therefore recommend eating a quarter-pound of beef or lamb liver per week; this provides 12 to 16 mg of copper, or 2 mg/day. (Other animal livers are not nearly as copper-rich. A quarter-pound of pork liver provides only 0.8 mg copper, and of chicken liver only 0.4 mg.)

Chromium

Little is certain about the need for and merits of chromium: there is no good measurement of bodily chromium status, and the chromium content of foods is not well-characterized, so researchers have had difficulty detecting chromium deficiencies. If researchers can't detect chromium deficiency, then it is difficult to link chromium deficiency to health problems.

BUT CHROMIUM IS PROBABLY IMPORTANT ...

Although it is hard to characterize the chromium status of *living* humans, it is possible to precisely quantify the amount of chromium in tissue samples from *dead* people. Thus, autopsies give a clue about the need for chromium.

Compared to the hearts of people who die from accidents, the hearts of people who die of heart attacks average 24% less magnesium, 17% less copper, 46% less chromium, and 26% *more* calcium. (Coronary calcification is a major risk factor for heart attacks and is largely attributable to vitamin D and K2 deficiencies.) The difference between the groups was 8 standard deviations in the case of magnesium, 4 in the case of copper, and 3.3 in the case of chromium.[463]

These data strongly suggest that these three minerals – magnesium, copper, and chromium – are needed for heart health, and that deficiencies synergistically promote fatal heart attacks. It is quite remarkable that nearly everyone who died from a heart attack was deficient in all three minerals.

Another hint of chromium's importance comes from the days when chromium was not included in total parenteral (i.e., intravenous) nutrition. Patients on parenteral nutrition developed unexplained weight loss, impaired glucose

---

[463] Anderson TW et al. Letter: Ischemic heart disease, water hardness and myocardial magnesium. *Can Med Assoc J.* 1975 Aug 9;113(3):199-203. *http://pmid.us/1139518.*

utilization, and peripheral neuropathy. Symptoms were cured by 2 weeks of chromium supplementation at 250 mcg/day.[464]

CHROMIUM AND IMMUNE FUNCTION

Chromium's primary function is to assist in the entry of glucose into cells. With increased chromium, more glucose finds its way into cells from the blood; thus in a Chinese study a group of diabetics taking 1,000 mcg/day of chromium picolinate had blood glucose levels 15% to 19% lower than those taking the placebo.[465]

Whether this is good for diabetics is not obvious. Chromium doesn't eliminate glucose poisoning, it only moves it into cells. Whether it is better to poison the inside or the outside of cells remains an open question.

Our interest in chromium is different. Chromium may be protective against chronic infections – which we believe cause most chronic disease and accelerate aging.

The cells which most need to be able to take in glucose quickly are immune cells, which use glucose to generate reactive oxygen species for the killing of fungi and bacteria. Without chromium, their ability to kill is impaired.

Experiments in animals have confirmed the importance of chromium for immune defense against fungal infections. Depriving goats of chromium causes them to contract systemic fungal infections.[466] Chromium is also directly toxic to fungi.[467] It is likely that chromium also aids immune defense against bacterial infections.

DEFICIENCY IS PROBABLY WIDESPREAD

Chromium intake in the U.S. has been estimated at 23-29 mcg/day for women and 39-54 mcg/day for men.[468] These intakes are probably severely deficient.

---

[464] Food and Nutrition Board, Institute of Medicine. "Chromium." *Dietary reference intakes for vitamin A, vitamin K, boron, chromium, copper, iodine, iron, manganese, molybdenum, nickel, silicon, vanadium, and zinc.* Washington, D.C.: National Academy Press; 2001:197-223. *http://www.nap.edu/openbook.php?record_id=10026&page=201.*

[465] Anderson RA et al. Elevated intakes of supplemental chromium improve glucose and insulin variables in individuals with type 2 diabetes. *Diabetes.* 1997 Nov;46(11):1786-91. *http://pmid.us/9356027.*

[466] Aupperle H et al. Experimental copper deficiency, chromium deficiency and additional molybdenum supplementation in goats--pathological findings. *Acta Vet Scand.* 2001;42(3):311-21. *http://pmid.us/11887391.*

[467] Poljsak B et al. Interference of chromium with biological systems in yeasts and fungi: a review. *J Basic Microbiol.* 2010 Feb;50(1):21-36. *http://pmid.us/19810050.*

[468] Food and Nutrition Board, Institute of Medicine. "Chromium." *Dietary reference intakes for vitamin A, vitamin K, boron, chromium, copper, iodine, iron, manganese, molybdenum,*

TOXICITY

The U.S. Food and Nutrition Board did not set a tolerable upper limit for chromium, because of a lack of evidence of toxicity.

Several studies have reported no ill effects from supplementation with 1,000 mcg/day for several months. On the other hand, there have been reports of kidney failure after use of 1,200 to 2,400 mcg/day for four to five months, and occasional reports of kidney failure on doses below 1,000 mcg/day.[469]

OUR TAKE

There is not enough information to clearly identify a plateau range for chromium, but we believe that supplementation with 200 mcg/day is safe and beneficial.

Vitamin C

Vitamin C is needed for the manufacture of critical body components:

- Collagen, the scaffolding on which all organs, bones, and tissues are built.

- Carnitine, which transports fats into mitochondria for energy production.

- Norepinephrine and epinephrine (adrenaline), hormones and neurotransmitters that control alertness, arousal, and motivation.

- Enzymes involved in creation of peptide hormones, tyrosine metabolism, and bile acid.

Vitamin C is also needed to maintain levels of glutathione, the immune system's primary antioxidant.

Symptoms of vitamin C deficiency may include a tendency toward cavities or fractures, hair or tooth loss, bruising, bleeding gums, muscle loss or difficulty gaining muscle, slow wound healing, and joint pain and swelling. Severe vitamin C deficiency results in death unless remedied.

VITAMIN C DEFICIENCY IS WIDESPREAD

Vitamin C deficiency is widespread. Analysis of the National Health and Nutrition Examination Survey (NHANES) found that 18% of US adults, and 14% of teenage males and 20% of teenage females, get less than 30 mg/day of vitamin C. This is far below the RDA of 90 mg for adult males, 75 mg for adult females and teenage males, and 65 mg for teenage females. Blood tests found that 34% of men and 27% of men were deficient or depleted in vitamin C, as indicated by

---

nickel, silicon, vanadium, and zinc. Washington, D.C.: National Academy Press; 2001:197-223. http://www.nap.edu/openbook.php?record_id=10026.

[469] "Chromium," Micronutrient Information Center, Linus Pauling Institute, http://lpi.oregonstate.edu/infocenter/minerals/chromium/.

circulating levels below 28 µmol/L. The elderly, the sick, alcoholics, smokers, the obese, and other persons under stress are most depleted in vitamin C, and probably have increased need for vitamin C.[470]

DEFICIENCIES CAN BE DEVASTATING

Vitamin C deficiency is devastating – and potentially fatal:

- Without carnitine, the body becomes fatigued and weak, and mitochondrial impairment accelerates aging.

- Without collagen, all tissues waste away – including the heart, blood vessels, muscle, gut, and bone – and wounds cannot be repaired.

- Without glutathione recycling, immune defenses are weakened, leading to infections and inflammation.

If vitamin C deficiency is combined with other nutrient deficiencies, effects are even more severe. For instance, combined selenium and vitamin C deficiency results in severe muscle cell death.[471]

400 MG/DAY OR MORE IS THE PLATEAU RANGE

Healthy young people need to supplement with at least 400 mg/day before blood cells – and, presumably, other cells – cease to take up vitamin C.[472]

This suggests that the body has beneficial uses for at least 400 mg/day of vitamin C – more in the elderly, sick, and stressed.

EVIDENCE FOR MORTALITY BENEFITS FROM VITAMIN C SUPPLEMENTATION

As always, our gold standard for measuring benefits is reduced mortality. Several studies have indicated that high-dose vitamin C supplementation reduces mortality, especially cardiovascular mortality.

- The First National Health and Nutrition Examination Survey (NHANES I) Epidemiologic Follow-up Study found that among those supplementing with vitamin C to achieve a total intake of 300 mg/day or more, the risk of death from all causes was decreased 35% in men and 10% in women. Cardiovascular disease mortality was 42% lower in men and 25% lower in women, and cancer mortality 22% lower in men and 14% lower in women.

---

[470] Hampl JS et al. Vitamin C deficiency and depletion in the United States: the Third National Health and Nutrition Examination Survey, 1988 to 1994. *Am J Public Health.* 2004 May;94(5):870-5. *http://pmid.us/15117714.*

[471] Hill KE et al. Combined selenium and vitamin C deficiency causes cell death in guinea pig skeletal muscle. *Nutr Res.* 2009 Mar;29(3):213-9. *http://pmid.us/19358936.*

[472] Levine M et al. A new recommended dietary allowance of vitamin C for healthy young women. *Proc Natl Acad Sci U S A.* 2001 Aug 14;98(17):9842-6. *http://pmid.us/11504949.*

Men who took 800 mg/day of vitamin C lived six years longer than those consuming only the recommended daily allowance.[473]

- The Nurses' Health Study (NHS), which followed the health of 85,000 women over 16 years, found that vitamin C supplementation was associated with a 28% lower risk of heart disease.[474]

- A pooled analysis of nine prospective cohort studies, which followed 290,000 adults for an average of ten years, found that those who took more than 700 mg/day of supplemental vitamin C had a 25% lower risk of CHD than those who did not take vitamin C supplements.[475]

These studies are supported by cellular and biochemical studies which have identified mechanisms by which vitamin C improves cardiovascular health.

They are also supported by some miraculous cures. We have blogged about the New Zealand man whose doctors considered his case hopeless and wanted to terminate life support; he was cured by 100 mg/day vitamin C.[476] Dr. Robert Cathcart treated over 12,000 patients with high-dose vitamin C, and found it was effective against many infections.[477]

No Toxicity

It has been remarkably difficult to find negative effects from high doses of vitamin C. Intravenous doses of 120 g/day are well tolerated and safe.[478] Oral doses in

---

[473] Enstrom JE et al. Vitamin C intake and mortality among a sample of the United States population. *Epidemiology*. 1992 May;3(3):194-202. *http://pmid.us/1591317*.

[474] Osganian SK et al. Vitamin C and risk of coronary heart disease in women. *J Am Coll Cardiol*. 2003 Jul 16;42(2):246-52. *http://pmid.us/12875759*.

[475] Knekt P et al. Antioxidant vitamins and coronary heart disease risk: a pooled analysis of 9 cohorts. *Am J Clin Nutr*. 2004 Dec;80(6):1508-20. *http://pmid.us/15585762*.

[476] "New Zealand Man Left For Dead By Doctors, Cured by Vitamin C," Aug 26, 2010, *http://perfecthealthdiet.com/?p=439*; "Vitamin C vs Modern Medicine," Sep 25, 2010, *http://perfecthealthdiet.com/?p=619*.

[477] "Fighting Viral Infections By Vitamin C at Bowel Tolerance," Sep 26, 2010, *http://perfecthealthdiet.com/?p=636*.

[478] Riordan HD et al. A pilot clinical study of continuous intravenous ascorbate in terminal cancer patients. *P R Health Sci J*. 2005 Dec;24(4):269-76. *http://pmid.us/16570523*. Hoffer LJ et al. Phase I clinical trial of i.v. ascorbic acid in advanced malignancy. *Ann Oncol*. 2008 Nov;19(11):1969-74. *http://pmid.us/18544557*.

excess of 4 g/day, however, may produce diarrhea. This is the basis for the Upper Limit (UL) of 2 g/day.[479]

A recent study reported that supplementing with 400 IU vitamin E and 1 gram vitamin C reduces the oxidative stress of exercise and may reduce its benefits.[480] This may argue for limiting vitamin C to 500 mg/day, for avoiding vitamin E, or for exercising more intensely if you take vitamin C in order to make exercise more stressful.

A CAUTION FOR CANCER PATIENTS

Vitamin C protects all human cells against injury – including cancer cells.[481] As vitamin C reduces the effectiveness of chemotherapy, cancer patients should obtain vitamin C intermittently, avoiding it while on chemotherapy.

OUR TAKE

It is perilously easy to become vitamin C deficient on modern, hurried diets. The consequences of chronic vitamin C deficiency are devastating but also insidious, since the negative effects accumulate gradually and a deficiency may persist for years before it is diagnosed.

Vitamin C supplementation in the range 500 mg to 1 g per day does no harm and appears to offer substantial benefits, including a possibly significant reduction of mortality risk. Therefore, we recommend that healthy people supplement vitamin C in this range.

Those who are sick or under stress should supplement with higher doses, possibly – as Dr. Robert Cathcart recommended – to the limit of bowel tolerance, indicated by a sensation of queasiness.

---

[479] Food and Nutrition Board, Institute of Medicine. "Vitamin C." *Dietary Reference Intakes for Vitamin C, Vitamin E, Selenium, and Carotenoids.* Washington D.C.: National Academy Press; 2000:95-185. *http://www.nap.edu/openbook.php?isbn=0309069351.*

[480] Ristow M et al. Antioxidants prevent health-promoting effects of physical exercise in humans. *Proc Natl Acad Sci U S A.* 2009 May 26;106(21):8665-70. *http://pmid.us/19433800.*

[481] Heaney ML et al. Vitamin C antagonizes the cytotoxic effects of antineoplastic drugs. *Cancer Res.* 2008 Oct 1;68(19):8031-8. *http://pmid.us/18829561.*

To B or Not to B

B vitamins are water-soluble and easily excreted in urine, which makes their toxicity risk low.

In this chapter, we treat the non-toxic B-vitamins. The following B vitamins are so non-toxic that the Food and Nutrition Board did not establish a tolerable upper level of intake (UL): thiamin (B1), riboflavin (B2), pantothenic acid (B5), biotin (B7), and vitamin B12. We include vitamin B6 in this chapter because its UL, 100 mg/day, is high – more than 50 times the recommended daily allowance (RDA).

Folic acid (UL of 1 mg/day) and niacin (UL of 35 mg/day) we'll discuss in the next chapter.

Deficiencies Are Common ... But Not on Our Diet

Most Americans do not take a multivitamin and eat a lot of "empty calorie" foods like sugary beverages. As a result they often develop B vitamin deficiencies. Some indicators of B vitamin deficiency rates:

- Thiamin deficiency was observed in 12% of healthy persons and 33% of heart failure patients.[482]

- Riboflavin deficiency afflicts somewhere between 25% and 75% of the population, as evidenced by: (1) Cataract rates in the bottom 20% in riboflavin status are nearly double those in the top 20%[483]; (2) 27% of heart failure patients were found to have deficient red blood cell function due to riboflavin deficiency[484]; and (3) The bottom 25% in riboflavin status is twice as likely to have advanced colorectal adenomas as the top 25%.[485]

- B6 deficiency was found in 38% of heart failure patients.[486]

---

[482] Hanninen SA et al. The prevalence of thiamin deficiency in hospitalized patients with congestive heart failure. *J Am Coll Cardiol.* 2006 Jan 17;47(2):354-61. *http://pmid.us/16412860.*

[483] Mares-Perlman JA et al. Diet and nuclear lens opacities. *Am J Epidemiol.* 1995 Feb 15;141(4):322-34. *http://pmid.us/7840110.*

[484] Keith ME et al. B-vitamin deficiency in hospitalized patients with heart failure. *J Am Diet Assoc.* 2009 Aug;109(8):1406-10. *http://pmid.us/19631047.*

[485] Figueiredo JC et al. Vitamins B2, B6, and B12 and risk of new colorectal adenomas in a randomized trial of aspirin use and folic acid supplementation. *Cancer Epidemiol Biomarkers Prev.* 2008 Aug;17(8):2136-45. *http://pmid.us/18708408.*

[486] Keith ME et al. B-vitamin deficiency in hospitalized patients with heart failure. *J Am Diet Assoc.* 2009 Aug;109(8):1406-10. *http://pmid.us/19631047.*

On the Perfect Health Diet, food and multivitamin deliver about triple the RDA of B vitamins. This is enough to eliminate known deficiency syndromes. So the benefits of supplementation, if any, are likely to be subtle, or associated with unusual needs due to disease conditions.

Few Benefits From High-Dose Supplementation

There are few or no clinically documented benefits to healthy people from high-dose supplementation of B vitamins.

However, high-dose B vitamins can bring therapeutic benefits in some diseases. Here are a few diseases against which high-dose B vitamins proved therapeutic:

- Thiamin reversed microalbuminuria in diabetics in a clinical trial.[487]
- Riboflavin reduced the frequency of migraines in a clinical trial.[488]
- Biotin and thiamin produced "spectacular clinical and radiologic improvement" in two patients with brain disorders.[489]

Our Take

The low toxicity of these vitamins means that they are safe to supplement. For healthy people, it is not necessary to supplement beyond a multivitamin, and any benefits would likely be undetectable. However, some diseased people may see significant benefits from B vitamin supplementation.

For those who do choose B vitamin supplementation, plausible daily doses are:

- Possible benefit, no risk: thiamin (100 mg), riboflavin (100 mg), biotin (1 mg), pantothenic acid (500 mg).
- Possible benefit, possible risk: B6 (50 mg), B12 (500 mcg).

People who severely restrict carbohydrates, to 200 calories or less, should probably supplement biotin and B6 to support gluconeogenesis.

In general, our take is that "to B or not to B" remains an open question, but probably not one of great significance for most people. But we'll be monitoring clinical trials and will report on our blog if evidence for supplementation grows.

---

[487] Rabbani N et al. High-dose thiamine therapy for patients with type 2 diabetes and microalbuminuria: a randomised, double-blind placebo-controlled pilot study. *Diabetologia.* 2009 Feb;52(2):208-12. *http://pmid.us/19057893.*

[488] Schoenen J et al. Effectiveness of high-dose riboflavin in migraine prophylaxis. A randomized controlled trial. *Neurology.* 1998 Feb;50(2):466-70. *http://pmid.us/9484373.*

[489] Debs R et al. Biotin-responsive basal ganglia disease in ethnic Europeans with novel SLC19A3 mutations. *Arch Neurol.* 2010 Jan;67(1):126-30. *http://pmid.us/20065143.*

Seven Temptations to Resist

Some micronutrients are toxic in high doses, and should be limited to the levels found in food plus a daily multivitamin. Strangely enough, seven that fall in this category are among the most popular supplements: **vitamin A, calcium, zinc, niacin, vitamin E, folic acid,** and **fish oil capsules**.

Vitamin A

Many studies have found negative effects from high doses of vitamin A and its precursor β-carotene. A review and meta-analysis of 7 high-quality clinical trials covering 131,727 persons found that supplementation with β-carotene and vitamin A together increased mortality by 29%; β-carotene alone increased mortality by 5%.[490]

A prospective observational study of 72,000 nurses found that those ingesting more than 10,000 IU/day of vitamin A from food and supplements had a 48% higher risk of hip fractures than those ingesting about 3,000 IU/day.[491] Unfortunately, this study did not report death rates.

The high-fracture group obtained about half their vitamin A from multivitamins. The low-fracture group took neither multivitamins nor beta-carotene supplements, obtaining almost all their vitamin A from food. Carrots supplied about two-thirds of the food-sourced vitamin A in the study, with liver and milk the next most abundant food sources.

VITAMIN A AND VITAMIN D BALANCE

The negative effects observed with high vitamin A intake – bone fractures and cancer – are health problems associated with vitamin D deficiency. The "vitamin A toxicity" which the clinical trials observed may be due to an exacerbation of vitamin D deficiency by a relative surplus of vitamin A.

Vitamin A and vitamin D need to be in balance for good health. It appears that Americans have an excess of vitamin A relative to vitamin D.[492] On this view, the reason vitamin A appears to be toxic in clinical trials is that supplemental vitamin A makes an already-too-high A-to-D ratio even higher.

---

[490] Bjelakovic G et al. Antioxidant supplements for prevention of gastrointestinal cancers: a systematic review and meta-analysis. *Lancet.* 2004 Oct 2-8;364(9441):1219-28. *http://pmid.us/15464182.*

[491] Feskanich D et al. Vitamin A intake and hip fractures among postmenopausal women. *JAMA.* 2002 Jan 2;287(1):47-54. *http://pmid.us/11754708.*

[492] Cannell JJ et al. Cod liver oil, vitamin A toxicity, frequent respiratory infections, and the vitamin D deficiency epidemic. *Ann Otol Rhinol Laryngol.* 2008 Nov;117(11):864-70. *http://pmid.us/19102134.*

This hypothesis is plausible, because vitamin D and vitamin A act in concert with one another to affect gene expression in the nucleus of human cells. Both vitamins interact with specific "nuclear receptors," proteins on the surface of the nuclear membrane:

- Vitamin D interacts with the Vitamin D Receptor (VDR).

- Vitamin A interacts with two receptors, the Retinoid-X Receptor (RXR) and Retinoid-A Receptor (RAR).

After the vitamins interact with their receptors, the receptors enter the nucleus and interact with each other to form "heterodimers," or combined molecules, that regulate the transcription of genes.   RXR combined with VDR is one such heterodimer, and RXR combined with RAR is another. Each heterodimer causes tens or hundreds of genes to manufacture proteins.

- If vitamin A is high and vitamin D is low, then the nucleus is filled with RXR and RAR but has very little VDR. There is a lot of RXR-RAR activity but very little RXR-VDR activity. *This is the unhealthy situation many Americans are in.*

- If vitamin A and vitamin D are in balance, there is both RXR-VDR and RXR-RAR activity. *This is the healthy state.*

- If vitamin A is low and vitamin D is high, then there is plenty of RXR-VDR activity but not much RXR-RAR activity. *This situation is common in Africa, and is associated with the symptoms of vitamin A deficiency.*

Support for this "balance" view is provided by a study by Tufts University researchers.   They followed up on a suggestion by Chris Masterjohn[493] and assessed the relation between vitamin A and vitamin D status and the activation state of the vitamin K-dependent protein MGP.

Their findings[494]:

- Vitamin A alone does nothing to improve the status of MGP.

- Vitamin D alone increases the amount of activated MGP, but increases the amount of uncarboxylated MGP – a probable toxin – even more.

---

[493] Masterjohn C. Vitamin D toxicity redefined: vitamin K and the molecular mechanism. *Med Hypotheses.* 2007;68(5):1026-34. *http://pmid.us/17145139.*

[494] Fu X et al. 9-Cis retinoic acid reduces 1alpha,25-dihydroxycholecalciferol-induced renal calcification by altering vitamin K-dependent gamma-carboxylation of matrix gamma-carboxyglutamic acid protein in A/J male mice. *J Nutr.* 2008 Dec;138(12):2337-41. *http://pmid.us/19022954.* Hat tip Chris Masterjohn, *http://www.facebook.com/note.php?note_id=112375358783617.*

- Vitamin A and D together increased the amount of activated MGP even more than vitamin D alone, but completely eliminated the increase in toxic uncarboxylated MGP.

Thus a balanced intake of vitamins A and D amplifies the benefits of vitamin D, while eliminating side effects.

Unfortunately, we don't know precisely what the proper "balanced" ratio of vitamin D to vitamin A should be. We know only that the typical intake of Americans who take multivitamins – 10,000 IU vitamin A and less than 2,000 IU vitamin D – is problematic: it is associated with high rates of bone fractures, cancer, and other diseases. This suggests that the optimal ratio of vitamin A to vitamin D is no more than 3 IU to 1 IU.

OUR TAKE

We believe that the maximum healthy A to D ratio is about 3 IU to 1 IU, and that, since optimal vitamin D provision by sun and supplements is about 4,000 IU/day, vitamin A intake should be limited to 12,000 IU or less.

Multivitamins have about 5,000 IU of vitamin A, and the Perfect Health Diet is rich in fat-soluble vitamin A and carotenoids. There is no need to supplement vitamin A or carotenoids beyond what the diet and multivitamin provide.

Good food sources of vitamin A are colorful vegetables such as carrots, pumpkin and squash, peppers, sweet potatoes, and green leafy vegetables (supplying mixed carotenoids), egg yolks (supplying alpha carotene, beta cryptoxanthin, lutein, and zeaxanthin), liver, giblets, and oily fish.

A diet rich in colorful vegetables and eggs, plus about a quarter-pound of liver per week (which we recommend for its copper, molybdenum, vitamin B12, choline, and other nutrients) will provide sufficient vitamin A even before the multivitamin.

Calcium

Calcium has become an extremely popular dietary supplement, especially among older women, due to the hope that it might prevent osteoporosis.

Unfortunately, calcium supplements seem to have been a mistake.

IF VITAMIN D IS NORMAL, CALCIUM SUPPLEMENTS HAVE NO BENEFITS

The evidence that calcium supplementation will help bones and teeth is weak. Calcium supplements do not clearly reduce fracture rates in older women, and might increase the rate of hip fractures.[495]

---

[495] Reid IR et al. Effect of calcium supplementation on hip fractures. *Osteoporos Int.* 2008 Aug;19(8):1119-23. *http://pmid.us/18286218.*

Some studies have looked into how the effects of calcium vary with vitamin D status. These have shown that in people with normal vitamin D levels (25OHD above 30 ng/ml), there is no benefit to calcium supplementation. Normal dietary intakes of calcium – 500 to 600 mg/day – maximize bone health.[496]

CALCIUM SUPPLEMENTS CAN BE HARMFUL

A systematic review found that calcium supplementation increases the risk of heart attack by 31%, the risk of stroke by 20% and the risk of death by 9%.[497]

Heart attacks aren't the only risk from calcium supplementation:

- Calcium intake is associated with brain lesions in the elderly.[498]

- In the Nurse's Health Study, supplementation of calcium increased the risk of calcium oxalate kidney stones by 20%.[499]

- Calcium promotes the formation of biofilms and can aggravate infections.[500]

- Those who supplement with vitamin D may develop a dangerous hypercalcemia when supplementing calcium at 1200 mg/day.[501]

OTHER NUTRIENT DEFICIENCIES ARE THE TRUE CAUSES OF OSTEOPOROSIS

Other nutrient deficiencies, not calcium deficiency, seem to be the true causes of bone weakness:

---

[496] Bischoff-Ferrari HA et al. Dietary calcium and serum 25-hydroxyvitamin D status in relation to BMD among U.S. adults. *J Bone Miner Res.* 2009 May;24(5):935-42. *http://pmid.us/19113911.*

[497] Bolland MJ et al. Effect of calcium supplements on risk of myocardial infarction and cardiovascular events: meta-analysis. *BMJ.* 2010 Jul 29;341:c3691. doi: 10.1136/bmj.c3691. *http://pmid.us/20671013.*

[498] Payne ME et al. Calcium and vitamin D intakes may be positively associated with brain lesions in depressed and nondepressed elders. *Nutr Res.* 2008 May;28(5):285-92. *http://pmid.us/19083421.*

[499] Curhan GC et al. Comparison of dietary calcium with supplemental calcium and other nutrients as factors affecting the risk for kidney stones in women. *Ann Intern Med.* 1997 Apr 1;126(7):497-504. *http://pmid.us/9092314.*

[500] Kierek K, Watnick PI. The Vibrio cholerae O139 O-antigen polysaccharide is essential for Ca2+-dependent biofilm development in sea water. *Proc Natl Acad Sci U S A.* 2003 Nov 25;100(24):14357-62. *http://pmid.us/14614140.* Geesey GG et al. Influence of calcium and other cations on surface adhesion of bacteria and diatoms: a review. *Biofouling* 2000; 15:195–205.

[501] Dr. William Davis, "Increased Blood calcium and Vitamin D," The Heart Scan Blog, June 21, 2010, *http://heartscanblog.blogspot.com/2010/06/increased-blood-calcium-and-vitamin-d.html.*

- Severe vitamin D deficiency reduces intestinal absorption of calcium by two-thirds and may cause a calcium deficiency.[502] Bone mineral density is maximized with serum 25OHD around 40 ng/ml.[503]

- Vitamin K2 supplementation brings about a 4-fold decrease in hip fractures and a 5-fold decrease in vertebral fractures. [504]

- Magnesium supplementation does much more to improve bone mineral density than calcium.[505]

If you're worried about bone health, supplement with vitamins C, D, K2, and magnesium – not calcium.

OUR TAKE

In an editorial for the *British Medical Journal,* Dr. John Cleland writes:

> Calcium supplements ... seem to be unnecessary in adults with an adequate diet. Given the uncertain benefits of calcium supplements, any level of risk is unwarranted.[506]

We concur. The Perfect Health Diet, especially if it includes green leafy vegetables and dairy foods, probably supplies a sufficiency of calcium, and a multivitamin with modest amount of calcium – 220 mg in ours – probably brings calcium toward the high (toxic) end of the plateau range. Therefore, we believe calcium should NOT be supplemented except as part of a multivitamin.

Zinc

Zinc is an essential mineral whose deficiency can be fatal. Before zinc supplements were available, babies with acrodermatitis enteropathica, a genetic disorder that impairs zinc absorption, died in infancy.

---

[502] Bouillon R et al. Intestinal calcium absorption: Molecular vitamin D mediated mechanisms. *J Cell Biochem.* 2003 Feb 1;88(2):332-9. *http://pmid.us/12520535.*

[503] Bischoff-Ferrari HA et al. Positive association between 25-hydroxy vitamin D levels and bone mineral density: a population-based study of younger and older adults. *Am J Med.* 2004 May 1;116(9):634-9. *http://pmid.us/15093761.*

[504] Geleijnse JM et al. Dietary Intake of Menaquinone Is Associated with a Reduced Risk of Coronary Heart Disease: The Rotterdam Study. *J Nutr.* 2004 Nov;134(11):3100-5. *http://pmid.us/15514282.*

[505] Abraham GE, Grewal H. A total dietary program emphasizing magnesium instead of calcium. Effect on the mineral density of calcaneous bone in postmenopausal women on hormonal therapy. *J Reprod Med.* 1990 May;35(5):503-7. *http://pmid.us/2352244.*

[506] Cleland JG et al. Calcium supplements in people with osteoporosis. *BMJ.* 2010 Jul 29;341:c3856. *http://pmid.us/20671014.*

Symptoms of severe zinc deficiency include dwarfism, delayed sexual maturation, skin rashes, hair loss, diarrhea, immune impairment, impaired wound healing, night blindness, depression, cognitive decline, and behavioral disturbances. Mild zinc deficiencies impair immune function.[507]

Zinc shares with copper a critical function – forming the essential cellular antioxidant, superoxide dismutase. Copper and zinc supplementation prevent atherosclerosis in one of the classic animal models of atherosclerosis, the cholesterol-poisoned rabbit.[508]

MANY PEOPLE ARE ZINC DEFICIENT

The US RDA is 8 mg/day for women, 11 mg/day for men. Median intake is about 9 mg/day for women, 14 mg/day for men. Perhaps one-third of Americans get less than the RDA.

BENEFITS OF SUPPLEMENTATION

Clinical trials have observed benefits from zinc supplementation, notably improved immune function and improved physical and neuropsychological development of children, confirming that most people are receiving less than the optimal levels of zinc. [509]

TOXICITY

The tolerable upper intake level (UL) for zinc is 40 mg/day. The reason is that high levels of zinc can induce copper deficiency: High levels of zinc impair copper absorption in the intestine. High intake of zinc therefore *reduces* levels of the essential cellular antioxidant, zinc-copper superoxide dismutase.[510]

BUT THERE MAY BE OTHER NEGATIVES TO ZINC ...

Zinc is a key nutrient for pathogens as well as humans. Our immune defenses take advantage of this: calprotectin, a protein released by white blood cells into abscess

---

507 Food and Nutrition Board, Institute of Medicine. "Zinc." *Dietary reference intakes for vitamin A, vitamin K, boron, chromium, copper, iodine, iron, manganese, molybdenum, nickel, silicon, vanadium, and zinc.* Washington, D.C.: National Academy Press; 2001:442-501. *http://www.nap.edu/openbook.php?record_id=10026.*

508 Alissa EM et al. The effects of coadministration of dietary copper and zinc supplements on atherosclerosis, antioxidant enzymes and indices of lipid peroxidation in the cholesterol-fed rabbit. *Int J Exp Pathol.* 2004 Oct;85(5):265-75. *http://pmid.us/15379959.*

509 Hambidge M. Human zinc deficiency. *J Nutr.* 2000 May;130(5S Suppl):1344S-9S. *http://pmid.us/10801941.*

510 Food and Nutrition Board, Institute of Medicine. "Zinc." *Dietary reference intakes for vitamin A, vitamin K, boron, chromium, copper, iodine, iron, manganese, molybdenum, nickel, silicon, vanadium, and zinc.* Washington, D.C.: National Academy Press; 2001:442-501. *http://www.nap.edu/openbook.php?record_id=10026.*

fluid, is a chelator whose purpose is to deprive pathogens of zinc. Zinc seems to be the most potent of all minerals in promoting fungal growth.[511]

OUR TAKE

Typical multivitamin levels of 15 mg/day, in addition to food intake of 10-20 mg/day, is likely to bring nearly everyone into the "plateau range" for zinc.

Especially in light of zinc's promotion of pathogen growth and the importance of copper to health, we would avoid megadoses of zinc and respect the Food and Nutrition Board's upper limit of 40 mg/day. Since dietary intakes on the Perfect Health Diet might easily reach 25 mg/day, zinc supplementation beyond a multivitamin is risky.

Niacin (vitamin B3)

There is a potentially fatal disease, pellagra, which is cured by vitamin B3. And in most people, high doses of niacinamide are tolerated with few observable negative effects.

Ordinarily these facts would strongly recommend niacinamide supplementation. A fatal deficiency disease suggests great benefits; great benefits with low toxicity recommend supplementation.

NIACIN VERSUS NIACINAMIDE

Niacin, but not niacinamide, has certain toxic effects. It causes uncomfortable skin flushing and, more seriously, liver damage. Slow-release niacin induces less skin flushing but causes much more severe liver damage.

The niacin detoxification process raises HDL levels and seems to reduce the risk of heart disease. Cardiologists frequently recommend niacin for this reason.

Niacin seems to achieve its beneficial effects by stimulation of certain ketone receptors. The same beneficial effects can be obtained by eating coconut oil, without any of the toxicity.

To us the combination of coconut oil with niacinamide makes more sense than niacin as a supplement. It achieves the cardiovascular benefits of niacin, and the vitamin effects of B3, without niacin's toxicity.

For that reason, we will consider niacinamide only from this point on. Niacin is converted in the body to niacinamide, so all the positive and negative effects of niacinamide accrue to niacin as well.

---

[511] Lulloff SJ et al. Fungal susceptibility to zinc deprivation. *J Lab Clin Med.* 2004 Oct;144(4):208-14. *http://pmid.us/15514589*. Sohnle PG et al. Effect of metals on Candida albicans growth in the presence of chemical chelators and human abscess fluid. *J Lab Clin Med.* 2001 Apr;137(4):284-9. *http://pmid.us/11283523*.

DEFICIENCY IS RARE ON THE PERFECT HEALTH DIET

We noted earlier that pellagra was unknown in Europe before the introduction of maize, and is primarily associated with corn or sorghum consumption. Perhaps pellagra should be classified as a grain toxicity disease, rather than a niacin deficiency disease.

Niacin deficiency is prevented by 11 mg/day. The RDA is 16 mg/day for adult men, 14 mg/day for adult women.

Nearly all foods contain niacin, with most meats having about 20 mg per pound and most plant foods about 5 mg per pound. Achieving a minimal sedentary person's calorie intake on the Perfect Health Diet requires 1/2 lb animal foods and 1.5 lb plant foods, and therefore provides at least 18 mg/day. More active people may obtain about twice the RDA.

NIACINAMIDE CAN PROMOTE BACTERIAL INFECTIONS

Niacinamide has little direct toxicity, but it has the potential to promote bacterial infections. Bacteria obtain energy from fermentation of glucose and its products like pyruvate, and niacinamide (in the form of a compound called NAD+) is the vitamin bacteria need for their metabolism. Niacin or niacinamide supplementation, therefore, gives an energy boost to bacteria in the body, helping them to reproduce and produce proteins that interfere with bodily functions.

Chronic bacterial infections are extremely common among the elderly and are a major cause of aging and age-related diseases. For instance, the "grumpy old man" syndrome, and the propensity of the elderly to fall, may be due to chronic bacterial infection of the brain or nerves.

DOES NIACINAMIDE PROMOTE OBESITY?

Recently, a group of Chinese researchers noticed that providing 300 mg niacinamide along with glucose during a glucose tolerance test exacerbated the subsequent swings in glucose and insulin. Those receiving the niacin had higher insulin one hour into the test, and a stronger hypoglycemia 3 hours into the test. That led to higher levels of hydrogen peroxide and a stronger appetite. They noted that the US obesity epidemic began about the same time as fortification of foods with niacin, and conclude, "Excess niacin consumption may be a major factor in the increased obesity prevalence in US children."[512]

While we don't believe that niacin fortification caused the obesity epidemic – vegetable oils and fructose are more plausible culprits – these changes in glucose and insulin levels are undesirable.

---

[512] Li D et al. Chronic niacin overload may be involved in the increased prevalence of obesity in US children. *World J Gastroenterol.* 2010 May 21;16(19):2378-87. *http://pmid.us/20480523.*

OUR TAKE

Food plus multivitamin will provide 40 to 50 mg/day of niacin to Perfect Health Dieters, about three times the RDA and probably within the plateau range.

Pharmacologic doses of niacinamide or niacin may have benefits in some diseases, but may also interfere with glucose metabolism and feed bacterial infections.

There is room for diverse opinion on this one, but our take is that niacin beyond levels contained in a multivitamin is unnecessary and too risky to recommend.

Vitamin E

A meta-analysis of 19 vitamin E clinical trials covering 135,000 people, of whom 12,504 died, showed that supplemental vitamin E of more than 400 IU/day increased a person's risk of dying during the study period by 4%.[513] In a later trial, death rates were the same in vitamin E and placebo groups.[514]

Two recent studies looked at vitamin E alone and in combination with vitamin C or selenium. In these studies, no benefit was seen:

- A clinical trial of almost 15,000 male doctors taking 200 IU/day vitamin E and 500 mg/day vitamin C for a decade found that total mortality was 8% higher in the vitamin E group and 7% higher in the vitamin C group.[515] The differences were not considered significant.

- The SELECT trial (Selenium and Vitamin E Cancer Prevention Trial) studied supplementation of 400 IU/day vitamin E and 200 mcg selenium in 35,000 men for five and a half years.[516] This time the placebo group had the highest mortality rate, but again the differences were not significant.

OUR TAKE

While the evidence is hardly conclusive, it may be dangerous to supplement with more than 400 IU/day of alpha-tocopherol. This could be due to vitamin E toxicity

---

[513] Miller ER 3rd et al. Meta-analysis: high-dosage vitamin E supplementation may increase all-cause mortality. *Ann Intern Med*. 2005 Jan 4;142(1):37-46. *http://pmid.us/15537682*.

[514] Effects of long-term vitamin E supplementation on cardiovascular events and cancer: a randomized controlled trial. *JAMA*. 2005 Mar 16;293(11):1338-47. *http://pmid.us/15769967*.

[515] Gaziano JM et al. Vitamins E and C in the prevention of prostate and total cancer in men: the Physicians' Health Study II randomized controlled trial. *JAMA*. 2009 Jan 7;301(1):52-62. *http://pmid.us/19066368*.

[516] Lippman SM et al. Effect of selenium and vitamin E on risk of prostate cancer and other cancers: the Selenium and Vitamin E Cancer Prevention Trial (SELECT). *JAMA*. 2009 Jan 7;301(1):39-51. *http://pmid.us/19066370*.

at high doses, or it could be due to an imbalance in the different vitamin E types – since vitamin E in foods comes as a mix of different tocopherols and tocotrienols.

We recommend obtaining vitamin E from foods only. If supplements are taken, they should supply **low doses** of mixed tocopherols and tocotrienols, not alpha-tocopherol only.

Folic Acid

Folic acid supplements have been linked to increased risk of cancer and cardiovascular disease. For instance:

- Although folate from vegetables appears to reduce cancer risk, 1 mg/day supplemental folic acid doubled the risk of prostate cancer.[517]

- In a Norwegian trial, persons receiving 0.8 mg/day folic acid and a small amount of vitamin B12 were 21% more likely to develop cancer and 38% more likely to die.[518]

- A Canadian trial supplied diabetics with 2.5 mg/day folic acid, and small amounts of vitamins B6 and B12. The folic acid group experienced 20% higher death rate, a doubled risk of heart attack or amputation, and a 6-fold higher rate of stroke, as well as greater kidney damage.[519]

OUR TAKE

Natural folate from foods seems to be beneficial, but the synthetic compound in supplements, folic acid, may not be. The body doesn't completely convert folic acid to natural folate[520], and the clinical trials may be telling us that unconverted folic acid is toxic.

Therefore, we recommend obtaining folate **entirely from foods** such as liver, giblets, egg yolks, seaweed, green leafy vegetables, and mushrooms. (These are the same foods which also provide vitamin A.) If a multivitamin is taken, it should contain 400 mcg folic acid or less.

---

[517] Figueiredo JC et al. Folic acid and risk of prostate cancer: results from a randomized clinical trial. *J Natl Cancer Inst.* 2009 Mar 18;101(6):432-5. *http://pmid.us/19276452.*

[518] Ebbing M et al. Cancer incidence and mortality after treatment with folic acid and vitamin B12. *JAMA.* 2009 Nov 18;302(19):2119-26. *http://pmid.us/19920236.*

[519] House AA et al. Effect of B-vitamin therapy on progression of diabetic nephropathy: a randomized controlled trial. *JAMA.* 2010 Apr 28;303(16):1603-9. *http://pmid.us/20424250.*

[520] Sweeney MR et al. Persistent circulating unmetabolised folic acid in a setting of liberal voluntary folic acid fortification. Implications for further mandatory fortification? *BMC Public Health.* 2009 Aug 18;9:295. *http://pmid.us/19689788.*

Due to the risk of birth defects from folate deficiency, pregnant women and women trying to become pregnant should consider folic acid supplements. However, 400 mcg/day may be a more prudent dose than the 800 mcg/day in prenatal vitamins.

Choline is a healthful supplement which can perform many of the functions of folate, and relieves folate deficiency.[521] Choline is especially desirable for pregnant mothers, as maternal choline deficiency leads to lifelong memory and learning deficits in the child.[522] We recommend that pregnant women and women trying to become pregnant supplement with choline.

Fish Oil Capsules

As we noted earlier, fish consumption has an excellent record in clinical trials, but fish oil capsule supplements do not. In the Diet and Angina Randomized Trial (DART-2), the group eating oily fish did well, but the group taking three fish oil capsules per day experienced a significant increase in sudden cardiac death.[523]

OUR TAKE

We recommend eating about 1 lb per week of fresh oily fish, like salmon, for omega-3 fats; **but do not take fish oil capsules**. Omega-3 fats in capsules are likely to become oxidized, rancid, and toxic long before the pills are ingested.

---

[521] Niculescu MD, Zeisel SH. Diet, methyl donors and DNA methylation: interactions between dietary folate, methionine and choline. *J Nutr.* 2002 Aug;132(8 Suppl):2333S-2335S. *http://pmid.us/12163687.*

[522] Zeisel SH. The fetal origins of memory: the role of dietary choline in optimal brain development. *J Pediatr.* 2006 Nov;149(5 Suppl):S131-6. *http://pmid.us/17212955.*

[523] Burr ML et al. Lack of benefit of dietary advice to men with angina: results of a controlled trial. *Eur J Clin Nutr.* 2003 Feb;57(2):193-200. *http://pmid.us/12571649.*

Summary: Micronutrient Recommendations

Supplementation can potentially deliver tremendous health benefits.

Here, in table form, is a summary of our recommended supplements, along with possible alternative sources.

Table: Our Recommended Supplement Regimen

Nutrient	Daily Amount	Alternative
Multivitamin	1	
Vitamin D	~2,500 IU	sunshine
Vitamin K2	1 mg	
Selenium	200 mcg	Brazil nuts, liver
Iodine	1 to 50 mg	seaweed
Magnesium chelate	200 mg	mineral water
Copper	2 mg	beef liver
Chromium picolinate	200 mcg	
Vitamin C	1 g	

In addition, there are nutrient-rich foods that we strongly recommend including in your diet. These foods are the topic of our next "Ideas" section.

Ideas for Micronutritious Eating

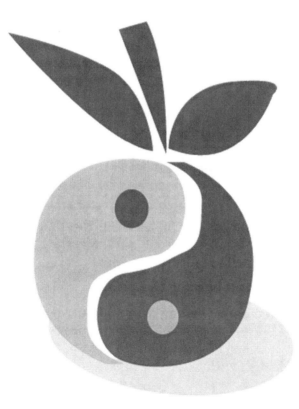

Micronutritious Cooking

Cooking should preserve the nutrient value of food, by (1) avoiding high heats and sugars that may denature foods, and (2) preserving drippings.

Avoid Damaging Chemical Reactions

In Step Two, we touched on the importance of cooking in ways that do not generate food toxins. The key steps are:

- **Avoid high heat**. High temperatures promote oxidation and other damaging chemical reactions that turn nutrients into toxins. Simmering and baking are good ways to keep temperatures from getting too high.

- **Avoiding mixing sugar with meats and polyunsaturated fats**. Sugars are highly reactive. Especially under heat, sugars react with proteins and polyunsaturated fats to create toxic endproducts. Sugar flavoring should be used only in PUFA-empty foods (such as the cream in ice cream) and at low temperatures (as in ice cream).

These are the first two principles of micronutritious cooking. The same chemical reactions that create toxins can denature nutrients, reducing the nutritional content of food. So, to preserve nutrition, avoid high heat and avoid mixing sugar with chemically fragile foods.

Preserve and Eat Juices and Drippings

Many cooking methods discard cooking juices or fat drippings. These residues are often nutrient-rich.

We recommend preserving and eating juices and drippings, except when the drippings are likely to be omega-6-rich, as when roasting duck. Drippings can be used to make gravies or sauces, mixed with starches like rice for flavor, or reserved for use as cooking oils in future stir-fries.

To preserve drippings without burning them:

- Roast meats in a ceramic baking dish and put vegetables and perhaps a bit of water in the bottom to prevent the drippings from burning. We typically seat the meat on a bed of vegetables, to elevate it above liquids and provide a vegetable side dish with little effort.

- Create soups, stews, and other dishes in which you eat the liquid in which meat and vegetables are cooked. Chicken cacciatore, seaweed soups, bone broth soups, beef rib stews, and beef tendon stews are good examples.

Micronutritious Foods

Supplements, though important, should not be your only source of nutrition. Nutrient-rich foods provide benefits supplements can't:

- They have nutrients like *folate* and *mixed carotenoids* that are superior to supplemental forms of *folic acid* and *vitamin A.*

- They are rich in organic compounds like *choline* or the raw materials for organic compounds like *gelatin (cooked collagen).*

- They are rich in *trace minerals.*

Nutrient-rich superfoods include egg yolks, liver and other organ meats, bone and joint soups, brain and bone marrow, seafood, seaweed, green leafy vegetables, and fermented vegetables.

Here are few pictures of nutritious foods, to help give you ideas.

Tendons and Connective Tissue

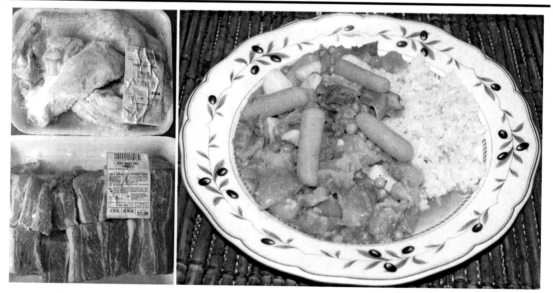

Left: Beef stew ingredients: beef tendon (top) and beef short ribs (bottom). Right: Finished beef stew with rice. The rib meat has fallen off the bones.

Food should supply the raw materials for all parts of the body – including bones and connective tissue as well as muscle. But most people eat only muscle, so they have a relative lack of the nutrients found in connective tissue. This can be remedied by including tendon or other connective tissue in stews or soups.

Asian supermarkets usually offer collagen-rich foods such as oxtail and beef tendon. Connective tissue has to be well cooked to render it digestible.

Seaweed and Bone Broth Soups

Seaweed is beneficial in any dish, but goes especially well in soups, as in the classic Japanese miso soup.

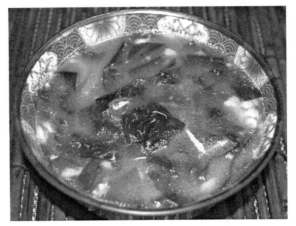

Beef bone and seaweed soup

Including bones in soups improves the taste. It's possible that minerals may leach from bones into bone-broth soups, providing nutrients like calcium, magnesium, manganese, and boron. Above is a miso-style soup with a beef bone broth.

Seafood

Like seaweed, seafood tends to be rich in iodine, selenium, and other minerals. Seafood also often contains high levels of vitamin B12 and omega-3 fats.

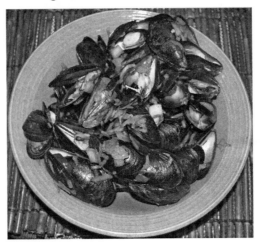

Mussels with onions, carrots, garlic, and shallots in a soy sauce.

Egg Yolks

Egg yolks are high in folate and carotenoids – the healthy natural forms of vitamins whose supplemental forms could be dangerous.

Egg yolks can substitute for fats or oils in many dishes. We previously showed how egg yolks could be added to chicken-and-rice soup to reproduce a 1 carb to 2 fat calorie ratio. We often add egg yolks and rice wine vinegar to rice, and then add meat and vegetables to make bibimbap, the classic Korean dish. Here is a classic summer egg dish. Cold potatoes provide gut-healthy resistant starch.

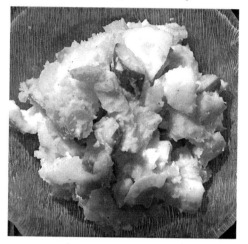

Egg-and-potato salad: Make mayonnaise from egg yolks, oil (we prefer coconut oil), vinegar and lemon juice. Mix diced potatoes, eggs, carrots, cucumber, and spices.

Variety Meats

Variety meats make beneficial additions to the diet. We especially recommend:

- Brain and bone marrow were prized foods among Paleolithic humans, and are rich in nutritious lipids and fat-soluble vitamins.

- Liver is famously nutritious. It is rich in enzymes, and thus contains many of the trace minerals needed for enzyme production; is a storage reservoir for vitamins such as B12 and A; and is rich in phospholipids.

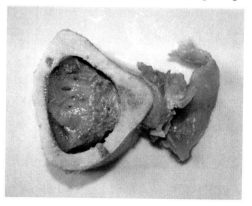

Bone marrow.

There is an old Chinese saying that you should "eat what ails you." If you have a stomach problem, for instance, then eat tripe; a kidney problem, eat kidney. This is a sure way of obtaining the micronutrients your ailing organ needs.

A Japanese Buffet

Quality ingredients make a nutritious meal. Any combination of a safe starch, seaweed, vegetables, and meat, eggs, or seafood makes a great meal.

A frequent meal for us, because it is so easy to prepare, is a Japanese buffet – a sort of homemade sushi. Here is how it looks:

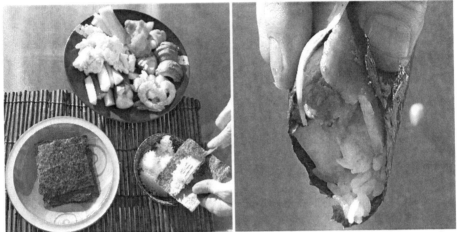

Left: A buffet: Eggs, bacon, shrimp, avocado, cucumber, and smoked gouda cheese; sushi nori seaweed; and white rice. Right: A homemade sushi roll.

Vegetable-Wrapped Finger Foods

A variation on the Japanese buffet is to use more conventional vegetables in place of the nori, and sautéed meat and vegetables in place of the buffet ingredients.

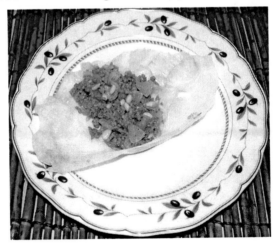

Beef with pine nuts and mandarin oranges in a boiled cabbage leaf. Add in rice or potato for a more complete meal.

Step Four: Heal and Prevent Disease

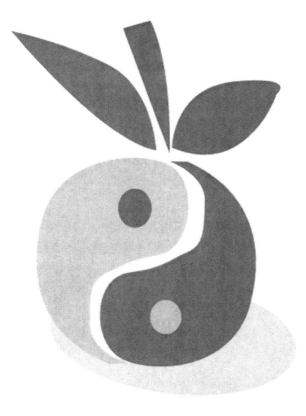

From Perfect Diet to Perfect Health

"All healthy people are alike; each unhealthy person is unhealthy in his own way." If *Anna Karenina* were a diet book, this is how it might have begun.

Apart from genetic conditions and injuries, diseases have three root causes:

- Malnutrition.
- Toxins.
- Pathogens – bacteria, viruses, fungi, and protozoa.

There are at least 44 essential nutrients whose lack produces malnutrition. There are thousands of toxins in most diets. There are at least 300 pathogens that produce human disease.

It doesn't take a mathematician to see that there are myriad possible combinations of nutrient deficiencies, toxicity syndromes, and infections. This is why *every sick person is sick in his own way*.

It is also why doctors are so poor at diagnosing and curing chronic disease. Since every disease is unique, and medications will address only one of many underlying causes, doctors will often lack an obvious diagnosis and have difficulty justifying a treatment.

How To Attack Disease With The Perfect Health Diet

It's best to start attacking any disease through diet and nutrition, because this will cure many problems and can do no harm. If you've implemented Steps 1, 2, and 3, you've eliminated malnutrition and toxins as contributing factors to ill health.

The next step is to deal with the third root cause of ill health, infections. In Step 4, we explore how to maximize immune function to prevent or cure infections.

Against entrenched diseases, antibiotics will generally be necessary for a cure. However, we believe that the Perfect Health Diet plus appropriate antibiotics can cure most chronic diseases.

A final complication is that diseases sometimes cause cellular changes or tissue damage that enduringly impair the ability to metabolize glucose or long-chain fats. Such diseases – which include diabetes, obesity, cancer, and a host of brain and nervous system afflictions – can be helpfully treated by a variant of the Perfect Health Diet: the "Herbivore Strategy" or ketogenic diet.

We therefore conclude Step 4 with a discussion of when and how to eat a "Herbivore Strategy" diet, and also – because many overweight people follow badly misguided weight loss strategies – how to lose weight.

Chronic Infections and Human Disease

Human beings are saturated in germs. Scientists have begun to carefully analyze the "human microbiome" and have established that at any one time, each person carries in the gut alone *100 trillion bacteria* weighing *2 to 3 pounds* from *over a thousand* species.[524] Trillions more bacteria line the skin, sinuses, lungs, and every other body surface.

At least 300 species of these pathogens are known to cause human disease.

Some infections are acute: they run their course within a few days or weeks. But many are chronic: the pathogens lodge in cells or biofilms, parasitize their hosts and steal glucose and nutrients for their own use, sabotage the immune system to ensure their survival, and gradually increase their numbers over decades.

Everyone Gets Chronic Infections

One way to estimate the prevalence of a given infection is by measuring how many people have antibodies to its pathogen.

Antibody studies have shown that many bacterial and viral infections are extremely common. One study of Alaskan Eskimos[525] found that:

- 94% had antibodies to cytomegalovirus (CMV), 90% to herpes simplex 1 (HSV1), 38% to herpes simplex 2 (HSV2), 80% to *H. pylori*, and 42% to *C. pneumoniae*.

- Over 70% had antibodies to at least 3 of the five pathogens tested.

- Seropositivity increased with age: a majority had antibodies to HSV2 and *C. pneumoniae* by age 45.

C. pneumoniae is associated with atherosclerosis, stroke, Alzheimer's, multiple sclerosis, arthritis, rosacea, and other diseases. Its infection rates are:

- Among Finns, the prevalence of antibodies is 70% in 15-19 year olds, and 100% in elderly men.[526]

---

[524] Fujimura KE et al. Role of the gut microbiota in defining human health. *Expert Rev Anti Infect Ther.* 2010 Apr;8(4):435-54. *http://pmid.us/20377338.*

[525] Zhu J et al. Prevalence and persistence of antibodies to herpes viruses, Chlamydia pneumoniae and Helicobacter pylori in Alaskan Eskimos: the GOCADAN Study. *Clin Microbiol Infect.* 2006 Feb;12(2):118-22. *http://pmid.us/16441448.*

[526] Tuuminen T et al. Prevalence of Chlamydia pneumoniae and Mycoplasma pneumoniae immunoglobulin G and A antibodies in a healthy Finnish population as analyzed by quantitative enzyme immunoassays. *Clin Diagn Lab Immunol.* 2000 Sep;7(5):734-8. *http://pmid.us/10973446.*

- Among Japanese, 59% to 73% have antibodies.[527]

- Among Israelis, 31% of children and 74% of adults are seropositive.[528]

- Among Italian schoolchildren, 29% have antibodies, and the prevalence increases steadily with age.[529]

- In Singapore, antibody prevalence is 75% in men and 65% in women. By age group, it is 46.5% at ages 18-29 and 78.9% above age 40.[530]

Infections with protozoa and fungi are also common. The protozoal parasite *Toxoplasma gondii* infects 20% to 60% of the population in most countries, forms cysts throughout the body including the brain, and influences behavior. Humans infected with *T. gondii* are 6 times more likely to get in traffic accidents.[531] Rats infected with *T. gondii* lose their fear of cats and are likely to get eaten.[532]

Diseases May Be Caused By Chronic Infections

Medicine is just beginning to link chronic infections to human diseases.

In 2005, Barry Marshall and J. Robin Warren won the Nobel Prize in Medicine for showing that *H. pylori* bacteria cause stomach ulcers. The 2008 Prize was awarded to Harald zur Hausen for linking human papilloma virus to cervical cancer.

Almost a dozen pathogens are now known to be causal factors in human cancers.

A recently discovered virus, Human Gamma Retrovirus, was isolated from prostate cancer tumors and is strongly associated with chronic fatigue syndrome.

---

[527] Miyashita N et al. Seroepidemiology of Chlamydia pneumoniae in Japan between 1991 and 2000. *J Clin Pathol*. 2002 Feb;55(2):115-7. *http://pmid.us/11865005*.

[528] Ben-Yaakov M et al. Prevalence of antibodies to Chlamydia pneumoniae in an Israeli population without clinical evidence of respiratory infection. *J Clin Pathol*. 2002 May;55(5):355-8. *http://pmid.us/11986341*.

[529] Dal Molin G et al. A population based seroepidemiological survey of Chlamydia pneumoniae infections in schoolchildren. *J Clin Pathol*. 2005 Jun;58(6):617-20. *http://pmid.us/15917413*.

[530] Koh WP et al. Seroprevalence of IgG antibodies against Chlamydia pneumoniae in Chinese, Malays and Asian Indians in Singapore. Int J Epidemiol. 2002 Oct;31(5):1001-7. *http://pmid.us/12435775*.

[531] Flegr J et al. Increased incidence of traffic accidents in Toxoplasma-infected military drivers and protective effect RhD molecule revealed by a large-scale prospective cohort study. *BMC Infect Dis*. 2009 May 26;9:72. *http://pmid.us/19470165*.

[532] Webster JP et al. Parasites as causative agents of human affective disorders? The impact of anti-psychotic, mood-stabilizer and anti-parasite medication on Toxoplasma gondii's ability to alter host behaviour. *Proc Biol Sci*. 2006 Apr 22;273(1589):1023-30. *http://pmid.us/16627289*.

DNA inserted into the human genome by this virus has been found in 86.5% of persons with chronic fatigue, but only 6.8% of controls.[533]

Atherosclerosis, stroke, Alzheimer's, multiple sclerosis, arthritis, and other diseases are linked to *C. pneumoniae*, which has been found:

- in the central nervous system of 97% of multiple sclerosis patients.[534]

- in the brains of 89% of Alzheimer's patients but only 5% of non-Alzheimer's elderly.[535]

- in 71% of atheromatous arteries and 67% of early atherosclerotic lesions but only 9% of nonatheromatous arteries.[536]

C. pneumoniae antibodies bring a 3.62-fold higher risk of hemorrhagic stroke.[537]

Parkinson's disease has been associated with the bacterium *Nocardia*.[538] Amyotrophic Lateral Sclerosis (ALS), also known as Lou Gehrig's Disease, has been linked to cyanobacteria.[539] *T. gondii* infection is associated with schizophrenia, mood disorders, and cognitive impairment.[540]

In almost every disease, evidence is building for pathogens as causal agents.

Infections Disable, Then Kill

Many chronic infections are permanent acquisitions. This is why antibody-positivity increases with age in all studies.

---

[533] Lo SC et al. Detection of MLV-related virus gene sequences in blood of patients with chronic fatigue syndrome and healthy blood donors. *Proc Natl Acad Sci U S A*. 2010 Aug 23. [Epub ahead of print]. *http://pmid.us/20798047*.

[534] Sriram S et al. Chlamydia pneumoniae infection of the central nervous system in multiple sclerosis. *Ann Neurol*. 1999 Jul;46(1):6-14. *http://pmid.us/10401775*.

[535] Balin BJ et al. Chlamydophila pneumoniae and the etiology of late-onset Alzheimer's disease. *J Alzheimers Dis*. 2008 May;13(4):371-80. *http://pmid.us/18487846*.

[536] Taylor-Robinson D, Thomas BJ. Chlamydia pneumoniae in atherosclerotic tissue. *J Infect Dis*. 2000 Jun;181 Suppl 3:S437-40. *http://pmid.us/10839732*.

[537] Yoneda H et al. Chlamydia pneumoniae infection as a risk factor for subarachnoid hemorrhage. *Cerebrovasc Dis*. 2005;19(4):209-13. *http://pmid.us/15703463*.

[538] Broxmeyer L. Parkinson's: another look. *Med Hypotheses*. 2002 Oct;59(4):373-7. *http://pmid.us/12208174*.

[539] Bradley WG. Possible therapy for ALS based on the cyanobacteria/BMAA hypothesis. *Amyotroph Lateral Scler*. 2009;10 Suppl 2:118-23. *http://pmid.us/19929743*.

[540] Fekadu A et al. Toxoplasmosis as a cause for behaviour disorders--overview of evidence and mechanisms. *Folia Parasitol (Praha)*. 2010 Jun;57(2):105-13. *http://pmid.us/20608472*.

As the number of chronic infections builds, people become increasingly disabled. Much of what we consider "aging" is not a natural degeneration of the human body, but increasing debilitation from chronic infections. Cardiovascular disease, dementia and memory loss, neuropathy and lost balance and falls, "grouchy old man" syndrome, cold intolerance, inflamed and arthritic joints – these are all symptoms of chronic infections.

But these pathogens are not content to merely disable. When the host becomes sufficiently diseased, these parasites may poison their host to create an acute disease that can infect others. Often the disease is pneumonia, since sneezing helps spread germs to new hosts. Acute diseases produced by chronic infections are a leading cause of death in the elderly.

The Good News

If, as we believe, chronic infections are the main cause of "aging" and disease, then we have good news!

Chronic infections can be cured by diet, nutrition, and antibiotics. It stands to reason, then, that *aging and most human diseases can be cured*.

Let's look now at dietary practices that aid the immune system.

Eleven Ways To Enhance Immunity

The human body has evolved powerful methods for defeating infections. Several dietary and nutritional steps can help **defeat chronic infections by cooperating with the body's immune defenses**.

Two Types of Pathogen

There are basically two types of pathogens the body has to confront:

- **Extracellular pathogens** – including fungi and some bacteria and protozoa – tend to live outside human cells. They circulate in the blood and live on surfaces, such as extracellular matrix, scar tissue, and the epithelial lining of the gut, urinary tract, lungs, sinuses, and vagina. On these surfaces, they form biofilms – meshworks of chained sugars that, rather like bone, are mineralized with calcium, iron, magnesium, and heavy metals. Biofilms are a sort of fortress that cannot easily be penetrated by immune cells or antibiotics. Pathogens shelter and reproduce within biofilms. Extracellular infections often begin in the gut, where food is available, and spread from the gut to the body.

- **Intracellular pathogens** – including viruses and some bacteria and protozoa – live inside human cells, except during temporary stages when they travel to new host cells. They are parasitic upon the cell they infect, and may need to be inside a cell to reproduce. Many intracellular bacteria are "cell wall deficient": in order to better hide from the immune system they shed their bacterial cell walls and hide within human vesicles. A single infected cell can host thousands of bacteria or viruses. When a cell becomes too crowded, pathogens may kill the cell, bursting its outer membrane, to facilitate their spread to new cellular hosts.

Most diseased people have both kinds of infections, but one type is usually dominant. As a rule, extracellular infections originate in the gut and most affect surface tissues (gut, urinary tract, sinuses), while intracellular infections most strongly affect the brain, nerves, and immune system.

Diet-Dependent Immune Defenses

The body has a variety of immune responses, some best-suited for extracellular pathogens, others for intracellular pathogens. To be fully effective, many of these need to be supported by diet.

Here are four critical human immune pathways that need dietary support:

1) **Antimicrobial peptides (AMPs).** AMPs are small proteins that can disrupt membranes, interfere with metabolism, and damage cell

components. The most important human AMPs, cathelicidin and defensins, are induced by vitamin D.[541] *Maintaining optimal 25OHD levels is essential to health; the body should be drenched in AMPs.*

2) **Respiratory bursts.** Phagocytic white blood cells, such as monocytes and neutrophils, engulf extracellular pathogens and destroy them with reactive oxygen species (ROS). The killing power of respiratory bursts begins with the generation of hydrogen peroxide using glucose by the enzyme glucose oxidase.[542] Next, myeloperoxidase, an iron-based enzyme, combines with a halide partner, preferably iodine, to turn the peroxide into a deadly acid.[543] For protection from their own respiratory bursts, white blood cells need the antioxidants glutathione, zinc-copper superoxide dismutase, and catalase. This myeloperoxidase-halide-hydrogen peroxide system is especially important against fungi, extracellular bacteria, and cancers. *Iodine supplementation increases phagocyte killing power; adequate glucose, iron, zinc, copper, and glutathione are also essential.*

3) **Autophagy.** Every human cell has organelles called lysosomes which are intracellular garbage collectors. Much like phagocytes outside the cell, lysosomes engulf intracellular pathogens (also junk cellular components) and digest them down to elemental amino acids and fatty acids that can be re-used for cellular purposes. Lysosome activity is called *autophagy* ("self-eating") and is upregulated during infections and when proteins and fatty acids are scarce. High levels of autophagy are associated with longevity and with immunity to disease. *Autophagy is strongly upregulated by fasting and by protein deficiency, making fasting and protein restriction essential tactics against intracellular infections.*

4) **Protein restriction.** Bacteria and protozoa such as *T. gondii* are highly dependent on certain amino acids, such as tryptophan, which they use for protein synthesis and manufacture of niacin, the vitamin that is essential to bacterial energy metabolism. The human immune response to intracellular infections generates high levels of interferons, and induces a compound called indoleamine 2,3-dioxygenase (IDO). The function of IDO is to strip the cell of as much tryptophan as possible, thereby preventing

---

[541] Wang TT et al. Cutting edge: 1,25-dihydroxyvitamin D3 is a direct inducer of antimicrobial peptide gene expression. *J Immunol.* 2004 Sep 1;173(5):2909-12. *http://pmid.us/15322146.*

[542] Babior BM. The respiratory burst of phagocytes. *J Clin Invest.* 1984 Mar;73(3):599-601. *http://pmid.us/6323522.*

[543] Klebanoff SJ. Myeloperoxidase-halide-hydrogen peroxide antibacterial system. *J Bacteriol.* 1968 Jun;95(6):2131-8. *http://pmid.us/4970226.* Klebanoff SJ. Iodination of bacteria: a bactericidal mechanism. *J Exp Med.* 1967 Dec 1;126(6):1063-78. *http://pmid.us/4964565.*

bacteria from reproducing and from synthesizing disease-promoting proteins.[544] (Many antibiotics are "protein synthesis inhibitors," so IDO is a natural antibiotic.) This has side effects for the human cell, of course – notably, deficiencies of serotonin and melatonin, which are made from tryptophan. This is why people with bacterial infections of the brain generally have symptoms of serotonin deficiency. (Bacterial infections of the brain often cause depression, and drugs which relieve the depression by increasing serotonin levels may backfire by providing bacteria with tryptophan.) However, overall the benefits of depriving bacteria of tryptophan far outweigh the costs. *Eating a low-protein diet, and resistance exercise to direct protein toward muscle, helps the immune system deprive bacteria of critical amino acids.*

To support these four immune pathways, anyone with a chronic disease should take the following dietary and nutritional steps.

First Way: Keep Blood Glucose and Insulin Low

We discussed this in Step 1. Keeping blood glucose low deprives bacteria, fungi, and protozoa of their favorite food, and avoids the immune-suppressing effects of glucose and insulin – for instance, their suppression of antimicrobial peptides.[545]

Second Way: Lower Omega-6 and Optimize Omega-3 Intake

As discussed in Step 1, omega-6 fats divert the immune response away from intracellular pathogens; at high levels they suppress all immunity.

Third Way: Avoid Toxic Foods

As discussed in Step 2, wheat interferes with vitamin D function, and sugar suppresses immunity. There are probably many other mechanisms by which toxic foods suppress immunity.

Fourth Way: Optimize Vitamin D Levels

Since vitamin D is so important for intracellular immunity and production of antimicrobial peptides, it's highly desirable to optimize vitamin D levels. For healthy people, this requires obtaining 3,000 to 5,000 IU/day from sun or supplements, reaching 25OHD levels around 40 ng/ml.

---

[544] Brown RR et al. Implications of interferon-induced tryptophan catabolism in cancer, auto-immune diseases and AIDS. *Adv Exp Med Biol.* 1991;294:425-35. *http://pmid.us/1722946*.

[545] Becker T et al. FOXO-dependent regulation of innate immune homeostasis. *Nature.* 2010 Jan 21;463(7279):369-73. *http://pmid.us/20090753*.

Unfortunately, pathogens have evolved ways to interfere with vitamin D function. This has several consequences which we've blogged about:

- Chronic diseases sufferers often have high serum levels of 1,25D and low levels of 25OHD.[546]

- Some disease sufferers appear to benefit from 25OHD levels double the normal optimum.[547]

Unfortunately research is currently inadequate to tell who might benefit from vitamin D levels different than the normal optimum. Disease patients may wish to self-experiment with vitamin D, but if no improvement is seen within a month, should aim for the normal optimum.

Fifth Way: Supplement With High-Dose Iodine

Iodine is the most effective halide for immune killing. We know this because:

- In experiments, addition of iodine greatly increases killing power.[548]

- When immune cells employ phagocytosis against infections, they strip iodine from thyroid hormone.[549] Not surprisingly, chronic disease patients often develop iodine deficiency hypothyroidism.

- High-dose iodine often cures infectious conditions, as the old doctor's mnemonic, recalled by Albert Szent Györgyi, suggests: "If ye don't know where, what, and why / Prescribe ye then K and I."[550]

A typical prescribed dose of iodine for acute infections in Szent Györgyi's time was 770 mg. We suggest 50 mg daily for chronic infections.

Sixth Way: Restrict Protein

Protein restriction benefits intracellular immunity in two ways:

---

[546] "Vitamin D Dysregulation in Chronic Infectious Diseases," August 21, 2010, *http://perfecthealthdiet.com/?p=421*.

[547] "The Amazing Curative Powers of High-Dose Vitamin D in Aging and Autism," August 30, 2010, *http://perfecthealthdiet.com/?p=448*.

[548] Sugar AM et al. The iron-hydrogen peroxide-iodide system is fungicidal: activity against the yeast phase of Blastomyces dermatitidis. *J Leukoc Biol.* 1984 Oct;36(4):545-8. *http://pmid.us/6592286*.

[549] Woeber KA, Ingbar SH. Metabolism of L-thyroxine by phagocytosing human leukocytes. *J Clin Invest.* 1973 Aug;52(8):1796-803. *http://pmid.us/4719661*.

[550] Szent-Györgyi, A. (1957) *Bioenergetics*. New York: Academic Press, p. 112.

(1) It cooperates with the body's intracellular immune strategy of depriving bacteria of amino acids. For example, *C. pneumoniae* needs tryptophan, tyrosine, and phenylalanine to grow.[551] The intracellular immune response induces interferon-gamma and IDO to deprive *C. pneumoniae* of these amino acids.[552]

(2) Reduced protein intake promotes lysosomal autophagy[553], which kills bacteria and viruses.

If you have a disease caused by an intracellular pathogen like *C. pneumoniae* or viruses, a low-protein diet is highly desirable.

Resistance exercise, which redirects protein toward muscle, helps deprive pathogens of amino acids. More importantly, it creates a protein reserve; muscle can be catabolized if needed to avert protein deficiency. Thus, resistance exercise makes low-protein diets safer.

Seventh Way: Regular Short Fasts

A short fast turns on autophagy throughout the body. Somewhat surprisingly, even neurons, which are sheltered from resource scarcity, benefit: "short-term fasting induces profound neuronal autophagy" and "sporadic fasting might represent a simple, safe and inexpensive means to promote this potentially therapeutic neuronal response."[554]

Neuronal autophagy has been found to be therapeutic for Alzheimer's.[555] This is no surprise – autophagy should be therapeutic for any intracellular infection, and Alzheimer's is likely caused by C. pneumoniae infection.[556] But it confirms that regular short fasts are likely to enhance immunity.

---

[551] Abromaitis S et al. Chlamydia pneumoniae encodes a functional aromatic amino acid hydroxylase. *FEMS Immunol Med Microbiol.* 2009 Mar;55(2):196-205. *http://pmid.us/19141112.*

[552] Kane CD et al. Intracellular tryptophan pool sizes may account for differences in gamma interferon-mediated inhibition and persistence of chlamydial growth in polarized and nonpolarized cells. *Infect Immun.* 1999 Apr;67(4):1666-71. *http://pmid.us/10085001.*

[553] Hipkiss AR. On methionine restriction, suppression of mitochondrial dysfunction and aging. *Rejuvenation Res.* 2008 Jun;11(3):685-8. *http://pmid.us/18593287.*

[554] Alirezaei M et al. Short-term fasting induces profound neuronal autophagy. *Autophagy.* 2010 Aug 14;6(6). *http://pmid.us/20534972.*

[555] Boland B et al. Autophagy induction and autophagosome clearance in neurons: relationship to autophagic pathology in Alzheimer's disease. *J Neurosci.* 2008 Jul 2;28(27):6926-37. *http://pmid.us/18596167.*

[556] "Is Alzheimer's Caused by a Bacterial Infection of the Brain?", June 28, 2010, *http://perfecthealthdiet.com/?p=126.*

WHAT IS THE PROPER LENGTH AND FREQUENCY OF "SHORT" FASTS?

Many of the benefits of fasting appear to be triggered as the liver starts to run short of glycogen. The liver's glycogen stores are 70 to 100 grams, or about 300 to 400 calories. Since the body consumes 500 to 600 glucose calories per day, liver glycogen stores become low about 12 to 16 hours into a fast. This suggests that *a 16 hour fast is sufficiently long to trigger autophagy*.

So a good way to implement short fasting is to confine eating to an 8-hour window each day – say, noon to 8 pm. This naturally creates a 16-hour fast from 8 pm to noon.

There is little danger from repeated 16-hour fasts, as long as liver glycogen stores are replenished by eating ~400 calories of starchy carbohydrates during the 8-hour feeding window. So it will be health-improving to engage in 16-hour fasts every day, or nearly every day.

CAN ANYTHING BE EATEN DURING A SHORT FAST?

Yes.

The key is to avoid carbs and protein, which would diminish the benefits of the fast. But *fat and fiber (vegetables)* can be eaten.

Coffee is an effective appetite suppressant, and may make the fast more comfortable. Paul, who doesn't care for the taste of coffee unless it is heavily diluted, drinks coffee mixed with an equal amount of heavy cream. Since the cream provides fat calories only, it doesn't interfere with the fast.

Eighth Way: "Herbivore Strategy" Diet Days

Ketogenic diets – the "Herbivore Strategy" of our Preview – also promote autophagy.[557]

Ketogenic diets have been successfully tested as Alzheimer's therapies. A placebo-controlled study found that those receiving supplemental coconut oil fats performed significantly better on a standard test for cognitive function.[558] Another randomized placebo-controlled trial also found substantially improved cognition on a ketogenic diet.[559] This success suggests an anti-bacterial effect.

---

[557] Finn PF, Dice JF. Ketone bodies stimulate chaperone-mediated autophagy. *J Biol Chem.* 2005 Jul 8;280(27):25864-70. *http://pmid.us/15883160.*

[558] Reger MA et al. Effects of beta-hydroxybutyrate on cognition in memory-impaired adults. *Neurobiol Aging.* 2004 Mar;25(3):311-4. *http://pmid.us/15123336.*

[559] Henderson ST et al. Study of the ketogenic agent AC-1202 in mild to moderate Alzheimer's disease: a randomized, double-blind, placebo-controlled, multicenter trial. *Nutr Metab (Lond).* 2009 Aug 10;6:31. *http://pmid.us/19664276.*

A simple way to turn the normal Perfect Health Diet into a ketogenic diet is to reduce carbs from 400 to 200 calories, and make up the glucose deficit by increasing coconut oil from 2 tablespoons to 12. The short-chain fats in coconut oil are readily converted to ketones.

We don't favor following a "Herbivore Strategy" diet every day, except in certain diseases, since it is less well protected against glucose deficiency than the normal Perfect Health Diet. However, as we'll see later, certain diseases may benefit from routine consumption of a "Herbivore Strategy" diet.

Ninth Way: Long Ketogenic Fasts

If short fasts are good, and ketogenic diets are good, then a hybrid of the two – long ketogenic fasts – may be even better.

It is hard to over-emphasize the importance of autophagy in fighting intracellular infections. Indeed, many pathogens have evolved ways to suppress autophagy. A much-cited review in *Nature* notes,

> [S]uccessful intracellular pathogens modulate the signaling pathways that regulate autophagy or block the membrane trafficking events required for autophagy-mediated pathogen delivery to the lysosome.... [M]icrobial evasion of autophagy may be essential for microbial pathogenesis.[560]

The danger in a long fast is glucose deprivation. This danger can be relieved by consuming copious amounts of coconut oil.

The short-chain fats in coconut oil are abundantly converted to ketones in the liver, and so high coconut oil consumption can reduce the glucose needs of brain and nerves by up to 300 calories per day. This relieves the liver from having to manufacture ketones and glucose from protein, which is a metabolically expensive process that may fail to generate enough calories.

About 12 tablespoons (6 fluid ounces) of coconut oil, supplying about 1500 calories, seems to meet a substantial part of the body's ketone needs.

WHAT IS THE PROPER LENGTH AND FREQUENCY OF "LONG" FASTS?

We suggest a monthly 36-hour fast, from dinner one day to breakfast on the day after next. However, scientist Thomas Seyfried believes that a 7-day to 10-day fast once or twice a year is optimal to achieve the full benefits of fasting.[561]

---

[560] Mizushima N et al. Autophagy fights disease through cellular self-digestion. *Nature.* 2008 Feb 28;451(7182):1069-75. *http://pmid.us/18305538.*

[561] Robb Wolf, "An Interview with Dr. Thomas N. Seyfried," *http://www.crossfit.com/cf-journal/seyfriedInterview.pdf.*

Since long fasts are stressful for the body, we recommend heavy consumption of coconut oil throughout the fast to supply ketones. Green leafy vegetables and seaweed may be added for a bit of calorie-free fiber.

SAFETY CONSIDERATIONS

A long fast should be terminated with any sign of nutrient deprivation, such as dry mouth, dry eyes, skin infections, irritability, anger, or anxiety.

Also, we recommend that you cease fasting if you feel hungry. Hunger on a fast, once you are adapted to the Perfect Health Diet, indicates a nutrient deficiency – possibly glucose, possibly protein, possibly a micronutrient such as vitamin C.

Tenth Way: Sleep and Melatonin

Sleep deprivation is dangerous. As one paper puts it: "[I]n the long run [lack of sleep] makes us sick. An increasing amount of scientific data indicate that sleep deprivation has detrimental effects on immune function."[562] Evidence:

- People getting less than 6 hours of sleep per night were 12% more likely to die over a 25-year period than people getting 6 to 8 hours per night.[563]

- Insomnia causes a progressive loss of gray matter from the brain.[564]

- People with sleep apnea experience shortened telomeres, a sign of premature aging; are more likely to develop high blood pressure, stroke, and heart attack; and are more likely to die.[565]

Some of the ill effects of lost sleep may result from deficient production of the hormone melatonin.

MELATONIN, THE HORMONE OF DARKNESS

If vitamin D is the daylight hormone, melatonin is the night-time hormone. Generated during sleep, its production normally peaks at about 2 a.m.

---

[562] Bollinger T et al. Sleep, Immunity, and Circadian Clocks: A Mechanistic Model. *Gerontology.* 2010 Feb 3. [Epub ahead of print] *http://pmid.us/20130392.*

[563] Cappuccio FP et al. Sleep duration and all-cause mortality: a systematic review and meta-analysis of prospective studies. *Sleep.* 2010 May 1;33(5):585-92. *http://pmid.us/20469800.*

[564] Altena E et al. Reduced orbitofrontal and parietal gray matter in chronic insomnia: a voxel-based morphometric study. *Biol Psychiatry.* 2010 Jan 15;67(2):182-5. *http://pmid.us/19782344.*

[565] Barceló A et al. Telomere shortening in sleep apnea syndrome. *Respir Med.* 2010 Apr 27. [Epub ahead of print] *http://pmid.us/20430605.* Selim B et al. Cardiovascular Consequences of Sleep Apnea. *Clin Chest Med.* 2010 Jun;31(2):203-220. *http://pmid.us/20488282.*

Melatonin is an antimicrobial hormone that has many benefits:

- Melatonin increases levels of growth hormone and amplifies the effects of resistance exercise, promoting muscle growth.[566]

- Melatonin kills tumor cells and prevents tumor growth.[567] Melatonin also extends cancer patient survival. In a trial of metastatic lung cancer, no patient survived two years on chemotherapy alone, but 6% of patients on the melatonin plus chemotherapy arm were still alive after five years.[568]

- Melatonin's anti-cancer effect is confirmed by higher-than-normal cancer rates among people who work at night, and lower-than-normal cancer rates among the blind.[569]

- Melatonin has antimicrobial functions, and protects against infections by the parasitic bacteria *Chlamydia*.[570]

- Clinical trials have shown melatonin to be effective against diseases such as irritable bowel syndrome, high blood pressure, macular degeneration, glaucoma, and diabetes.[571]

SLEEP IN A TOTALLY DARKENED ROOM

Even a small amount of light blocks production of melatonin.[572] To assure adequate melatonin, **sleep should occur in total darkness**: windows covered by an opaque curtain, LCD clocks turned face down, and lights turned off. Just one

---

[566] Nassar E et al. Effects of a single dose of N-Acetyl-5-methoxytryptamine (Melatonin) and resistance exercise on the growth hormone/IGF-1 axis in young males and females. *J Int Soc Sports Nutr*. 2007 Oct 23;4:14. *http://pmid.us/17956623*.

[567] Blask DE et al. Putting cancer to sleep at night: the neuroendocrine/circadian melatonin signal. *Endocrine*. 2005 Jul;27(2):179-88. *http://pmid.us/16217131*.

[568] Lissoni P et al. Five years survival in metastatic non-small cell lung cancer patients treated with chemotherapy alone or chemotherapy and melatonin: A randomized trial. *J Pineal Res*. 2003 Aug;35(1):12-5.. *http://pmid.us/12823608*.

[569] Schernhammer ES et al. Night-shift work and risk of colorectal cancer in the nurses' health study. *J Natl Cancer Inst*. 2003 Jun 4;95(11):825-8. *http://pmid.us/12783938*. Feychting M et al. Reduced cancer incidence among the blind. *Epidemiology*. 1998 Sep;9(5):490-4. *http://pmid.us/9730026*.

[570] Rahman MA et al. Serotonin and melatonin, neurohormones for homeostasis, as novel inhibitors of infections by the intracellular parasite chlamydia. *J Antimicrob Chemother*. 2005 Nov;56(5):861-8. *http://pmid.us/16172105*.

[571] Sánchez-Barceló EJ et al. Clinical Uses of Melatonin: Evaluation of Human Trials. *Curr Med Chem*. 2010 Apr 28. [Epub ahead of print], *http://pmid.us/20423309*.

[572] "Melatonin," Wikipedia, *http://en.wikipedia.org/wiki/Melatonin*.

'pulse' of artificial light at night impairs cell division in mice brains, and promotes patterns of gene expression associated with cancer.[573]

INFECTIONS OF THE BRAIN CALL FOR MELATONIN SUPPLEMENTATION

In chronic infections of the brain, the intracellular immune response sequesters tryptophan. This prevents serotonin and melatonin manufacture.

Since melatonin is so important for health and immune function, any melatonin deficiency should be remedied by supplementation. Time-release melatonin tablets can maintain a relatively even level of melatonin through the night, preventing early waking from a drop in melatonin levels. Melatonin is non-toxic.[574]

Eleventh Way: Relieve Stress

Chronic stress increases the risk of nearly every health problem. It accelerates aging and suppresses immune function.

Scientists have begun to figure out how stress does harm. The stress hormone cortisol prevents telomeres, a stabilizing end cap on DNA, from being maintained. Shorter telomeres bring impaired cellular function, unstable DNA, and shortened lifespan. Immune cells with shortened telomeres lose their effectiveness against viral infections.[575]

Sleep and cortisol affect each other. Cortisol levels follow a circadian rhythm, high during the day and low at night. When sleep is impaired, cortisol levels rise.[576] Cortisol levels are higher in insomniacs than in normal sleepers.[577]

Two excellent ways to relieve stress and improve sleep quality are exercise and slow, deep breathing:

---

[573] Ben-Shlomo R, Kyriacou CP. Light pulses administered during the circadian dark phase alter expression of cell cycle associated transcripts in mouse brain. *Cancer Genet Cytogenet.* 2010 Feb;197(1):65-70. *http://pmid.us/20113839.*

[574] Seabra ML et al. Randomized, double-blind clinical trial, controlled with placebo, of the toxicology of chronic melatonin treatment. *J Pineal Res.* 2000 Nov;29(4):193-200. *http://pmid.us/11068941.*

[575] Effros RB. Kleemeier Award Lecture 2008--the canary in the coal mine: telomeres and human healthspan. *J Gerontol A Biol Sci Med Sci.* 2009 May;64(5):511-5. *http://pmid.us/19228779.*

[576] Balbo M et al. Impact of sleep and its disturbances on hypothalamo-pituitary-adrenal axis activity. *Int J Endocrinol.* 2010;2010:759234. *http://pmid.us/20628523.*

[577] Vgontzas AN et al. Chronic insomnia is associated with nyctohemeral activation of the hypothalamic-pituitary-adrenal axis: clinical implications. *J Clin Endocrinol Metab.* 2001 Aug;86(8):3787-94. *http://pmid.us/11502812.*

- For every additional hour of physical activity during the day, children fall asleep three minutes quicker and sleep 20 minutes longer.[578] The same pattern holds in adults.[579]

- Diaphragmatic breathing – slow, relaxed, deep breaths, as practiced in many yoga disciplines – is a proven method for reducing cortisol and increasing melatonin.[580]

These are both techniques that can be practiced throughout the day. Taking the stairs rather than the elevator; standing or squatting rather than sitting; and being mindful to breathe deeply and slowly throughout the day, can significantly reduce stress.

[578] Nixon GM et al. Falling asleep: the determinants of sleep latency. *Arch Dis Child.* 2009 Sep;94(9):686-9. *http://pmid.us/19633062.* Hat tip Anahad O'Connor, *New York Times, http://www.nytimes.com/2009/12/01/health/01really.html.*

[579] King AC et al. Moderate-intensity exercise and self-rated quality of sleep in older adults. A randomized controlled trial. *JAMA.* 1997 Jan 1;277(1):32-7. *http://pmid.us/8980207.*

[580] Martarelli D et al. Diaphragmatic Breathing Reduces Exercise-induced Oxidative Stress. *Evid Based Complement Alternat Med.* 2009 Oct 29. [Epub ahead of print] *http://pmid.us/19875429.*

The "Herbivore Strategy" for Metabolic Diseases

The Perfect Health Diet, we stated in the Preview, is a hybrid of the various mammalian diets. With 400 carb calories a day (Omnivore strategy), ketogenic short-chain fats from coconut oil and fiber (Herbivore strategy), and slight under-eating of glucose to force synthesis of a little bit of glucose from protein (Carnivore strategy), the Perfect Health Diet eliminates risk of glucose deprivation while retaining the benefits of low glucose and insulin. Probably 90% to 95% of the population will optimize their health by following the regular Perfect Health Diet.

Unfortunately, some people have metabolic damage that impairs the normal pathways of glucose or fat metabolism. Both glucose and fats require complex transport systems to reach mitochondria and generate energy. In some diseases, these transport systems don't work properly.

People with metabolic diseases often benefit from a ketogenic diet – as we call it, a Herbivore strategy diet. Ketones don't need transport systems: they are water-soluble small molecules that diffuse throughout the body. They can feed mitochondria when other nutrients can't.

Diseases That May Benefit from a Herbivore Strategy

Any disease in which high levels of glucose or glutamate are problematic may benefit from a Herbivore strategy. Such diseases include:

- **Epilepsy** and other brain conditions, probably including **schizophrenia, bipolar disorder, depression, psychoses,** and **migraines**. Here the benefit comes from providing a neuron-nourishing energy source other than glucose (ketones) and from reducing brain glutamate levels.

- **Solid tumor cancers.** Cancer cells are metabolically impaired and can only metabolize glucose, a phenomenon known as the Warburg Effect. A ketogenic diet starves cancer cells, slowing tumor growth.

- **Diabetes, metabolic syndrome,** and **obesity**. In these diseases, damage to the liver, mitochondria, pancreatic beta cells, and adipose cells impairs handling of dietary carbs and long-chain fats. Ketones provide an alternative non-toxic energy source.

- **Bacterial infections of the brain and nerves**, causing such diseases as Alzheimer's, Parkinson's, multiple sclerosis, Lyme disease, fibromyalgia, and neuropathies.

Implementing A Ketogenic Diet

Each disease may have its own optimal compromise between too little glucose (resulting in glucose deprivation to healthy tissues), and too much. Unfortunately, we have little research to guide us except in the case of epilepsy, a disease for which ketogenic diets have long been used.

The Epilepsy Experience: Don't Eliminate Carbs, Do Increase Protein

Experience with epilepsy patients suggests that modest shifts toward lower carbs, higher protein, and more short-chain fats are sufficient to make the Perfect Health Diet a ketogenic diet.

In epilepsy, and probably all other diseases, it's better to include carb calories in a ketogenic diet. A study using a blinded crossover design switched 20 epileptic children between (1) a zero-carb ketogenic diet and (2) the same diet with 240 glucose calories. On both diets, ketones were produced. The glucose group had fewer seizures.[581]

With decreased carb intake, it's prudent to increase protein intake, in case protein is needed for manufacture of glucose and ketones. For no good reason, however, the classic ketogenic diet for epilepsy patients has been a low-protein diet.

The most beneficial amino acids are likely to be ketogenic branched-chain amino acids like leucine which support both muscle synthesis and ketone synthesis. A 2009 study among epileptics seems to confirm this: adding branched chain amino acids to the classic ketogenic diet reduced seizures and did not reduce ketone production.[582]

Macronutrient Recommendations

We suggest the following food intake for a ketogenic diet:

- Eat 200 carb calories per day, as much as possible from fiber-rich safe starches like taro and sweet potato.

- Eat 400 protein calories per day, to reach the minimum 600 calories of carb plus protein in case the remaining glucose deficit has to be made up from protein. Ketogenic branched-chain amino acids, perhaps from whey, are preferable.

- Eat some fiber and copious short-chain fats. Up to 1,500 calories (12 tbsp / 6 fluid ounces) coconut oil is desirable.

Some diabetics find that even 200 calories of carbs is too much. Dr. Richard Bernstein in his *Diabetes Solution* recommends limiting carbs to 30 grams, or 120 calories. Just remember: The lower carb intake goes, the more important it is to

---

[581] Freeman JM et al. A blinded, crossover study of the efficacy of the ketogenic diet. *Epilepsia.* 2009 Feb;50(2):322-5. *http://pmid.us/18717710.* Hat tip Pål Jåbekk, *http://ramblingsofacarnivore.blogspot.com/2010/05/ketogenic-diets-and-treatment-of.html.*

[582] Evangeliou A et al. Branched chain amino acids as adjunctive therapy to ketogenic diet in epilepsy: pilot study and hypothesis. *J Child Neurol.* 2009 Oct;24(10):1268-72. *http://pmid.us/19687389.*

provide ketogenic substrates from coconut oil, fiber, and ketogenic amino acids such as leucine.

MINIMIZING RISKS

On any extreme low-carb diet, major risks are:

1. Glucose deficiency may lead to insufficient production of mucus in the digestive tract, increasing risk of bowel cancers or gut infections.

2. Vitamin deficiencies can arise. With low insulin, vitamin C is not recycled and more vitamin C is needed. Compensating nutrients for glutathione support, like selenium, are also needed. Needs for vitamins involved in gluconeogenesis, such as B6 and biotin, may be higher.

3. Since glucose is needed to generate hydrogen peroxide for immune respiratory bursts, immune function against extracellular pathogens like fungi may be impaired.

Fungal infections or signs of dry mouth, dry eyes, or dry sinuses (indicating impaired glycoprotein production) indicate a glucose deficiency. Unexplained weight loss, bleeding, or slow wound healing indicate a vitamin C deficiency. Any deficiencies should be repaired immediately by eating starch or taking vitamins.

Healthy Weight Loss

Although we have avoided discussing specific diseases in this book, we will make an exception for obesity. So many overweight people follow misguided weight loss strategies that it seems important to provide some guidance.

The modern obesity epidemic does not arise from overeating or lack of exercise. Gluttony and sloth have always been with us, but obesity has not.

Consider this photo. It is of Chauncy Morlan, who in the 1880s and '90s toured with the Barnum & Bailey Circus as their fat man.[583]

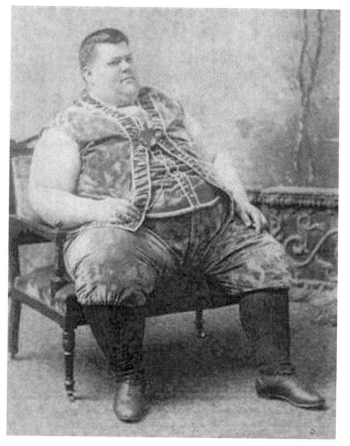

In the 1800s people paid money to gawk at Chauncy; he was a sideshow freak. Today no one would give him a second glance.

What has changed since the 19th century? New food toxins:

---

[583] Hat tip Adam Ozimek, *http://modeledbehavior.com/2010/04/15/americas-obesity-epidemic-bringing-sideshow-freaks-into-the-discussion/.*

- Vegetable seed oils entered the human diet in the 20th century, as industrial processing methods were invented to remove unpalatable flavors and the deadliest toxins from the oils of major seed crops. Its use soared after doctors began recommending it as a way to reduce cholesterol levels.

- Fructose consumption greatly increased in the 20th century, driven in part by the invention of high-fructose corn syrup.

In Step One, when discussing omega-6 fats, we mentioned that in animal studies obesity is readily produced by combining a fat toxin (such as omega-6 fats in vegetable oils) with a carb toxin (such as fructose, wheat, or alcohol).

The 20th century invention of vegetable seed oils and new fructose sources could plausibly be considered *the invention of obesity*.

The Causes and Pathology of Obesity

Obesity in general results from the same causes as other health problems – food toxicity, malnourishment, and infections. Briefly:

- **Toxins:** Fructose and PUFA readily induce obesity in lab animals by poisoning the liver. Wheat toxins also promote obesity. The recent sharp rises in fructose and vegetable oil consumption, and a mild rise in wheat consumption, are probably the major drivers of the obesity epidemic.

- **Malnourishment:** Obesity can be induced in mice and rats via choline deficient diets.[584] Since choline is a methyl donor, and supports silencing of gene expression via DNA methylation, it's likely that improper gene regulation due to nutrient deficiencies is a cause of obesity in humans too.

- **Infection:** We mentioned earlier that the level of bacterial endotoxins in the liver predicts metabolic syndrome and obesity. Recently, researchers have connected viruses to obesity. The adenovirus AD-36 has been shown to cause fat cells to proliferate; people infected with AD-36 are three times more likely to become obese and obese people infected with AD-36 are much fatter than non-infected obese.[585]

Obese people generally have damage to organs involved in metabolic control – the liver, the thyroid, hormonal control centers of the brain, and adipose cells. These cause hormonal problems, such as insulin resistance in the liver and leptin resistance in the brain.

---

[584] Veteläinen R et al. Essential pathogenic and metabolic differences in steatosis induced by choline or methione-choline deficient diets in a rat model. *J Gastroenterol Hepatol.* 2007 Sep;22(9):1526-33. *http://pmid.us/17716355.*

[585] See our post "Obesity: Often an Infectious Disease," September 22, 2010, *http://perfecthealthdiet.com/?p=606.*

Once these "resistances" occur, hormones no longer properly control blood sugar, insulin, appetite, or metabolism.

Obesity is actually the *healthiest* response to these resistances: it results from adipose cells removing toxic glucose from the blood. Conversion of glucose to fat rescues the body from its failure to properly control blood glucose levels.

However, adipose cells can only rescue the body for so long. Eventually, they reach their limit, and no longer add fat. At this point weight plateaus and **obesity gives way to diabetes**. Devastating health problems begin to develop from chronic glucose poisoning.

Calorie Restriction Is Dangerous

Most people think of a "weight loss diet" as a calorie-restricted diet. They think the recipe for weight loss is temporary starvation.

But this is a dangerous strategy. Malnourishment is one of the causes of obesity, and *reduced food intake aggravates malnourishment*. So **a starvation diet may cause more obesity**.

Experience bears this out:

- People who lose weight through starvation diets usually end up *more obese than when they started*. UCLA researchers analyzed 31 long-term diet studies and found that a majority of people who "diet" to lose weight subsequently regain even more weight than they lost.[586]

- When we look at countries that have suffered famines, we find that *people become obese once the famine is over*. Malnourished people tend to become obese as soon as they have sufficient calories. [587]

Since starvation continued long enough results in death, the period of calorie restriction must come to an end. If at that time the liver, brain, and thyroid have not healed, then faulty hormones will drive the body back to its previous weight. If the liver, brain, and thyroid have become even more damaged due to malnourishment during the "diet," then **the obesity problem has now become even more severe and intractable**.

Calorie Restriction Is Unnecessary

Weight can be lost, and body shape normalized, *without ever reducing calories below a normal person's intake*.

---

[586] Mann T et al. Medicare's search for effective obesity treatments: diets are not the answer. *Am Psychol.* 2007 Apr;62(3):220-33. *http://pmid.us/17469900*.

[587] Caballero B. A nutrition paradox – underweight and obesity in developing countries. *N Engl J Med.* 2005 Apr 14;352(15):1514-6. *http://pmid.us/15829531*.

The reason is that caloric expenditure increases with body weight. The obese burn more calories per day than the slender. It's a lot of work to carry that extra weight around; and extra surface area means more energy lost as heat.

In one representative study, slender persons (average weight 146 pounds) used 2,481 calories per day, while obese persons (average weight 288 pounds) used 3,162 calories per day.[588]

So an obese person can eat a normal, 2,481-calorie-per-day diet and still lose weight at a steady pace. At an expenditure of 3,162 calories per day and consumption of 2,481 calories per day, fat loss would be about 75 g per day, 1.2 pounds per week, sixty pounds per year.

The Best Weight Loss Diet is a Diet for Life

Some gurus advocate different diets for weight loss and maintenance.

This is unnecessary. Since it's possible to lose weight fairly rapidly eating the same calories as a normal person, it's not necessary to eat a diet different than a normal person's to lose weight.

We think it's also a mistake. After all, an obese person got that way by being inclined toward an unhealthy diet. Adopting a new diet is hard. Making an obese person learn **TWO** new diets – a "weight loss" and a "maintenance" diet – imposes an unnecessary burden.

We think it's much better to train yourself in healthy eating from the beginning, while the motivation to lose weight is strong. Use the Perfect Health Diet for weight loss from the beginning, and the odds of long-term success will be higher.

The Proper Fix For Obesity

Here are key steps for curing obesity:

FIRST STEP: Eliminate omega-6 containing oils; reduce omega-6 fats by eating red meats and oily fish.

Do not eat any oil which has 15% omega-6 fats or more. Be sure to read food labels closely; do not buy any products made with soybean oil, corn oil, safflower oil, or canola oil. Olive oil is acceptable, but butter and coconut oil are better.

Among meats, beef, lamb, and salmon are lowest in omega-6.

Including coconut oil or coconut milk will increase metabolism and promote weight loss. But reducing omega-6 intake is the most important step.

---

[588] Leibel RL et al. Changes in energy expenditure resulting from altered body weight. *N Engl J Med.* 1995 Mar 9;332(10):621-8. *http://pmid.us/7632212.*

SECOND STEP: Cut fructose intake. Do not eat sugar, high fructose corn syrup, or products containing them, except occasional lightly-sweetened desserts like high-fat ice cream. Do eat fruit, but not too much.

Fructose is particularly dangerous in combination with omega-6 fats. Because omega-6 levels in the body take four to five years to return to low levels after vegetable oils are removed from the diet, fructose avoidance is needed to prevent toxic "fructation" of omega-6.

Fructose avoidance also helps to limit chronic infections and gut bacterial overgrowth, which have been implicated in metabolic syndrome and obesity.

THIRD STEP: Remove wheat and other cereal grain products from the diet; replace them with fatty foods.

Wheat and other grain toxins damage the thyroid, produce chronic inflammation, and derange hormone levels to promote weight gain. The notorious "beer belly" is really a "grain belly."

Replacing grains with fatty foods will bring macronutrient ratios near the optimum "Perfect Health Diet" ratios. This will keep blood glucose and insulin levels close to the healthy range and reduce glucose toxicity.

Eating a fat-rich, low-carb diet is important for weight loss. As Gary Taubes points out in *Good Calories, Bad Calories*, high-carb diets are the only effective strategy for **intentional** weight gain. Sumo wrestlers eat diets with only 9% to 16% fat in order to gain weight.[589] "Every woman knows that carbohydrate is fattening," as a *British Journal of Nutrition* article noted in 1963.[590] The reverse practice of carb limitation is the heart of the most rapid weight loss diets, such as the Atkins diet.

FOURTH STEP: Normalize thyroid function.

This is extremely important; it is impossible to be healthy, and difficult to lose weight, with a malfunctioning thyroid. We place it fourth only because steps one, two, and three will fix many thyroid problems. Wheat toxicity and omega-6 toxicity are both causes of hypothyroidism.

The first step toward normalizing thyroid function is toxin removal and supplementation of iodine, selenium, and vitamin D. If these are not sufficient to restore thyroid function, then supplemental thyroid hormone (obtainable with a doctor's prescription) should be considered. The reason is that tissues – including the thyroid – cannot heal if they lack thyroid hormone. So it pays to normalize

---

[589] Nishizawa T et al. Some factors related to obesity in the Japanese Sumo Wrestler. *Am J Clin Nutr*. 1976 Oct;29(10):1167-74. *http://pmid.us/973605*.

[590] Passmore R, Swindells YE. Observations on the respiratory quotients and weight gain of man after eating large quantities of carbohydrate. *Br J Nutr* 1963; 17: 331–9. *http://pmid.us/14045336*.

thyroid hormone levels artificially while you wait for your body to heal. Aim for a TSH of 1.0 or below.

FIFTH STEP: Eat a sufficiency of nourishing foods. Supplement vitamins and minerals. When hungry, eat. Frequent snacking is OK, as long as snacks are nutritious and toxin-free.

Malnourishment is a cause of obesity. Nutrition must be sufficient to enable all bodily tissues to heal and function properly.

A nutrient-dense diet reduces appetite. So, for good health and rapid weight loss, be sure to **make nutrient-rich foods such as bone broths, liver, and green leafy vegetables a part of your diet.** Follow our supplement recommendations to get every major nutrient into its plateau range.

SIXTH STEP: Intermittent fasting and other immune-enhancing steps. Inducing autophagy by fasting will help defeat any obesity-inducing bacterial and viral infections, and will also promote beneficial metabolic adaptations. A 23 hour fast, dinner to dinner, is excellent for weight loss; confining food to an 8-hour window each day, for a daily 16-hour fast, is another excellent strategy.

These six steps will enable metabolic control organs to heal, and over time restore normal hormonal function, decrease hunger, and make weight loss easy.

Be Patient

Obese people should try to **optimize health, not speed of weight loss.**

A diet with 400 calories from carbs, 300 calories from protein, and 1300 calories from fats – the Perfect Health Diet for slender people – is also a weight loss diet for obese people. As long as toxins are removed, nutrition is good, and carbs are restricted, hunger disappears, the liver, brain and thyroid heal, and weight loss becomes easy and natural.

Your focus should be on restoring health, not on rapid weight loss. A healthy body loses excess weight easily. In an unhealthy body, weight lost by calorie restriction is soon regained.

A good measure of the quality of a weight loss diet is whether it builds muscle. Starvation diets cause loss of both lean mass (muscle) and adipose mass. Healthy diets, on the other hand, *move fats from adipose tissue to newly-generated muscle.* As we discussed earlier, muscle, not fat, is the body's natural storage reservoir for excess calories.

Other Tricks for Rapid Weight Loss

If you really want to lose weight quickly, here are a few tricks that can help:

1. **Expose yourself to cold.** In winter, go for a walk outside wearing short pants. (Be sure to cover your heart, and if your circulation is poor, your hands and ears.) In summer, take an extra five minutes at the end of your

shower, turn the water temperature down and turn yourself around under the cold water. In general, under-dress for the temperature, though not to the point of discomfort, just to the point that you feel awake and obliged to move a little more than usual.

2. **Spend as much time as possible on your feet**. The tiny muscle movements required to maintain balance while standing or walking have been shown to trigger fat burning and weight loss.

3. **Exercise at high intensity twice per week**. Sprint; jump; lift heavy weights. Resistance exercise will help migrate fats from adipose tissue to muscle, and promote a healthy metabolism.

4. **Eat coconut oil**. Short-chain fats are surprisingly effective at promoting weight loss.

5. **Get a good night's sleep**. Impaired sleep causes weight gain. Allow yourself at least eight hours for sleep, sleep in a totally darkened room, and experiment with melatonin supplementation if you're not sleeping well.

6. **Drink lots of water**. Dehydration reduces the rate of weight loss.

7. **Consider a "fecal transplant" from a healthy slender person**. Bad gut flora may be a cause of obesity. Restocking commensal species from a slender person may help restore normal metabolism.

Conclusion: Becoming a Healthy Centenarian

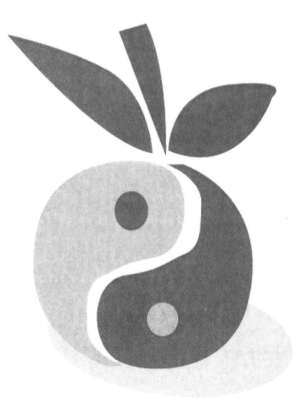

Achieving Long Life and Vitality

As we noted earlier, animal studies have shown that the key to extending lifespan is keeping glucose and insulin levels low. Animals live 20% to 30% longer when their blood glucose and insulin levels are kept consistently low.

There are two ways to achieve low glucose and insulin levels: (1) eating a high-fat diet, and (2) eating a calorie-restricted diet. Both dietary strategies extend the lifespan of animals.

What Do Supercentenarians Do?

Supercentenarians – those who live to 110 and beyond – are an elite group. There are only 600 supercentenarians in the world.

Two patterns are common in the diets of supercentenarians:

1. High-fat, low-carb diets.

2. Calorie restriction and intermittent fasting.

These practices go together. Calorie restriction and fasting are easy on a high-fat diet, since there is little hunger and, since the diet mimics the composition of human tissue, the body can easily transition between food and the fasting mode of self-cannibalization. The Okinawans are a famously long-lived people who, in addition to eating a high-fat diet that closely resembles the Perfect Health Diet, also practiced calorie restriction.[591]

Here are some examples of longevity diets.

Luigi Cornaro (1464-1566) was a Venetian nobleman who, sick and dying in his thirties, asked the doctors what to do. One told him, "Cut down on your riotous living, stop the drinking, cut out the rich food, eat as little as you can, and don't abuse your body. You can get well." **Luigi reduced his diet to 12 ounces of solid food, including one egg, and 14 ounces of wine per day**. He lived to 102.[592]

Gertrude Baines "lived to be the world's oldest person on a steady diet of crispy bacon, fried chicken and ice cream." She died at age 115 in 2009.[593]

---

[591] Willcox DC et al. Caloric restriction and human longevity: what can we learn from the Okinawans? *Biogerontology*. 2006 Jun;7(3):173-7. *http://pmid.us/16810568.*

[592] *http://en.wikipedia.org/wiki/Luigi_Cornaro. http://drbass.com/cornaro.html.* Hat tip Mike O'Donnell, *http://www.fitnessspotlight.com/2008/7/15/lessons-from-luigi-how-to-live-to-102/.*

[593] "World's oldest person dies in L.A. at 115," *Associated Press*, Sept 11, 2009, *http://www.msnbc.msn.com/id/32799091/ns/us_news-life/.*

Edna Parker, an Indiana schoolteacher, was the world's oldest person when she died at age 115 in November 2008. From her obituary:

> Parker lived by herself on the family farm until she was 100. At that lofty age, she could still climb a ladder to fix a light....
>
> **Parker especially enjoyed eggs, sausage, bacon and fried chicken. "I guess we'll have to rethink lard," Daniels quipped after hearing about her high-fat diet.**[594]

Jeanne Calment, who lived to 122, took up fencing at age 85 and was still riding a bicycle at age 100. According to Wikipedia, "**she ascribed her longevity and relatively youthful appearance for her age to olive oil, which she said she poured on all her food** and rubbed onto her skin." She also drank wine and ate chocolate – both recommended foods on the Perfect Health Diet.[595]

Larry Haubner of Fredericksburg, Virginia recently celebrated his 107th birthday in good health. News stories highlighted his avoidance of grains and sugars:

> Ask Larry Haubner for the secret to living 107 years, and the Fredericksburg man flexes his biceps, flashes a mostly toothless smile and growls. "Nutrition!" he bellows. "Exercise! I think we should all exercise more than we do."...
>
> "Well, I ate the cake," he said of his latest birthday celebration. "But I don't believe cake is a good food."[596]
>
> [H]e told me he was a "picky eater." Not finicky, but choosy.
>
> That was underscored when Heim, who enjoys visiting and befriending the elderly in area homes, told me that she once brought candy for Haubner. "The first thing he did was to read the fine print in the ingredients!" she said.
>
> She has visited since then, she said, and remembered his reaction to the candy: "The next time, I took him fruit," she said.[597]

Mr. Haubner also took a lot of vitamins, until his doctor took them away:

---

[594] Elaine Woo, "Edna Parker dies at 115; former teacher was world's oldest person," *Los Angeles Times*, Nov. 28, 2008, *http://www.latimes.com/news/obituaries/la-me-parker28-2008nov28,0,3824201.story*.

[595] *http://en.wikipedia.org/wiki/Jeanne_Calment*.

[596] Emma Brown, "Va. Man, 107, Finds Blessings And Burdens In Longevity," *Washington Post*, July 2, 2009, *http://www.washingtonpost.com/wp-dyn/content/article/2009/07/01/AR2009070103861.html*.

[597] "A Few Curly-isms for a Long Life," *Fredericksburg.com*, July 7, 2007, *http://fredericksburg.com/News/FLS/2007/072007/07072007/297776/printer_friendly*.

He takes no medicines. His only pills are a vitamin C tablet, some calcium and a multivitamin.

He brought many other vitamins with him to Greenfield, but [Dr. Robert] Prasse threw them away.[598]

Walter Breunig of Great Falls, Montana is the world's oldest man and recently celebrated his 114th birthday. He restricts calories and practices a daily 16-hour fast, eating only breakfast and lunch. Based on his choice of birthday lunch, he seems to favor healthy foods:

So what does the world's oldest man eat? The answer is not much, at least not too much.

Walter Breuning … eats just two meals a day and has done so for the past 35 years.

"I think you should push back from the table when you're still hungry," Breuning said.

At 5 foot 8, ("I shrunk a little," he admitted) and 125 pounds, Breuning limits himself to a big breakfast and lunch every day and no supper….

"You get in the habit of not eating at night, and you realize how good you feel. If you could just tell people not to eat so darn much."…

And for his birthday lunch he got his favorite: liver and onions.[599]

There are a few long-lived vegetarians, such as Marie-Louise Meilleur.[600] The "vegetarian strategy" for centenarianism is to avoid grains and other calorie-rich plant foods, and eat fiber-rich but calorie-restricted diets. A large share of calories comes from short-chain fats released by gut bacteria as they digest vegetable fibers, and longer-chain fats from oils such as olive oil; so the diet is strongly fat-dominant, not carb-dominant. Protein is severely restricted. Eggs and dairy substitute for animal foods.

However, there are far fewer vegetarian centenarians than most people presume. Longevity researcher Nir Barzilei notes of centenarians:

The most common thing this group had is that they did not reveal any particular lifestyle secret for their own longevity. When asked

---

[598] "He has health, if not wealth," *Fredericksburg.com*, June 16, 2007, *http://fredericksburg.com/News/FLS/2007/062007/06162007/292471/printer_friendly.*

[599] Sydne George, "Two-meal diet aids in oldest man's longevity," *USA Today*, Sept 24, 2009, *http://www.usatoday.com/news/nation/2009-09-24-oldest-man-diet_N.htm.*

[600] *http://en.wikipedia.org/wiki/Marie-Louise_Meilleur.*

specifically, none has exercised. **None was a vegetarian**. Not a single one ate yogurt throughout his life.[601]

It's possible to eat a vegetarian version of the Perfect Health Diet; we explain how in the Appendix. However, it's probably difficult to adhere to such a diet.

If there are few long-lived vegetarians, there are surprisingly many long-lived fast-food entrepreneurs. French-fry king J.R. Simplot died at 99; Carl Karcher, founder of Carl's Jr., died at 90; Troy Smith, founder of Sonic drive-thrus, died at 87; Lovey Yancey, founder of Fatburger, died at 96; Wilber Hardee, founder of Hardee's, died at 89; Ray Kroc, founder of McDonald's, died at 81; and Irvine Robbins, founder of Baskin-Robbins, died at 90.[602]

We don't recommend eating at fast food restaurants, especially now that vegetable oils have replaced beef tallow and coconut oil as cooking and dressing fats. But the longevity of fast-food moguls suggests that eating healthy does not mean abjuring taste, or speedy food preparation. A high-fat diet covers for a multitude of health sins.

---

[601] Claudia Dreifus, "A Conversation With Nir Barzilai; It's Not the Yogurt: Looking for Longevity Genes," *New York Times*, Feb 24, 2004, *http://www.nytimes.com/2004/02/24/health/a-conversation-with-nir-barzilai-it-s-not-the-yogurt-looking-for-longevity-genes.html*.

[602] Hamilton Nolan, "Grease is Good," *http://gawker.com/5393529/grease-is-good*.

Parting Thoughts

Contemporary medicine has failed at curing chronic disease. Doctors regard most diseases as incurable, and are content to palliate symptoms.

Drugs and medical care do little to halt disease or extend lifespan. Perhaps they shorten lifespan: Research based on the Dartmouth Atlas of Health Care found that chronically ill patients who receive the most intensive treatments often fare worse than those who receive minimal care.[603]

But Disease and Early Aging Can Be Eradicated

We believe that suffering from chronic disease is unnecessary. We believe that nearly all diseases can be cured, if they are attacked at their root causes: toxic foods, malnutrition, and chronic infections.

We believe that a revolution in medicine is on the way:

- Diets like the Perfect Health Diet will eliminate food toxins and malnutrition and enhance immunity against pathogens.

- New diagnostic methods will detect the pathogens that cause disease, and new antibiotics will specifically target those pathogens.

With diet and antibiotics, doctors will finally learn how to cure chronic disease. This will enable nearly everyone to become a healthy centenarian.

An Invitation To Explore Natural Healing With Us

Having had chronic diseases ourselves, we are eager to share all we know and help others avoid needless suffering. Especially if you have a chronic disease, please explore our blog at *http://perfecthealthdiet.com*.

If you do try the Perfect Health Diet, please tell us and our readers about your experiences, good or bad. By sharing experiences, we can hope to hasten the arrival of that happy day when chronic disease will be a thing of the past, and good health and long life will be everyone's birthright.

Thank you, dear reader, for your time with us. We wish you a long life, free of disease, and the best of health always!

---

[603] "The State of the Nation's Health," Dartmouth Medicine, Spring 2007, *http://dartmed.dartmouth.edu/spring07/html/atlas.php*.

Appendix: For Our Vegetarian Friends

We have several friends who are vegetarian for moral reasons. We respect this choice. It is possible to maintain good health while refraining from contributing to the death of animals, though it requires extra care.

First and most important, it is extremely desirable to eat eggs and whole-fat dairy. No animals are killed to obtain these foods. Without these foods, it is difficult to obtain balanced nutrition.

Vegetarians can relax our advice to restrict carbs to less than 600 glucose calories per day. In the absence of food toxins from grains and vegetable oils, it is possible to obtain a large share of calories from "safe starches" such as taro, yams, sweet potatoes, and white rice without much risk of diabetes, obesity, or heart disease. The experience of the Kitavans supports this.

However, we strongly recommend respecting the advice to eliminate toxins:

- No grains.
- No vegetable oils; minimal omega-6 PUFA.
- Limit fructose; 4 fruit portions per day is a reasonable maximum.

Some foods which we have advised eliminating can be eaten with careful preparation. Certain beans become reasonably low in toxins if soaked overnight and then thoroughly cooked. Vegetarians should become familiar with traditional methods of food preparation. The cookbook *Nourishing Traditions* by Sally Fallon and Mary Enig may be useful.

Coconut oil or coconut milk should be a central part of any vegetarian diet. It is an excellent oil and low in omega-6 fats. Palm oil, cocoa butter, and nutmeg butter are other desirable vegetarian sources of fat; tree nut butters, olive oil, and avocado oil are healthy in moderation but imperfect due to their omega-6 content. Avoid any oil or fatty vegetable food that is above 15% LA.

In general, the more tropical the plant, the healthier. Macadamia nuts are the healthiest nuts, and coconut oil the healthiest oil.

Fatty dairy products are excellent ways to obtain fat without PUFA, and to improve the macronutrient ratio of the diet. We recommend drinking whole-fat milk or cream, preferably unpasteurized.

Flaxseed oil, also known as linseed oil and commonly used as a wood varnish, can be a source of omega-3 ALA. However, this is adequate only if levels of omega-6 LA are low; high levels of LA block the elongation and desaturation of ALA to produce EPA and DHA. For this reason, and because of potential flaxseed toxicity, we recommend consuming sources of the long-chain omega-3s EPA and DHA. Microalgae oils, from zooplankton and phytoplankton such as Spirulina, are a vegetarian source. An animal source which may be acceptable to those who are vegetarian on moral grounds is fish eggs, such as caviar. Inclusion of microalgae oils, fish eggs, or other long omega-3 sources is more effective than flaxseed oil at raising tissue long omega-3 levels.[604] Consumption of long omega-3s is especially important for pregnant and breastfeeding mothers.[605]

Supplementation is strongly recommended for vegetarians. In addition to our recommended supplements, extra supplementation of choline (and, perhaps, inositol) is recommended. Animal fats are rich in phospholipids such as phosphatidylcholine and phosphatidylinositol; but plant and dairy fats are comparatively deficient. It would be difficult to get close to the US Recommended Daily Allowance of 500 mg choline on a vegetarian diet.

Vitamin B12 is another nutrient that all vegetarians should supplement. Also, fat-soluble vitamins commonly obtained from animal foods, such as vitamin K2, should be supplemented.

We recommend that vegetarians weigh and document their own diet for a week and use sites like nutritiondata.com or fitday.com to assess their micronutrient intake. Any deficiencies should be remedied through supplementation.

Finally, for vegans who wish to avoid eggs and dairy, we suggest Lierre Keith's book *The Vegetarian Myth*. We believe there is no moral reason to avoid eggs or dairy; there are certainly good health reasons to include them.

---

[604] Geppert J et al. Docosahexaenoic acid supplementation in vegetarians effectively increases omega-3 index: a randomized trial. *Lipids*. 2005 Aug;40(8):807-14. *http://pmid.us/16296399*. Anderson BM, Ma DW. Are all n-3 polyunsaturated fatty acids created equal? *Lipids Health Dis*. 2009 Aug 10;8:33. *http://pmid.us/19664246*. Hat tip Rhonda Perciavalle, *http://www.fitnessspotlight.com/2010/06/14/microalgae-oil/*.

[605] Francois CA et al. Supplementing lactating women with flaxseed oil does not increase docosahexaenoic acid in their milk. *Am J Clin Nutr*. 2003 Jan;77(1):226-33. *http://pmid.us/12499346*.

CPSIA information can be obtained at www.ICGtesting.com
Printed in the USA
LVOW052106070212

267612LV00003B/9/P